Precision Cancer Medicine

Bharat Jasani • Ralf Huss • Clive R. Taylor

Precision Cancer Medicine

Role of the Pathologist

Springer

Bharat Jasani
Discovery Life sciences Global
Biomarker Services
Kassel, Hessen
Germany

Clive R. Taylor
Department of Pathology
University of Southern California
Los Angeles, CA
USA

Ralf Huss
Institute of Pathology and Molecular
Diagnostics & Institute for Digital
Medicine
University Hospital Augsburg
Augsburg, Bavaria
Germany

ISBN 978-3-030-84086-0 ISBN 978-3-030-84087-7 (eBook)
https://doi.org/10.1007/978-3-030-84087-7

This Springer imprint is published by the registered company Springer Nature Switzerland AG
The registered company address is: Gewerbestrasse 11, 6330 Cham, Switzerland

Foreword

Significant progress in the prevention, early detection, and treatment of cancer continues to be made and the death rate from cancer continues to decline. In fact, for each of the last 2 years, we have seen the steepest single-year decline in the cancer death rate on record. Cancer drug therapies have become more precise, surgical treatments less invasive, radiation more targeted, and we are learning additional ways to unleash a patient's immune system against their cancer. At the same time, scientists are unlocking the increasingly complex mechanisms tumor cells use to escape treatment and developing sophisticated diagnostics and drugs to find and treat them. The completion of the human genome sequencing project in 2003 accelerated the ability to determine genetic abnormalities in tumors that can be used to design precision therapeutics. This technological advance has been accompanied by rapid progress in multi-omic technologies, complemented by evolving artificial intelligence and machine learning capabilities. Clearly, there is a bright path forward for further interception and successful treatment of cancer.

As these evolving technologies and therapeutics move forward, the pathologist sits at command central, playing an ever-increasing and critically important role in their application. Of course, the pathologist is always the arbiter of a diagnosis of cancer and an important adjudicator of clinical treatment plans. In the multidisciplinary tumor board, the final word of the pathologist with their real-time review of the tumor histology and its inked margin dictate the next steps in the patient's care. As a practicing surgical, medical, or radiation oncologist, effective relationships with the surgical pathologists are critical for success and are foundational parts of an educational curriculum for trainees.

However, the increasing diagnostic complexity with shifts toward more molecular and morphological-based analytics has created their own set of challenges for the pathologist. In fact, when coupled with the declining pathology workforce, it is becoming increasingly difficult to integrate the latest advances into the routine care of cancer patients. Nonetheless, with challenges, there are always opportunities. For pathologists, the opportunity lies in their position at the tip of the spear of the Fourth Industrial Revolution.[1] This digital revolution started in the middle of the twentieth century and represents the fusion of the physical, digital, and biological worlds with a wide range of new technologies. The speed of breakthroughs already seen in this

1. https://www.weforum.org/agenda/2016/01/the-fourth-industrial-revolution-what-it-means-and-how-to-respond/

revolution is unprecedented and it is both transformational and disruptive. For pathologists, it means moving onward from the light microscope into the myriad of evolving analytic technologies and correlating them with the massive amounts of clinical and outcomes data on cancer patients. For cancer patients, it means better diagnostics, improved precision-based therapeutics, and most importantly, continued improved outcomes.

Finally, as we relish the prospects of what this industrial revolution will bring to the patient with cancer, it is important to remember that we still have widespread disparities in cancer care and cancer outcomes. Sadly, a patient's zip code frequently has a better prediction of their outcome than their genetic code and these disparities are currently widening. However, through existing digital approaches, pathologists can directly solve some of these disparities. In fact, this is already happening. For example, in sub-Saharan Africa, by providing hospitals with tissue processing protocols and slide scanners, central pathological analysis is happening. Pathologists are working together digitally to ensure that accurate diagnoses are rendered to patients in widespread areas. This is one example of how the technological revolution can and will provide positive solutions to cancer disparities, with the pathologist, again, at the center of patient care.

So, there are many reasons to be optimistic about progress in understanding, preventing, diagnosing, and treating cancer. Given the pace of discovery, we likely have little idea of how this will evolve during these transformative times. But one thing appears crystal-clear: the multidisciplinary approach to oncology will have an ever-expanding importance, and the pathologist will remain a critical force behind increasingly successful patient outcomes.

William G. Cance, MD, FACS
American Cancer Society, Inc.
Kennesaw, GA, USA

Preface

Pathologists represent an increasingly scarce healthcare resource worldwide. Optimization of their role is thus critical to sustaining modern cancer diagnosis and patient care. Machine learning/artificial intelligence (ML/AI) is a powerful complementary tool that could aid the pathologists to improve efficiency and provide next-generation interpretation that includes analysis of complex biomarker and genomics data. For this approach to succeed, pathologists must be active in all phases of ML/AI development, from early design and testing through implementation. The alternative is to risk the pathologist being bypassed by non-medical data mining experts, leading to compromised outcomes for the patient due to lack of integration with the complete pathological information. The current increase in automation should lead pathologists to reassess their roles and their true value to the healthcare team, across the entire spectrum of biomarker testing as part of what is essentially a new field of precision oncology.

Part I introduces precision cancer medicine as founded on the principle of providing a highly specific molecularly targeted treatment that, based upon appropriate validated companion tests, is judged to be the most effective therapy for the particular cancer type or subtype affecting the individual patient. This approach has required the development of assays that are capable of identifying as accurately and precisely as possible those actionable molecular target(s) in the cancer cells that are present in the sample or biopsy available for analysis.

In Part II, such assays are described as based on the use of a variety of molecular probes referred to as predictive cancer biomarkers. The specificity and sensitivity of the biomarker-based cancer test, although largely determined by the accuracy and the precision of the analytical method used, are also critically influenced by the quality of the tissue sample and the method used for reading or scoring of the results, both areas of responsibility for the pathologist as described and exemplified in Part III.

Part IV presents the factors that influence the adoption of digital pathology as a complementary aid for patient care purpose. They include the mind-set of the pathologists as well as legal, financial, and technological challenges. The barriers to adoption are gradually breaking down. Digital pathology is gaining momentum, as evidenced by the approval of the first whole slide imaging system for primary diagnosis, recent advances in computational and imaging systems, and the fact that more pathology labs are incorporating digital pathology in their practice. Helpful practical resources, such as guidelines, validation, and accreditation requirements, will support the implementation of clinical grade digital pathology. Ultimately, however, the pathologist must help to integrate the rapidly moving fields of computer science and medical science. The end goal is to develop a new way of practicing pathology, which we in this book have termed 'precision pathology', suited to meet the demands of precision oncology, which itself is continually being reshaped by these very same scientific advances.

Regulatory bodies and expert opinion groups have introduced guidelines to reduce the overall variability of the total test process described in Part II, through recommendations for standardization of the pre-analytical phase involving handling of the tissue material, and the post-analytical phase of interpretation, namely scoring and reporting the results. However, the variability associated with an individual patient sample analysis still must be checked and quality controlled to ensure that the correct result is provided to the cancer physician or the oncologist. As emphasized in Part III, it has increasingly become the role of the pathologist to manage this complex process from bench to bedside, based on their detailed knowledge and unique experience of how predictive cancer biomarker tests are analytically and clinically validated, and exactly what measures are required to implement and run these tests safely and sustainably in routine diagnostic practice.

As we move toward the era of digital and computational pathology, this role continually is being extended, as well as changed, to include management of more stringent quality control of tissue sample handling and new analyses based on more complex biomarker tests as alluded to in Part IV. While many of these responsibilities are grounded in traditional pathology and clinical laboratory practice, the inevitable computer-driven ML/AI interface is largely new to anatomic pathology. Successful adoption will require that the surgical pathologist acquires new skills and new competencies, both through newly developed training programs and by on-the-job interactive experience, as part of an ever evolving learning process.

AI has permeated almost every aspect of our daily lives, from driving across town, to researching for a manuscript, to finding a restaurant, and virtual reality entertainment, in much of which the role of AI is largely subliminal and unnoticed. Surely, it is not beyond the compass of the present generation of pathologists to adopt and shape these powerful ML/AI tools into routine pathology practice, to the benefit of the pathologist, the oncologist, and ultimately the patient: precision medicine begets and demands precision pathology.

Kassel, Germany — Bharat Jasani
Augsburg, Germany — Ralf Huss
Los Angeles, CA — Clive R. Taylor

Contents

Part I

The Evolution of Pathology and Precision Medicine

Introduction: From 'Tissue Diagnosis' to Biomarkers

1

1.1 A Brief History of Pathology: The Progression to Precision Cancer Medicine

Cancer has been recognized from ancient times as an intractable disease process. Surgery, like all the other treatments available in the deep past, failed to cure the cancer once it had spread. It is true that Galen wrote of surgical cures for breast cancer, if the tumour could be completely removed at an early stage. However, this ideal was so rarely achievable that surgical intervention was often considered more harmful than no treatment at all, a viewpoint that ancient physicians extended to many other forms of treatment that, if not curative, might arguably slow the course. If there was any general agreement, it was that cure of cancer was not possible in most established cases, a general tenet that has held true to the present day.

1.1.1 Cure as a Generic Rationale for Cancer Treatment

Giovanni Morgagni (1682–1771) of Padua was one of the first to lay the foundation for the role of pathology in oncology (the study of cancer) through the systematic post-mortem examination of patients presumed to have died of cancer (Van den Tweel and Taylor 2010, 2013; Van den Tweel et al. 2016). From the perspective of surgery, John Hunter (1728–1793) in London advanced the notion that some cancers might be cured by surgery, advocating the removal of tumours from the body to save the patient; if a tumour is judged to be "moveable" then "there is no impropriety in removing it." (Taylor 2010; Van den Tweel et al. 2016). The pain, trauma and morbidity of surgery hampered progress for another 100 years pending the introduction anaesthesia and antisepsis, that facilitated the development of the classic major operations for grossly diagnosed cancers, such as radical mastectomy and gastrectomy, which were attempts at cure as opposed to palliation. The missing element necessary for the birth of what today is considered 'scientific oncology' was the development of the foundations of histopathology, which only occurred when microscope became available to study diseased tissues at the cellular level. The impact on medical practice was dramatic, leading to a transition from gross clinical diagnosis to direct microscopic examination of the cancerous lesion (the "tissue diagnosis") (Van den Tweel and Taylor, 2010, 2013; Van den Tweel et al. 2016).

1.2 The Microscope Invents Pathology and Pathologists

Rudimentary microscopes were in use in the 17C, pioneered by Antonie van Leewenhoek (1632–1723) and evidenced by the detailed botanical illustrations in *Micrographia* by Robert Hooke (Royal Society, London, 1665) (Fig. 1.1). However, it was not until the decades from around

B. Jasani et al., *Precision Cancer Medicine*, https://doi.org/10.1007/978-3-030-84087-7_1

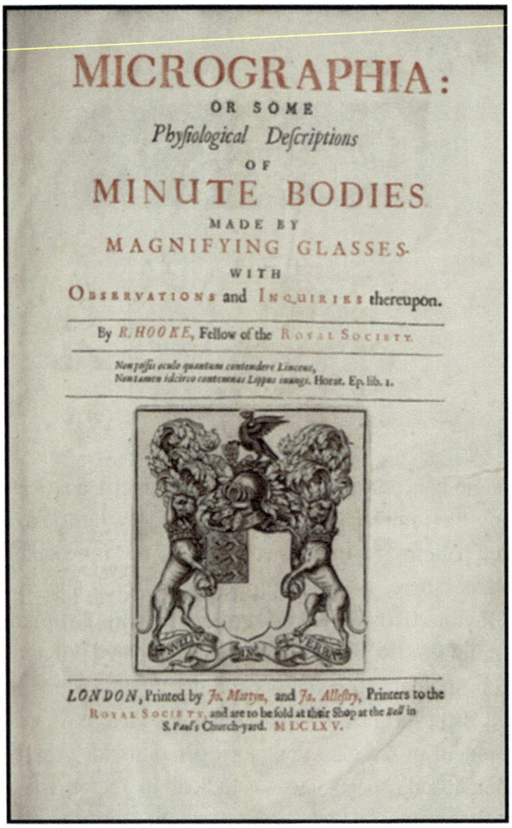

MICROGRAPHIA:
OR SOME
Physiological Descriptions
OF
MINUTE BODIES
MADE BY
MAGNIFYING GLASSES.
WITH
OBSERVATIONS and INQUIRIES thereupon.

By R. HOOKE, Fellow of the ROYAL SOCIETY.

Non possis oculo quantum contendere Linceus,
Non tamen idcirco contemnas Lippus inungi. Horat. Ep. lib. 1.

LONDON, Printed by Jo. Martyn, and Ja. Allestry, Printers to the ROYAL SOCIETY, and are to be sold at their Shop at the Bell in S. Paul's Church-yard. M DC LX V.

Fig. 1.1 Title Page. Micrographia. Robert Hooke. Royal Society 1665. Public Domain. British Library. Accessed 31 Dec 2020. https://www.bl.uk/collection-items/micrographia-by-robert-hooke-1665#

1830–1850 that improvements in lens design and manufacture at last rendered the microscope a useful tool in biology and medicine, heralding the advent of a new branch of medical practice as the *"first pathologists emerged from the treacherous swamps of medieval practice onto the relatively firm ground that histopathology seemed to offer with respect to the diagnosis of disease."* (Taylor 2011; Taylor & Cote, 2005).

A select number of physicians and surgeons were lured away from their clinical practice to experience the use of the microscope in medical diagnosis, with particular impact upon the field of cancer. The record of their experiences resulted in several texts that appeared across Germany, Italy, France and Britain, among which two had major lasting impact (Fig. 1.2).

Sir James Paget (1st Baronet, 1814–1899) and Rudolf Virchow (1821–1902) both published a series of highly influential lectures and came to share similar views, together providing huge impetus to microscopic pathology (Van den Tweel et al. 2016). Paget continued to practice primarily from the perspective of the surgeon, while Virchow is held by many to be the "Father of Pathology." Certainly Virchow's "*Cellularpathologie*" provided much of the scientific basis for the modern pathologic study of cancer. Somewhat in parallel to Morgagni systematic autopsy observations, made with the unaided eye and related to the clinical course of the illness, Virchow correlated microscopic pathological findings with clinical outcome to investigate the nature of cancer as an illness. The experiences of Virchow, Paget and those who followed generated numerous publications and new journals, such as '*Virchows Archiv,*' (founded 1847), which described the microscopic features of disease and laid the foundation for histopathology and the 'tissue diagnosis' as the 'Gold Standard' for cancer 200 years.

Histopathological examination led inevitably to new ideas about cancer, to fierce debate and eventually to a better understanding how the tissue damage caused by cancer ultimately was responsible for the death of the patient. Virchow, while he was central to the development of microscopy, held the view that cancer arose by transformation from connective tissue (called '*metaplasia*' in the concept of that time). Paget, however, concluded that cells from a primary tumour could spread through the bloodstream and could grow in distant organs. William Halsted (1852–1922), who pioneered radical mastectomy, tended to support the view that adequate local removal of the cancer would cure it and that if the cancer appeared later elsewhere, it was due to a new process. This process of spread, referred to as metastasis, became a key element in recognizing the limitations of cancer surgery. While debate was ongoing it resulted in the development of more rational and effective methods for surgical removal of the tumour. In addition, tissues removed by the surgeon could now be exam-

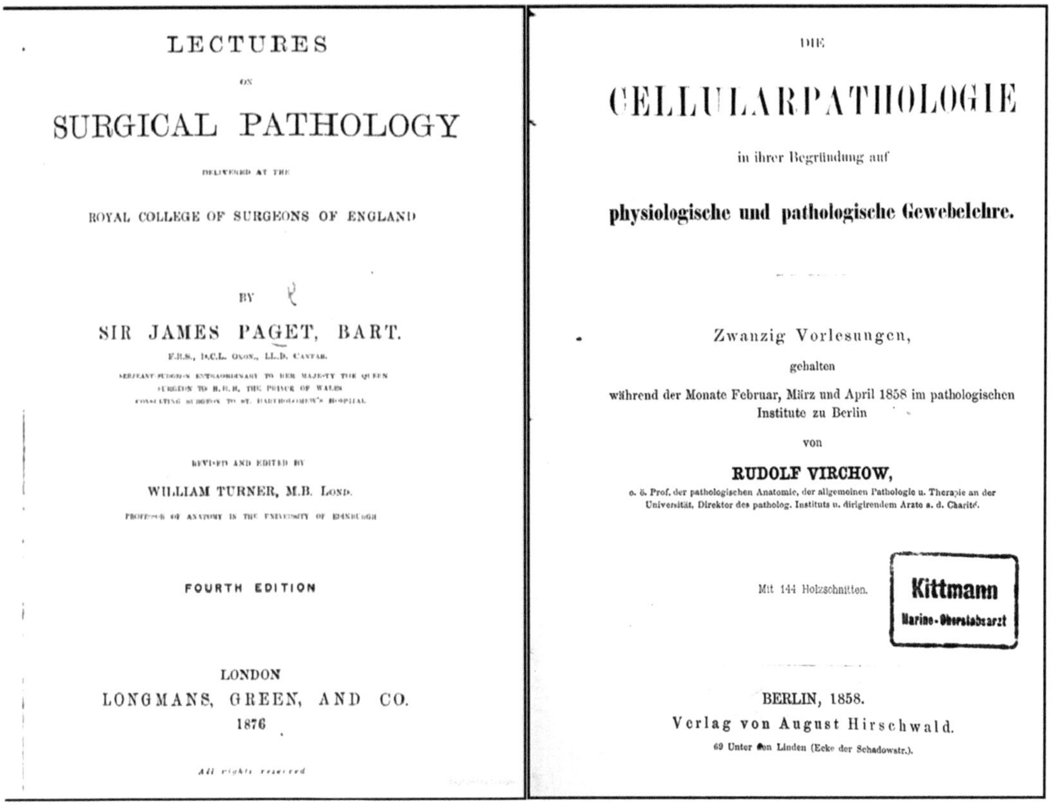

LECTURES
ON
SURGICAL PATHOLOGY
DELIVERED AT THE
ROYAL COLLEGE OF SURGEONS OF ENGLAND
BY
SIR JAMES PAGET, BART.
F.R.S., D.C.L. OXON., LL.D. CANTAB.
SERJEANT-SURGEON EXTRAORDINARY TO HER MAJESTY THE QUEEN
SURGEON TO H.R.H. THE PRINCE OF WALES
CONSULTING SURGEON TO ST. BARTHOLOMEW'S HOSPITAL
REVISED AND EDITED BY
WILLIAM TURNER, M.B. LOND.
PROFESSOR OF ANATOMY IN THE UNIVERSITY OF EDINBURGH
FOURTH EDITION
LONDON
LONGMANS, GREEN, AND CO.
1876
All rights reserved

DIE
CELLULARPATHOLOGIE
in ihrer Begründung auf
physiologische und pathologische Gewebelehre.
Zwanzig Vorlesungen,
gehalten
während der Monate Februar, März und April 1858 im pathologischen Institute zu Berlin
von
RUDOLF VIRCHOW,
o. ö. Prof. der pathologischen Anatomie, der allgemeinen Pathologie u. Therapie an der Universität, Direktor des patholog. Instituts u. dirigirendem Arzte a. d. Charité.
Mit 144 Holzschnitten.
Kittmann
Marine-Oberstabsarzt
BERLIN, 1858.
Verlag von August Hirschwald.
69 Unter den Linden (Ecke der Schadowstr.).

Fig. 1.2 The Foundations of Histopathology. Title Pages of the seminal texts. (**a**) Sir James Paget. Lectures on surgical pathology: delivered at the Royal College of Surgeons. First Edition 1853: title page from Fourth Edition, 1876 (Google books: digital). (**b**) Rudolf Virchow. Cellularpathologie: a series of lectures at the Institute zu Berlin, 1858. (collection of author, CRT)

ined to define more accurately both the type and the extent of the spread of cancer. The pathologist could also tell the surgeon whether the operation had been able to completely remove the cancer.

1.3 Seeking a Cure for Non-Symptomatic Early Stage Cancer; Cancer Screening

An alternative to attempting the cure established disease was, as suggested by Galen, to detect the cancer in its early stage before it had spread, to allow the surgical removal of the localised tumour in order to effect a cure. This idea led to the development of screening tests to detect the presence of cancer, in individuals who did not have symptoms.

The first screening test to be widely used for cancer was the Pap test, developed initially by George Papanicolaou (1883–1962) (Fig. 1.3) as a research method in understanding the menstrual cycle. Papanicolaou soon recognized the potential of the method for identifying cervical cancer early in its course. He presented his findings in 1923, but it was not until the American Cancer Society (ACS) promoted the test during the early 1960s that the Pap smear test became widely used. Subsequently the cervical cancer death rate in the United States has declined by about 70%.

Mammography was developed late in the 1960s as a screening method for breast cancer, and was first officially recommended by the ACS in 1976. Current American Cancer Society guidelines include a range of methods for early detection (screening) of cancers of the cervix, breast,

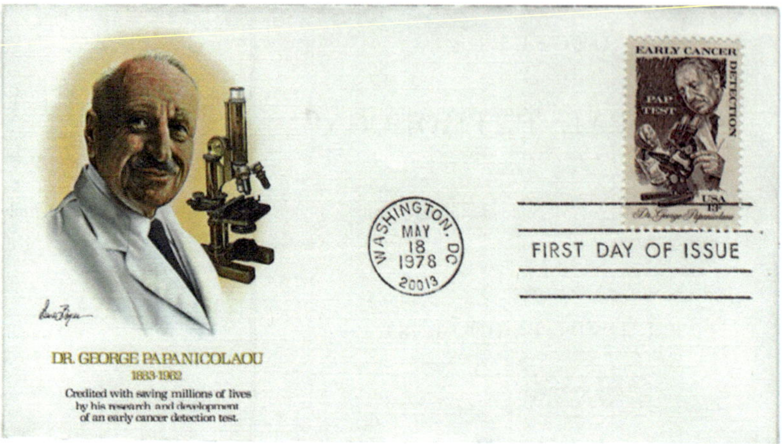

Fig. 1.3 George Papanicolaou; commemorative cover. First published in 1942, the PAP smear was in essence a morphologic biomarker for cervical cancer. (collection of the author, CRT)

colon and rectum, endometrium, lung, and prostate, in addition to cancer-related 'check-ups' which, depending on a person's age and gender, might include tests for cancers of the thyroid, mouth, skin, lymph nodes, testes, and ovaries.

Some of these tests in fact represent the early application of biomarkers for the detection and monitoring of cancer (e.g. CEA; PSA). In most of these approaches, pathologists play a key role by establishing laboratory-based assays, or more often by the examination of biospecimens using the microscope for cytologic or histologic examination.

1.4 Development of Targeted Therapies

An early example of therapy that targets a known characteristic of a specific type of tumour, relates to the realisation by Sir George Beatson (Colonel 1848–1933) that breast tissue was essentially "held in control" by the ovaries. On this basis Beatson decided to test removal of the ovaries (bilateral oophorectomy) in advanced breast cancer. The result was an improved survival rate. Conversely, and quite remarkably, he surmised that "the ovaries may be the exciting cause of carcinoma" of the breast. This hypothesis led eventually to realisation of the stimulatory effect of female ovarian hormone(s) on growth of breast cancer, even before the hormone, estrogen, itself was discovered. The idea launched a search for a mode of therapy designed specifically to oppose the growth effect of the hormone (i.e. a targeted therapy), thereby serving to inhibit growth of breast cancer. The metabolic pathways involved in the growth of breast cancer cells were studied with an intensity and focus hitherto not seen in the cancer field. Drugs such as tamoxifen and the aromatase inhibitors were developed, along with the corollary of developing tests to determine which patients would or would not be likely to respond. The precedents set for breast cancer and targeted therapy were to have far reaching implications.

The realisation that a better understanding of the growth and progression of cancer at the cell and molecular level could be used as a springboard for discovery of targeted methods to inhibit or treat cancer, was an additional practical powerful stimulus for accelerating research into genes and genetic alterations suspected to be at the root of causation of cancer. Following this paradigm, established long known 'cancer genes' have been better characterised and many new ones identified. Collectively termed 'oncogenes' and 'tumour suppressor genes,' when abnormal may lead to cancer. The presence of these abnormal genes, and the presence or alteration of their products, therefore qualify as biomarkers for cancer, and in some cases of specific cancer types.

Mutations of these genes may be inherited, but more often are acquired, spontaneously or as a result of damage by radiation, viruses or chemicals (carcinogens). In the vast majority of tumours of adults several gene abnormalities occur over time and act in concert in the develop-

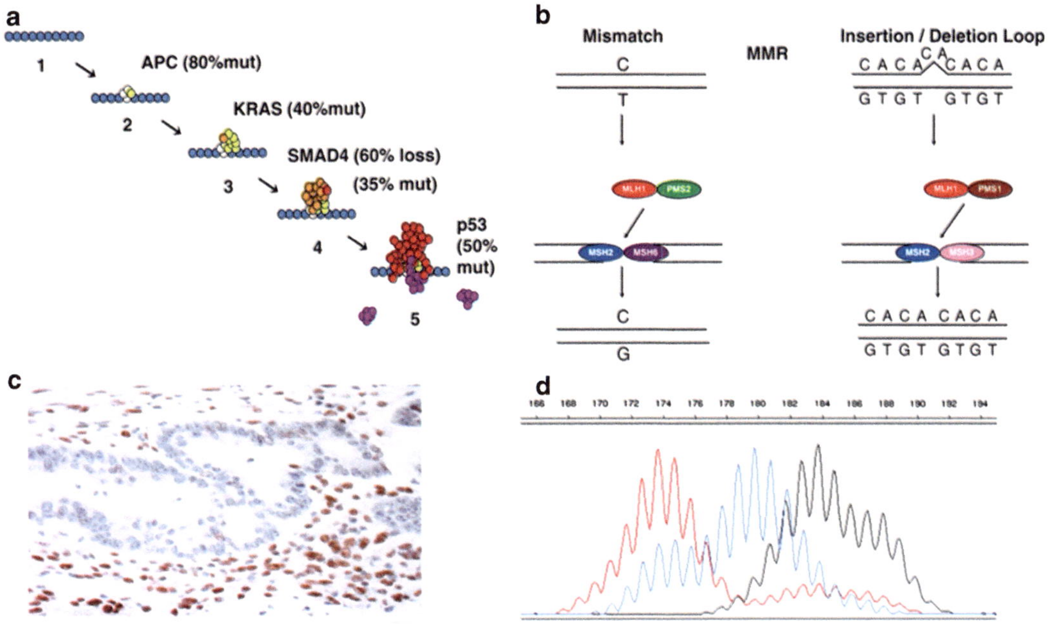

Fig. 1.4 Colorectal cancer as the prototypic model of sequential mutations in the genesis of cancer, showing the transitions of abnormal signalling pathways that drive cancer development. (**a**) Shows the sequence through hyperplasia, adenoma, dysplasia and carcinoma; (**b**) An alternative mechanism of failed mismatch repair; (**c**) shows loss of MLH1 by IHC; (**d**) shows microsatellite instability detection by fluorescent DNA analysis. From Pathways of Colorectal Carcinogenesis (Arends 2013; invited review Ed. Taylor CR)

ment of clinical cancer. This 'multi-hit phenomenon' has been beautifully demonstrated by the work of Arends and Vogelstein and others (Arends 2013; Vogelstein et al. 2013), initially in colon cancer, which lends itself to study over time by availability of sequential colonoscopic biopsies (Fig. 1.4), but it is now accepted as a common principle for most cancer types.

Abnormal, or mutated, genes may number from a few to more than 1000 in different cancer types. While many or most of these mutations are non-functional with respect to cell growth (harmless in the context of cancer), some so called 'driver genes' affect critical cell growth pathways, leading to over production of growth factors or receptors (oncogenes) or suppression of the same (suppressor genes). Typically, in adult cancers multiple abnormalities act together in cancer causation and progression (reviews: Vogelstein et al. 2013; Gu and Taylor 2014).

Over the past decade the presence of these abnormal genes or their products has been established as a key characteristic of cancer as a disease, providing many molecular lesions as possible targets for Precision Therapy (Chap. 2).

Identification of these mutational changes by molecular methods (PCR, Sequencing) or abnormal expression of their protein products (proteomics, IHC) represent examples of molecular biomarkers. A discussion of relative advantages and disadvantages of the different methods for detection and analysis of these biomarkers forms a major part of this book.

References

Arends MJ. Pathways of colorectal carcinogenesis. Appl Immunohistochem Mol Morph. 2013;21:97–102. https://doi.org/10.1097/PAI.0b013e31827ea79e.

Gu J, Taylor CR. Practicing pathology in the era of big data and personalized medicine. Appl Immunohistochem Mol Morph. 2014;22:1–9.

Taylor CR. From anatomy to surgery to pathology: eighteenth century London and the Hunterian schools. Virchow Archiv. 2010;457:405–14.

Taylor CR. From microscopy to whole slide digital images: a century and a half of image analysis. Appl Immunohistochem Mol Morph. 2011;19:491–3.

Taylor CR, Cote RJ. Immunomicroscopy: a diagnostic tool for the surgical pathologist. 3rd ed. Saunders, PA: Elsevier; 2005. (also 1st edition, Taylor 1986; 2nd edition, Taylor, Cote 1994)

Van den Tweel JG, Taylor CR. A brief history of pathology. Virchow Archiv. 2010;457:3–10. https://doi.org/10.1007/s00428-010-0934-4.

Van den Tweel JG, Taylor CR. The rise and fall of the autopsy. Virchow Archiv. 2013;462:371–80.

Van den Tweel JG, Gu J, Taylor CR. From magic to molecules: an illustrated history of disease. Beijing: Beijing University Press; 2016.

Vogelstein B, Papadopoulos N, Velculescu VE, Zhou S, Diaz LA Jr, Kinzler KW. Cancer genome landscapes. Science 29. 2013;339(6127):1546–58. https://doi.org/10.1126/science.1235122.

2 The Advent of Biomarker Testing

2.1 Biomarkers in Medicine and Cancer

The definition of biomarkers varies with context, ranging across many fields of science from 'bio-signatures,' such as geyser plumes on Europa and phosphine traces in the clouds of Venus, to the more earthly biomarkers sought by geochemical and chromatographic analysis in oil exploration. In Medicine, while the use of biological markers for diagnosis of disease is not new, the term 'biomarker' itself entered general usage only in the last 50 years or so.

In the context of this book the following broad NIH derived definition, will be used:

- a characteristic that is objectively measured and evaluated as an indicator of normal biological processes, pathogenic processes, or pharmacological responses to therapeutic intervention. Current usage within this definition is expanded in the accompanying table (Table 2.1).

The use of 'biomarkers' in general medical practice is not new (review: Taylor 2018). Many aspects of the general clinical examination, such as examination of urine or stool, fall under a broad definition, as do most clinical laboratory tests. Indeed, the definition may reasonably be extended into the realm of anatomic pathology: a PAP smear (Fig. 1.4) or a tissue diagnosis of prostate cancer, plus or minus grading (e.g. Gleason grades for

Table 2.1 Current application of molecular biomarkers in cancer

Biomarker: General definition.	• Intervention a characteristic that when measured may serve as an indicator of normal or diseased biological processes, and may be used for defined clinical purposes, including diagnostic, prognostic and predictive applications
Clinical purposes	
Diagnostic	Design and usage; primarily to assist diagnosis; commonly in IHC on tissue sections, but also sometimes indicative in serum assays
Prognostic	Design and usage; primarily as a guide to prognosis, namely the course and progress of disease—therapy unspecified
Predictive	Design and usage; for classification of responders vs. non-responders for a specified (usually targeted) therapy; assay and threshold typically developed in conjoint clinical trial with the specified drug
• Companion (diagnostic)	Predictive; co-developed with a specified therapy and 'required' prior to use of said therapy
• Complementary (diagnostic)	Predictive; co-developed with a specified therapy; accepted as providing guidance for therapy but not required
Pharmacodynamic	Definitional within the pharmaceutical field, such as providing a surrogate marker for disease status, as in disease remission or progression
Monitoring	Design and usage; for evaluation of status, progression and or recurrence of established disease process

B. Jasani et al., *Precision Cancer Medicine*, https://doi.org/10.1007/978-3-030-84087-7_2

prostate), is a morphologic biomarker of disease that is clinically actionable in a very real sense. In the clinical lab examples of commonly employed biomarkers include hormone levels for endocrine disorders, a succession of enzymes and proteins for renal or liver function, up to present day troponin for myocardial infarction and, in oncology, prostatic acid phosphatase, followed by PSA (prostate specific antigen), for prostate cancer. These tests represent the beginnings of application of biomarkers to the molecular level.

2.1.1 Biomarkers in Cancer

Among the first biological markers purposed for the diagnosis of malignant disease was the test for Bence-Jones protein in urine (Henry Bence-Jones, 1813–1873) (Fig. 2.1) associated with Kahler's disease (Otto Kahler, 1849–1893), a surrogate in part for the detection of monoclonal (malignant-M) proteins in the disease that we now know as multiple myeloma.

In more modern times the specific use of molecular biomarkers for cancer may be traced back to the use CEA (carcino-embryonic antigen) as a serum protein biomarker for colon cancer, and to the Philadelphia chromosome (Nowell and Hungerford 1960) as the first specific genetic marker of malignancy, in chronic myeloid leukemia.

Although serum testing for CEA fell short of diagnostic utility in terms of sensitivity and specificity, it did serve to advance the notion of using biomarkers for the monitoring established disease, and along with many other serum and tissue proteins, such as CA-125 and PSA, found a variable role as a diagnostic biomarker when demonstrated *in situ* in tissues by immunohistochemistry (IHC). Thus context matters.

The development of prognostic and predictive biomarkers owed much to the study of hormone receptors in breast cancer (ER and PR). Technical considerations as to assay method resulted in the original cytosol based competitive assays giving way to detection of ER (and or PR) in situ within tissue sections by labeled antibody methods, by IHC (immunohistochemistry) using FFPE (formalin fixed paraffin embedded) sections. This change occurred over objections raised against the use of IHC and FFPE tissue, because of the unknown effects of protein 'masking' and concerns regarding subjectivity in interpretation and variability in scoring (of IHC). The efforts of Jules Elias, Craig Allred and others led to the development of defined (but semi-quantitative) scoring methods, which showed that the results of IHC were clinically more relevant than the

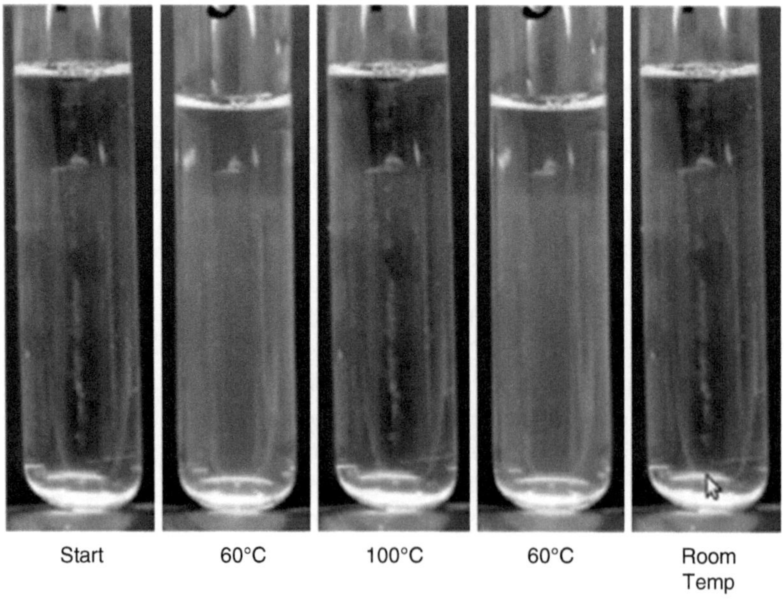

Fig. 2.1 An early biomarker test. The test for Bence Jones protein, by heating urine; a precipitate that appears at 60C, becomes soluble on further heating, and reappears on cooling is a biomarker for multiple myeloma. The test is not highly specific, especially when conducted on the ward by a resident physician at 2.00 AM (Personal collection, CRT)

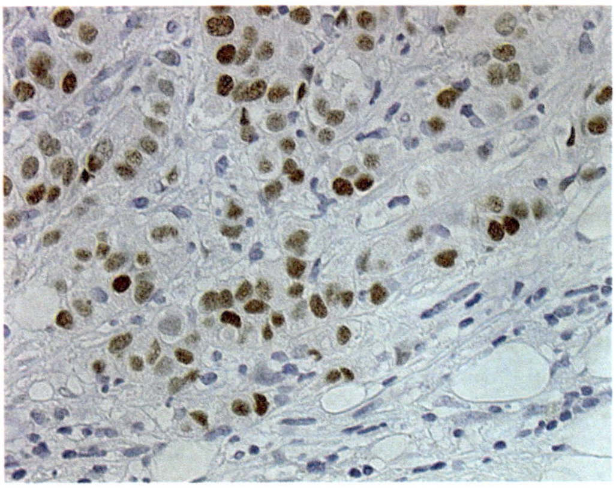

Fig. 2.2 An early tissue biomarker: Estrogen Receptor (ER) in breast cancer demonstrated by an IHC method on an FFPE tissue section. ER positive cancer cells show a brown nuclear stain pattern (Personal collection of author, CRT)

cytosol assays they replaced. The IHC ER 'test' (Fig. 2.2) may be rightly considered to represent the beginning of the current era of employment of biomarkers in tissue sections for cancer, for prognostic and predictive purposes (Taylor 2020).

This experience with testing for ER had other important consequences. It served as an important stimulus to careful re-evaluation of the mode of performance of the IHC method; tacit recognition that the traditional IHC method, when applied in its customary mode as a stain, lacked rigor in selection of reagents, controls, adherence to protocol and interpretation. For IHC to be used as an assay, with a quantitative result, it required a more rigorous protocol, validation and objective reporting, all of which are common practices for many clinical laboratory assays. It became apparent that the entire IHC process must be repurposed for this new and different goal; in reality, the difference between a qualitative stain and a quantitative assay. The concept of the Total Test that is followed throughout this book is borrowed from the clinical laboratory (Taylor 1992), where there is a long history of high quality test performance and control. This contrast in the rigour of test performance between the histology laboratory and the clinical laboratory is well reviewed by Bogen (2019) and is a central theme of Part II of this book. Notably, in addressing the goal of improved performance of IHC in the context of biomarker testing, the IHC method when applied as a stain also has benefited.

In the presence of validated reagents, protocol, proper controls of assay performance and accurate counting (see Part II), the IHC method applied to an FFPE tissue section has exquisite specificity; a trained pathologist is able to score only the specifically labelled cancer cells, distinct from any residual normal cells and stroma. In addition, the technical sensitivity is extraordinary, with the ability to detect one ER positive cell among a 100 identifiable cancer cells (1% is the current threshold for a positive ER IHC test), or in fact 1 positive cell among 1000 or 10,000 or more cancer cells. Expressed in these terms, namely detection of cells that display a positive reaction with reference to controls, the level of sensitivity is far beyond anything that can be achieved by any method that relies upon an extract of tissue, which is necessarily an imperfectly known extract of an imperfectly known mixture of normal and cancer cells, themselves imperfectly identified.

The further development of genetic biomarkers was initially less rapid, pending major technical advances in molecular and sequencing methods (Part III). BRCA1 and BRCA2 were discovered in 1990s as inheritable factors that contribute to causation of breast cancer, serving as potential biomarkers to identify women who have a higher risk of developing breast cancer. Therapy was modified accordingly; patients bearing mutated BRCA1 or BRCA2 genes were offered pre-emptive double mastectomies to prevent their cancers as a life-saving procedure. In this example the mutated BRCA1 and 2 serve as biomarkers for a patient risk group, but are not directly predictive of responders versus non-responders after the manner of the specific targeted therapies that followed.

Subsequently many other oncogenes and tumour suppressor genes, including some that run in families have been discovered and are instrumental in the causation of many types of cancer, including those of colon, rectum, kidney, ovary, thyroid, pancreas and skin (melanoma), many of which by the middle of the decade had been recognised to be clinically useful biomarkers (Table 2.2). Familial cancer is not nearly as common as spontaneous cancer (cancer that is caused by DNA damage occurs during a person's lifetime), accounting for less than 15% of all cancers. However, investigation of these families has been disproportionately important in leading to a better understanding of the complex interplay of these genes, not only in hereditary cancer but across the whole field of oncogenesis, as is well shown by the work of Vogelstein and colleagues alluded to previously (see Fig. 1.4).

Table 2.2 Selected biomarkers, both as approved tests and as LDTs*

Test	Commonly applied tumor types
HER2	Breast, gastric
PD-L1	Melanoma, lung, kidney, head & neck, uterus, breast
CTLA-4	Melanoma
CD 20	B lymphoma, CLL
CD 30	ALCL, Hodgkin L
ALK	Lung
TOPO1	Bladder, breast, colon, uterus, overy
MMR (MLH1, MSH2, MSH6, PMS2)	Colon, stomach
EGFR	Colon, lung, pancreas, thyroid
VEGF	Lung, kidney, glioboastoma, colon
TUBB3	Lung, bladder, uterus, kidney, prostate
PTEN	Breast, uterus, head & neck, lung, prostate
ER, PR	Breast, uterus, ovary
K-ras	Lung, colon
myc	Lymphoma
BCR-ABL 1	CML, (Ph chromosome)
BRCA 1	Breast, ovary, others
c-KIT protein ERCC1	GIST Bladder lung
BRAF	Melanoma, lung, colon, others
EZH2	Follicular lymphoma
IDH1,2	Acute myeloid leukemia
CLL FISH	Chronic lyphocytic leukemia
D816V	Mastocytosis
PDGFRB FISH	Myelodysplastic disease
POIK3CA	Breast
Immune cell profile CD3, CD4, CD8, CD20, CD68, FoxP3 and others	Melanoma, lung, colon, breast, others
IHC 'stains' PSA, CEA, p53, p21, Ki67 Multiple tissue biomarkers	Various tumours, prognostic mainly. Several hundred molecules demonstrated by IHC are use in diagnostic surgical pathology*

Those markers listed lend themselves to testing in cell preparations or tissue sections by IHC or IF and related methods; but many also may be tested by molecular methods in FFPE tissue extracts (Part III)

- IHC when employed as an aid to the surgical pathologist is classified by FDA as Class I; similarly by CIQC and other certifying agencies. IHC when used for ER in conjunction with pathology interpretation is Class II, and when used in 'stand alone' mode, as for PD-L1, is Class III. LDT, Lab developed test.

(Selected from US FDA 2021 U.S. Food and Drug Administration. List of Cleared or Approved Companion Diagnostic Devices (In Vitro and Imaging Tools). Accessed February 2021.

On a broader front, recognition of the key roles of specific genetic changes in the progression to cancer, led directly to the development of therapies that are designed to correct or oppose the effects of the specific mutation(s) that lead to abnormalities of cell growth control. Identification of the associated biomarkers already has become a necessary adjunct to the tissue diagnosis of many tumours, and in some instances emerges as the most important test result for determining therapy (Gu and Taylor 2014) (Fig. 2.3).

As discussed below, this approach employed clinical trials in a manner that differed from traditional multiple chemotherapy trials in two principal ways. First the trials were focused upon the presence (or absence) a specified mutational lesion (a biomarker) in the patient (and control) population. Second, they were designed to incorporate a specific biomarker test in an attempt to separate (probable) responders from non-responders (a companion diagnostic or predictive biomarker). The design of these combined trials increasingly was based upon scientific knowledge of the function and effect of mutations, the design of 'drugs' (antibodies or other molecules) to counteract the mutational change, and the co-

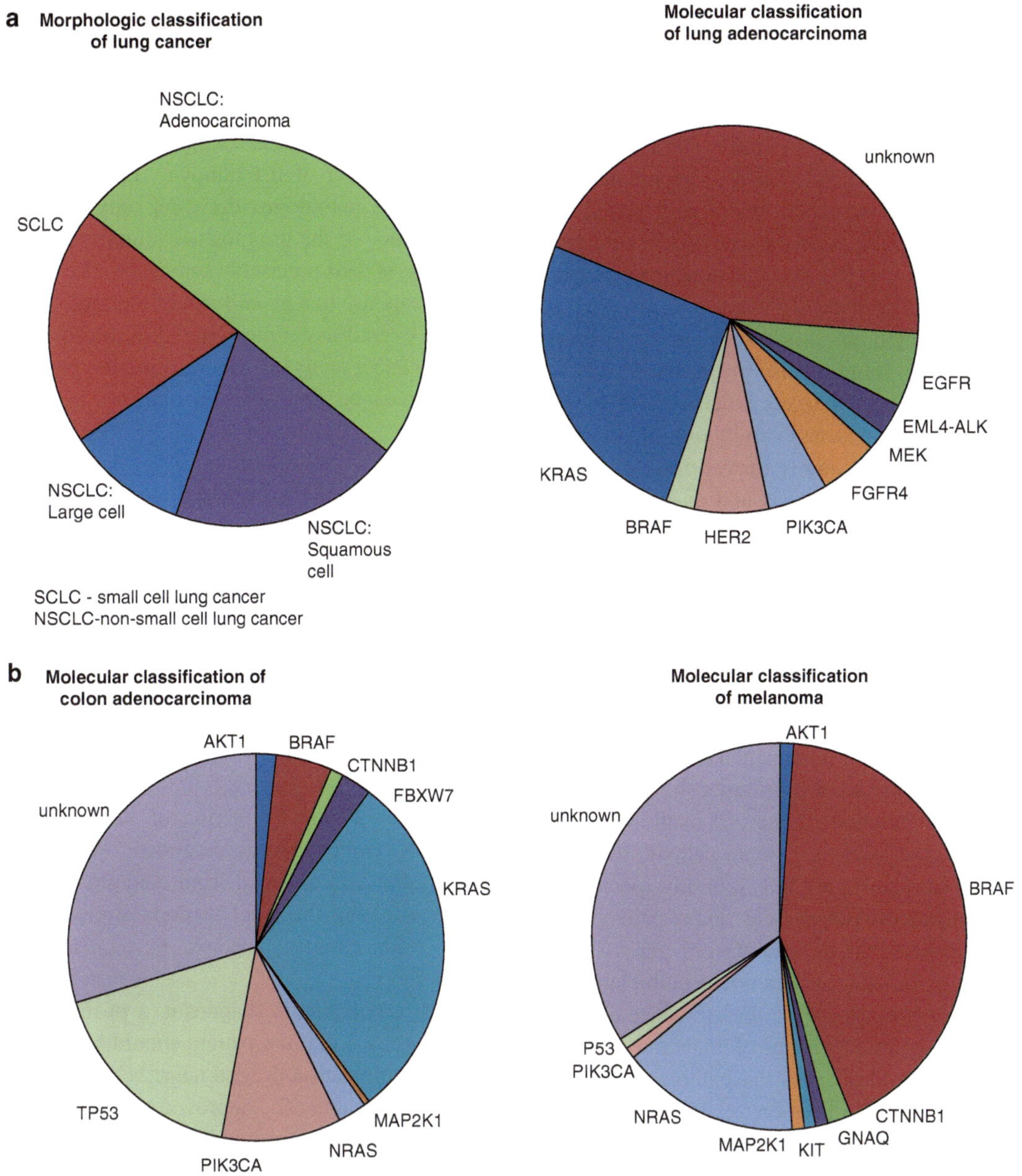

Fig. 2.3 The 'molecular' classification of these tumour types is superseding traditional morphologic classification as shown for lung cancer in (**a**); molecular profiles are shown for colon cancer and melanoma in (**b**). From Gu and Taylor (2014). With permission Lippincott, Williams and Wilkins

development of tests to detect whether or not the mutation is present. The ultimate interest of the cancer sufferer and oncologist alike is to maximize the chance of an objective response to treatment leading to a progression free survival up to the point of a cure, while avoiding side effect of treatment that are unlikely to be effective. The aim of predictive cancer therapy is to achieve this goal with high precision and high accuracy, as described next.

2.2 Basis of Prediction of Response to Therapy

The starting point for initiation of treatment and selection of therapy in solid tumours remains a "tissue diagnosis," increasingly supplemented by new knowledge of the underlying genetic and molecular changes. In the case of leukaemias this precept extends to blood and bone marrow examination, supplemented increasingly by IHC and/or flow cytometric studies using phenotypic markers for more precise diagnosis. In this context phenotypic markers (such as CD3, CD20, CD30 etc.) represent a variety of biomarkers that are employed primarily for cell recognition with the purpose of diagnosis and disease classification. While these biomarkers are often critical for determination of treatment regimens in these diseases, they do not stand alone as predictive or prognostic biomarkers exemplified by HER2 and PD-L1, the presence or absence of which predicates choice of therapy.

Predictive biomarkers evolved hand in glove with the concept of molecularly targeted therapy, with the purpose of translating the effectiveness of cancer treatment observed at the population level to the level of a single patient. To achieve this goal requires not only a highly specific drug action, but also precise selection of patients likely to respond to the targeted drug therapy. The role of the pathologist is paramount in the latter context, for the choice of therapy increasingly is determined by the results of a laboratory test.

For several decades the pathologist has contributed key information relating to prognosis and choice of therapy, through determination of cancer type, grade and stage of the cancer and integration with demographic features such as the age, gender, medical and social history. This type of information is derived from the collective experience of pathologists and oncologists over decades and from large scale chemotherapy trials that examined relative survival data in cancer populations. Predictive or prognostic value for an individual patient was inferential, dependent upon using the above information to place a patient within a particular population graphic. The goal of precision medicine is to take prognosis and prediction directly to the level of a single patient by combining choice of targeted therapy with a test that reliably predicts response or lack thereof. Such tests are termed companion or complementary diagnostics. By combining traditional subtyping of the tumour with molecular analysis the pathologist does not only improve the accuracy of the prognostic evaluation, but in many cases also precisely predict the likelihood of the response to a given form of therapy.

The overall assessment is referred to as predictive cancer analysis, which forms the basis of precision cancer therapy.

2.3 Role of Pathology and the Pathologist in the Advent of Precision Cancer Medicine

2.3.1 New Types of Tests: Companion and Complementary Diagnostics

The definition and distinction of 'Companion' versus 'Complementary' diagnostic biomarker tests (Table 2.1) emerged from conjoint clinical trials, reflecting the level of correlation of test result with clinical response to the drug in question.

With a companion diagnostic a positive test result signifies that the patient should be treated with the companion drug; a negative result indicates no treatment. The approved test is required before use of the corresponding approved drug.

With a complementary diagnostic a positive result may be considered to indicate treatment, and a patient having a negative result may or may not be treated according to an informed clinical decision. The test is, therefore, not required for use of the drug.

Whether or not a test is classified as a 'Companion' or 'Complementary' diagnostic is a function not only of the nature of the biomarker, but also of how the test itself is established and validated. For example, in conjoint clinical trials of various therapies for PD-1 and PD L-1 some of the associated PD L1 'tests' emerged as companion diagnostics, and others as complementary, varying according to which method was employed for testing, including in IHC which anti-PD-L1 antibody was used (Gu and Taylor 2014; Taylor 2018; Lu et al. 2019), as well as by specified tumor type.

An FDA approved companion diagnostic falls under the FDA definition of an approved IVD (in vitro diagnostic) with the following conditions—"it provides information that is essential for the safe and effective use of a corresponding therapeutic product"—and its use is "stipulated in the instructions for use in the labeling of both the diagnostic device and the corresponding therapeutic agent" (Table 2.2) (Taylor 2018, 2020; US FDA 2021). The EU definition is evolving, but similar and interestingly admits both "quantitative and qualitative determination of specific markers identifying subjects." It specifically excludes monitoring. The quantitative versus qualitative aspect of the test is considered further in Part II, particularly Chaps. 9 and 11, with evolution in the direction of a strictly quantitative assay.

The FDA definition assigns biomarker testing by IHC to Class III (the highest level), which requires PMA (Pre-market approval) in a co-development mode with the drug as described above. EU regulations are evolving and should be consulted directly. Also, these comments apply to companion diagnostics. Corresponding guidelines for so called complementary diagnostics are at present governed by precedent and usage.

While IHC applied to breast cancer was the prototypic method employed for the first companion diagnostic, the field has expanded rapidly in types of cancers evaluated, individual biomarkers and methods of testing.

The IHC HER2 test served as the model for a multitude of IHC based biomarker tests that were developed to accommodate the burgeoning repertoire of targeted therapies. Other available technologies also were rapidly adapted to companion diagnostic arena (Table 2.3), including ISH (in situ hybridization), PCR (polymerase chain reaction) and sequencing (Sanger or NGS—next generation sequencing), plus RNA expression methods and proteomics (usually mass spectrometry or Reverse Phase Protein Array). These methods were variously designed to detect DNA (mutations), RNA (expression), or proteins (receptors, ligands, enzymes), either singly, or in exploratory panels, initially the 40 plus mutation screens included in some NGS 'tests', but now expanded to screens of more than 200 potential markers.

Table 2.3 Principal technologies deployed for biomarker testing

Extraction based (usually FFPE)
Sequencing; sanger, and NGS (next generation)
Epigenetic differentiation
Laser capture microscopy
T & B cell receptor deep sequencing
Mass spectroscopy
Reverse phase protein arrays
RNA expression arrays
Tissue section based (FFPE)
In situ hybridization (ISH)
Multiplex immunofluorescence (IF)
Immunohistochemistry (IHC)
RNAscope
MIBI microscopy
Raman microscopy
Digital AI derived virtual biomarkers (AI VB)

FFPE, formalin fixed paraffin embedded tissue specimen (Comparative advantages of these methods are discussed further in Chap. 14)

This explosion in technology and testing, much of which had immediate clinical application, has presented huge challenges for pathologists involved in cancer diagnosis. Whereas for 200 years pathology has changed by evolution, the recent changes represent a revolution.

2.3.2 Evolution to Revolution: The Changing Role for Pathology

As described in Chap. 1, the treatment of cancer patients is based upon long established principles that attempt to correlate a tissue diagnosis with the observed clinical experience of therapeutic outcome. This approach is applied to surgical treatments, to radiotherapy and to drug treatments following the introduction, first of single chemotherapeutic agents, then of multiple drug regimens. In the very beginning selection of treatment was anecdotal, often based upon the experience of a single practitioner, and might therefore vary greatly from place to place. The advent of prospective studies that were designed to compare proposed therapeutic approaches with existing best methods, represented the first clinical trials.

Improvements in outcome were dependent not only upon the availability of new therapeutic approaches, but also upon improvements in diagnostic accuracy, coupled with selection of optimal therapy to fit that diagnosis. In meeting this goal clinical trials became essential, clearly exceeding the capabilities and experience of any single surgeon or physician.

The cancer pathologist played a crucial role with respect to diagnosis, expanding the 'Gold Standard' tissue diagnosis to include not only the major type of cancer, but also to such sub-types as were shown to have clinical relevance, and were agreed upon in international diagnosis and classification schemata such as those of the WHO. Uniform international grading and staging systems were developed *pari passu*. Integration of these pathologic data allowed more precise categorisation of patients for entry into clinical trials that were designed to compare different therapeutic choices.

Entry of patients into clinical trials and selection of treatment regimens that resulted from them, still was predicated upon clinical judgement, that because of the complexities of data for each patient, was increasingly made by a multidisciplinary team (Tumour Board) that included surgery, medical oncology, radiology and pathology. The charge was to integrate the various clinical and diagnostic data sets, including clinical examination, radiologic and pathologic staging, as well as the tissue diagnosis, which was rendered as precisely (and as narrow) as possible by well-developed morphologic criteria and such ancillary methods as IHC, and flow cytometry if appropriate. The integrated results for the patient were used as the basis for a clinical judgement for therapy.

The morphologic 'tissue diagnosis' was a major part of the multiparameter decision process, but it was by no means the sole arbiter of therapy.

Exactly what cancer patients themselves expect, and indeed want from this process should not be overlooked. When asked directly, their expressed needs include precise and accurate information on a range of issues concerning their condition; the type of cancer that they are suffering from, the most effective and the least harmful (both physical and psycho-social) therapy for their disease and information regarding their overall chances of survival (see 'ecancer' 2018, 12: 873 https://doi.org/10.3332/ecancer.2018.873'). Added to these individual needs, population focused health care systems worldwide increasingly are looking to maximise efficiency, while reducing overall costs.

Recognition of uniqueness of each cancer at the molecular level, and the uniqueness of its behaviour in each different patient have forced a revision of this paradigm, and driven the development of diagnostic and treatment protocols that are designed for the specifically characterised cancer in each individual patient, meeting the definitional requirement of Precision Medicine.

The traditional double-blind clinical trials in which patient entry was predicated on multiple factors including tissue diagnosis (cancer type/subtype), grade and stage (plus other factors such as response to existing therapies) has been quite suddenly supplanted by a new type of trial in which therapy is directed to a specified genetic lesion in the cancer, precision therapy targeted to a defined tumour and characterised by the relevant biomarker.

2.4 The Development Pathway for Targeted Therapeutics and Precision Diagnostics

As discussed in the preceding paragraphs, testing for estrogen receptor (ER) and progesterone receptor (PR) have become important in selection of the treatment program for women with a tissue diagnosis of breast cancer. Over a period of several decades ER and PR testing have evolved technically, and have grown in clinical significance, acquiring both prognostic and predictive importance, the latter in the context of whether or not the patient is likely to respond to hormonal manipulation (such as estrogen suppression by tamoxifen, (Nolvadex™, AstroZeneca™). Clinical trials tested this hypothesis, leading to clear recommendations for linking an ER test result with a defined mode of therapy—"A high degree of correlation between response and positive estrogen-receptor assay suggests the value of the diagnostic test as a means to select patients for tamoxifen treatment" (Lerner et al. 1976).

In the example of ER test and tamoxifen the acceptance of a clinical connection between the test and the specified mode of therapy developed over several decades, and was retrospective. On September 25th 1998 everything changed, consequent upon issuance of letters from the FDA to Dako (now Agilent, CA, USA) (Fig. 2.4) and Genetech (now Roche) giving joint approval to the HercepTest and the drug (Herceptin) targeted to the corresponding biomarker (HER2) and their combined use in selecting treatment.

From this action of the FDA, shortly mirrored by regulatory bodies in other countries, the concept of a Companion Diagnostic emerged, together with several very important precedents that subsequently have governed the development of this class of therapeutic agents.

1. The concept was introduced of linking a test to a drug in order more accurately to select individual patients as responders vs. non-responders; in contrast to the traditional multi-drug chemotherapy trials, which identified populations having survival advantages rather than individual patients
2. The importance of performing conjoint clinical (double blind) trials of test and drug together, was established, generating outcomes data that defined and validated the predictive value of the test, in the context of effectiveness of the drug.
3. The notion that the biomarker test result should be actionable in a defined clinical setting was introduced.
4. Further it was established that the biomarker test should have a scientific background of evidence including clinical significance, and must be performed in a test system having well established performance characteristics (i.e. validation), in a 'fit for purpose' approach.

In practice, the HercepTest/Herceptin process also established a fifth precedent, namely that conjoint development of drug and predictive biomarker should begin at the R&D stage, ahead of the actual clinical trial (Fig. 2.5).

This new process of biomarker based targeted drug development, as well as its implementation and routine application for cancer patient's management, required additional critical steps in specimen acquisition and handling, and additional new types of pathological analysis of biopsy samples. Pathology and the pathologist thereby acquired new responsibilities in managing the proper performance, interpretation and integration a rapidly expanding new range of tests, in the context of available tissue samples and relative test performance (Lu et al. 2019).

"*Pathologists are at the heart of cancer prevention through screening, diagnosis, monitoring*

a

DAKO Corporation
6392 Via Real
Carpinteria California 93013 SEP 25 1998

Re: P980018
DAKO Hercep Test
Filed: May 18, 1998
Amended: June 2, June 4, August 4, August 10, August 18, August 24, August 31 and September 25, 1998.

Dear Dr. Murray:

The Center for Devices and Radiological Health (CDRH) of the Food and Drug Administration (FDA) has completed its review of your premarket approval application (PMA) for the DAKO Herceptest. This device is a semi-quantitative immunohistochemical assay to determine HER2 overexpression in breast

b

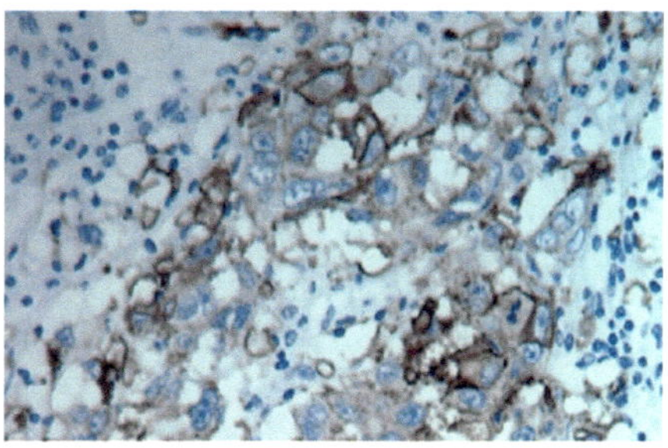

Fig. 2.4 (**a**) The crucial FDA approval letter. (**b**) The HercepTest:showing HER2 in breast cancer (Personal collection of author, CRT)

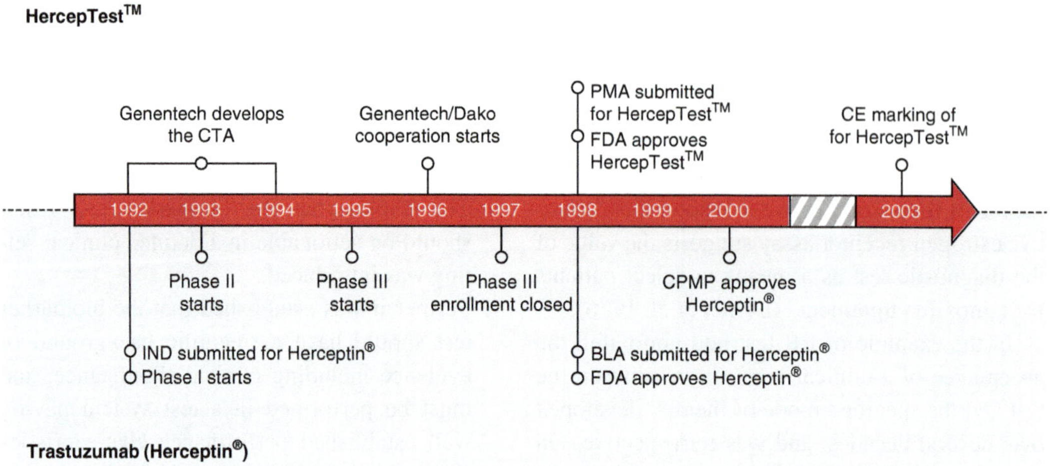

Fig. 2.5 Co-development of the drug Herceptin® and the companion diagnostics, HercepTest™. (From Pedersen and Jørgensen 2013). (Courtesy of Dako, now Agilent). CTA: Clinical Trial Assay; PMA: Premarket Approval; CE: Conformité Européene; IND: Investigational New Drug; BLA: Biologic License Application; CPMP: Committee for Proprietary Medicinal Products. FDA. US Food and Drug Administration. Dako, now Agilent; Genentech, now Roche. Reproduced with Permission, Courtesy of Agilent Technologies, Inc. ©Agilent Technologies, Inc. 2013

and treatment. Pathology is the service that handles the blood samples and the cells and tissues removed from suspicious 'lumps and bumps'. They identify the nature of the abnormality and, if malignant, provide evidence to the clinician on the type of cancer, its grade and, for some cancers, the likely profile of responsiveness to certain treatments." (https://www.rcpath.org/discover-pathology/public-affairs/cancer-diagnostics.html

References

Bogen SA. A root cause analysis into the high error rate in clinical immunohistochemistry. Appl Immunohistochem Mol Morph. 2019;27:329–38.

Gu J, Taylor CR. Practicing pathology in the era of big data and personalized medicine. Appl Immunohistochem Mol Morph. 2014;22:1–9.

Lerner HJ, Band PR, Israel L, Leung BS. Phase II study of tamoxifen: report of 74 patients with stage IV breast cancer. Cancer Treat Rep. 1976;60:1431–5.

Lu S, Stein JE, Rimm DL, Wang DW, Bell JM, Johnson DB, Sosman JA, Schalper DA, Anders RA, Wang H, Hoyt C, Pardoll DM, Danilova L, Taube JM. Comparison of biomarker modalities for predicting response to PD-1/PD-L1 checkpoint blockade a systematic review and meta-analysis. Jama Oncol. 2019; https://doi.org/10.1001/jamaoncol.2019.1549.

Nowell PC, Hungerford DA. Chromosome studies on normal and leukemic human leukocytes. J Natl Cancer Inst. 1960;25:85–109.

Pedersen HC, Jørgensen JT. Companion diagnostics, Chapter 11. In: Taylor CR, editor. Immunohistochemistry staining methods. Copenhagen: Dako Publications; 2013.

Taylor CR. Quality assurance and standardization in immunohistochemistry. A proposal for the annual meeting of the biological stain commission, June, 1991. Biotech Histochem. 1992;67:110–7.

Taylor CR. Introduction to predictive biomarkers: definitions and characteristics. In: Badve S, Kumar G, editors. Predictive biomarkers in oncology: applications in precision medicine. Springer Sciences; 2018.

Taylor CR. Milestones in immunohistochemistry and molecular morphology. App Immunohistochem Mol Morph. 2020;28:83–94.

U.S. Food and Drug Administration. List of Cleared or Approved Companion Diagnostic Devices (In Vitro and Imaging Tools). Other nucleic acid based tests are listed separately under an included link. 2021. http://www.fda.gov/MedicalDevices/ProductsandMedicalProcedures/InVitroDiagnostics/ucm301431.htm. Accessed 02 Apr 2021.

3 The Practical Challenges for Pathology: Multiple Rapidly Evolving Methods

Pathologists must rise to the challenges of precision cancer medicine by becoming:

"knowledge engineers capable of incorporating the new possibilities offered by artificial intelligence with automated and human expert systems, molecular oncology, to determine the best course of action for each patient with cancer." (https://www.ascopost.com/issues/april-25-2019/evolving-role-of-pathologists-in-the-diagnosis-and-treatment-of-cancer/)

These challenges are multifaceted and require that the surgical pathologist extends his or her knowledge and effort beyond the intellectual confines of the microscope and the surgical pathology sign out process, to ensure that a broader range of appropriate pathology expertise is involved, beginning with the earliest steps of biomarker development, and carrying through to the final crucial stages of interpretation and integration into the clinical plan.

3.1 Role in the Development Pathway for Targeted Therapeutics and Precision Diagnostics

The generic process summarised in the accompanying figure (Fig. 3.1) was born of the co-development process pioneered by Genentech and Dako (Fig. 2.5) and is well reviewed in a recent National Policy Workshop (Nass et al. 2015). Pathologists should take note that the approved biomarker tests that emerge, if morphologic in nature, require interpretation by none other than 'a pathologist.' It is incumbent, therefore, upon Pathology as a discipline to ensure that interpretation and scoring guidelines utilised by pathologists, are easy to teach, easy to learn, and reproducible in routine practice.

3.1.1 Pre-Clinical Research

The journey towards developing a reliable predictive assay begins with preclinical research that seeks to identify and select worthy drug candidates for entry into a double-blind clinical trial. This type of bench research may occur in Academia or in the laboratories of Pharma companies, large and small. It includes the pre-clinical discovery phase, identifying a potential drug that specifically targets a potentially actionable biomarker, which then is conjoined to a prototypic test for expression of that biomarker. Clinical trials establish that this so called 'companion diagnostic' is capable of selecting those patients who are most likely to respond to the specified drug therapy.

Conjoint clinical trials, Phases I, II and III; targeted drug and companion diagnostic test.

Completion of a satisfactory pre-clinical process is followed by a Phase I trial to test for the safety of the proposed drug therapy, but at the same time to monitor any objective clinical and/or biochemically measurable responses to the

B. Jasani et al., *Precision Cancer Medicine*, https://doi.org/10.1007/978-3-030-84087-7_3

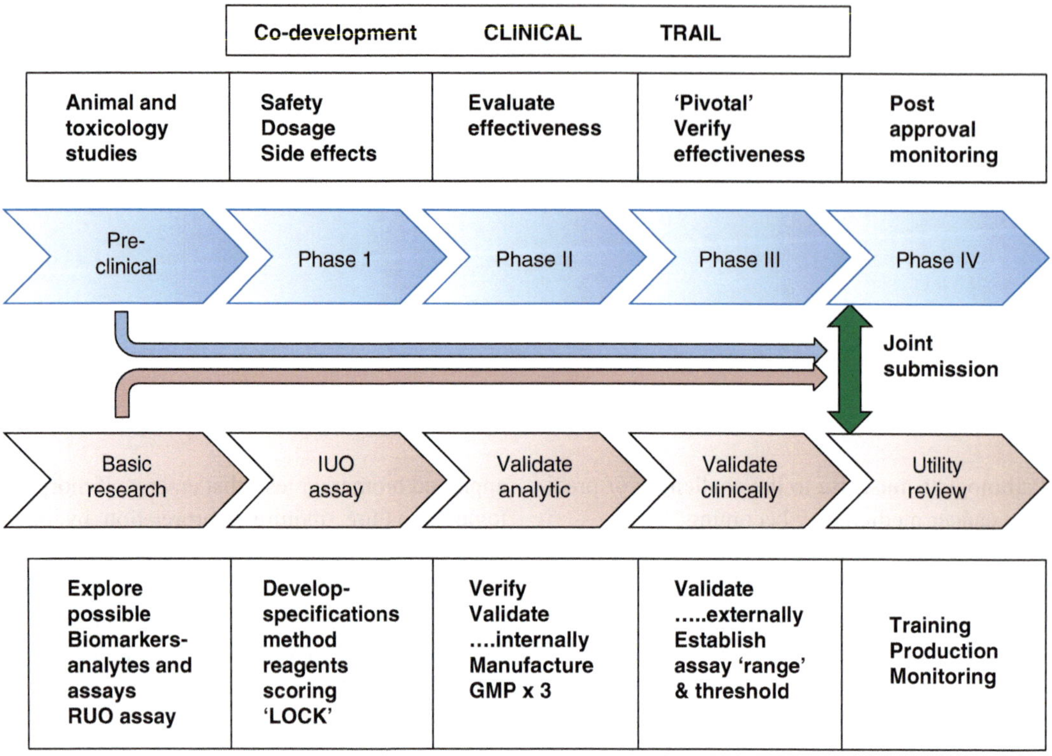

Fig. 3.1 The generic co-development process for targeted therapeutic and precision diagnostic. (Modified from Taylor 2018). With Permission of Springer Sciences

treatment. This discovery process incorporates further development of the companion test using reagents that pass through several stages of discovery and validation; typically through a research period using Analyte Specific Reagents (ASRs), leading to Investigative Use Only (IUO) test, which in the instance of a successful conjoint clinical trial (*vide infra*) with the associated targeted drug becomes a candidate for an approved IVD by FDA, European or other agencies (European Parliament 1998; US FDA 2010; Mahoney and Atkins 2014; Nass et al. 2015), a category which includes all companion and complementary diagnostics (Table 3.1) (Taylor 2018). Other regulatory bodies in other countries follow similar procedures.

If Phase I trial is successful according to above parameters, there follows a Phase II Trial which is designed set up to validate and extend the results of Phase I trial by examining a larger number of patients and establish drug dose and regimen, selected with more stringent selection and exclusion criteria. The achievement of statistically significant results allows progress to a subsequent Phase III with the goal of establishing clinical effectiveness of the test/drug combination for the defined purpose. Approval defines not only the drug and dosage, but also the test (as an approved test or IVD—Table 3.1), including all reagents and all aspects of test performance (method, platform, controls, and interpretation or scoring). Any departure, even slight, from the approved test protocols results in a non-valid test, as is discussed in detail in Part II of this book.

As will be described, there are instances in which clinical laboratories, for reasons of expediency, cost, or available equipment, may separately develop biomarker assays for clinical use, purport to replicate the performance of the corresponding approved IVD (Yaziji and Taylor 2017). Such tests are often referred to as 'home brew' or Laboratory Developed Tests (LDTs). LDT's require extensive internal validation

Table 3.1 Summary of categories of diagnostic test according to use and risk. Drawn from FDA 2010; 2021

ASR	RUO	IUO	IVD	LDT
Analyte specific reagent	Research use only	Investigational use only	In vitro device	Lab developed test
No diagnostic claims	No diagnostic claims	No diagnostic claims	Specified claims FDA approved	Lab responsible for any claims[a]
FDA regulations	FDA regulations	FDA regulations	FDA regulations	CLIA[b] regulations. FDA discretion
May be used as reagents for RUO, IUO, IVD and LDT tests	Not for clinical use	Use restricted to specified study	Intended use define by trial. Specified in labeling	For use only in the lab that developed the test

[a]LDTs potentially may require FDA approval if used as predictive markers; clinical utility must be validated by the user lab

[b]CLIA. Clinical Laboratory Improvement Amendments. https://www.cms.gov/Clia/

(beyond the capabilities of many routine laboratories) (Chaps. 9 and 12), which, in the US, falls under CLIA (Clinical Laboratories Improvement Act) regulations. The use of an LDT is restricted to the laboratory in which it is developed; it cannot be sold or transferred. The position of regulatory authorities with respect to this practice varies widely in different countries. The FDA has provided written notice that it has authority to regulate LDTs, and has published guidelines, but to date not enforced them. The critical impact of these guidelines for modern laboratory practice and for the role of the pathologists as arbiters of this process is examined at length in Parts II and III.

Following the introduction of HercepTest/Herceptin and the seminal work of basic science in uncovering regions of mutations in many (all) cancer types as described in the preceding chapters, targeted therapies have proliferated, and so of course have the corresponding biomarkers, and the methods applied for their detection (Tables 2.2 and 2.3). Surgical pathologist and pathology laboratories have scrambled to set up new manifold biomarker assays, often requiring new equipment and new methods and new skills, in an attempt to meet these burgeoning new demands. An important derivative effect has been the growing recognition of the need for higher standards of testing in the surgical (anatomic/histology) laboratory to meet the exacting requirements of a quantitative assay (as opposed to a biological tissue stain), in particular higher level of control and reproducibility of test results from lab to lab which is the primary theme of Part II.

In short, the practice of surgical pathology as a whole already has been forced to change in an attempt to meet these new demands, converting tissue specimens, most critically the FFPE tissue block to an ever increasing variety of testing pathways, in addition to the time honoured H&E section. (Fig. 3.2). At long last the anatomic or surgical pathology laboratory that performs these tests, or at a minimum is involved in providing and preparing the tissues for these tests, is being held to the standards of the clinical laboratory.

3.2 Conversion of IHC from a 'Qualitative' Stain; to a Quantitative Assay

HercepTest, the first companion diagnostic, as noted previously, is an IHC—FFPE based test for HER2. The FDA approved tests for HER2 included cell line based technical controls, a defined protocol and a defined scoring method derived from conjoint clinical studies. Here the challenge for Pathology was to upgrade an existing routinely used test method, namely the IHC 'stain,' to create what essentially is a newly purposed test, namely, IHC deployed in the form of an assay with at least a semi-quantitative function (Taylor 2014). This challenge is illustrated in Fig. 3.3 and discussed at length in Part II, III and IV.

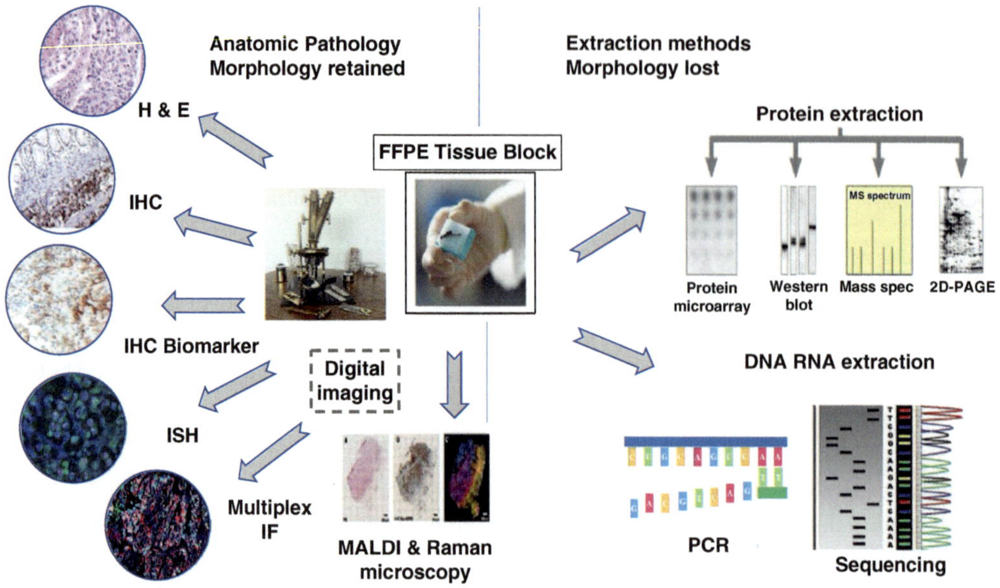

Fig. 3.2 Managing multiple testing modalities. For genesis of this concept see Taylor and Becker (2011)

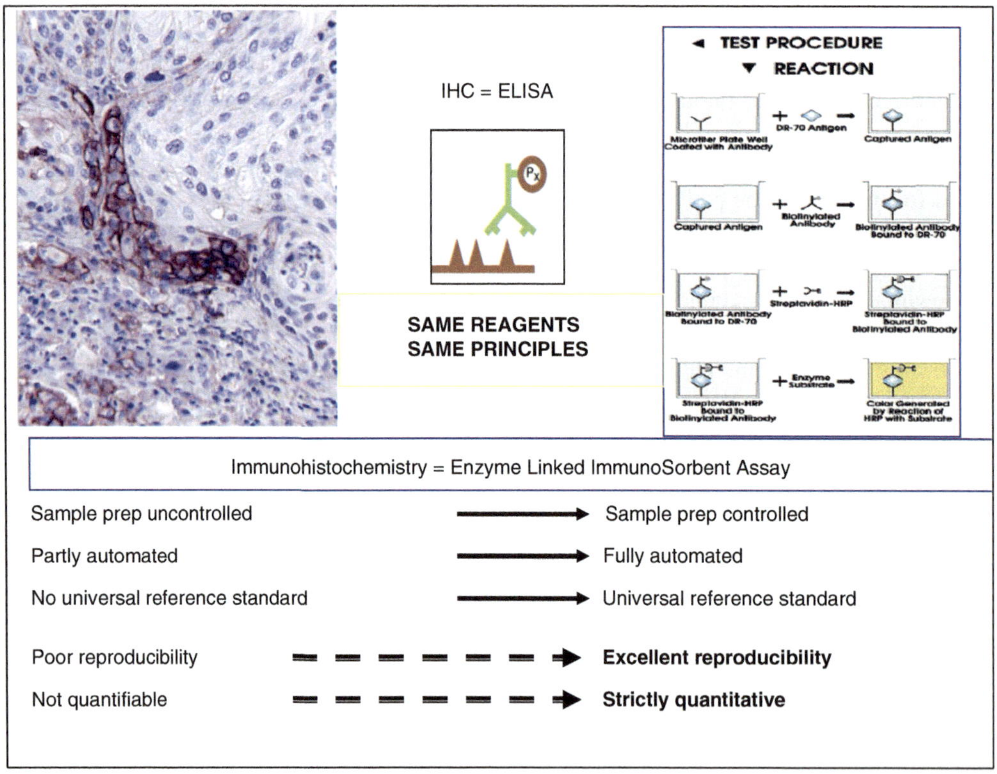

Fig. 3.3 IHC stain compared with ELISA (Enzyme Linked ImmunoSorbent Assay). The extent of antibody binding to the target antigen (protein) is revealed by reaction with a chromogen system (peroxidase plus substrate) that generates a coloured reaction product. This reaction takes place in situ in the slide in IHC, where it is scored subjectively by the pathologist, or is released into the solution (ELISA), where it may be quantified accurately using a standardised calibration curve

In addition, this first approved IHC HER2 biomarker test served as the prototypic model for a rapidly growing range of new IHC based predictive biomarker tests, the approved versions of which were each rigorously defined in terms of primary antibody, labelling reagents, protocol, staining platform and method of scoring for each separate tumor type. To meet this need for IHC alone a pathology laboratory would be required to set up and validate more than a dozen different biomarker tests on several different staining platforms, each of which must be performed exactly to approved protocol. Admittedly the basic methodology is familiar with some equipment in place, but the more rigorous mode of performance is not, for IHC when fitted to a newly purposed assay, presenting a challenge beyond most hospital laboratories and pathologists, both technically and economically (Yaziji and Taylor 2017).

Parts II and III discuss the responses of pathologists and laboratories in detail, in the context of which type of test is 'fit for purpose' with respect to the patient, the tumour type, the available laboratory resources and the clinical environment as a whole.

3.3 ISH and Multiplex Immunofluorescence Methods for Multiple Biomarkers

As will be discussed in Part III, determination of the immune profile of the cancer is now believed to be an important response indicator for a broad range of new therapies, for which patient selection is critical to outcome (e.g. EGFR, PD-L1) (Fig. 3.4) (Table 2.2).

Information on the nature and extent of any immune response may be obtained by several methods. Extraction of FFPE tissues for genomic sequencing and proteomics studies, yields extensive data as to the presence of an immune reaction in the extracted material, but the accuracy is compromised by extraction methods which may not contain representative tumor cells, in both small and large biopsies. Also, the immune cell

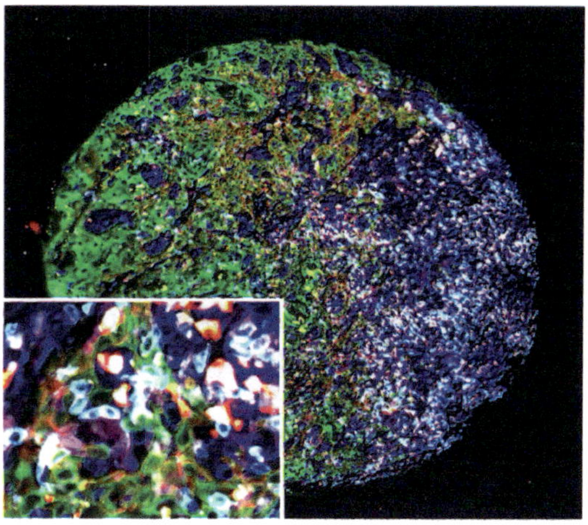

Fig. 3.4 Multiplex Immunofluorescent stain for biomarker and immune profile. This decaplex (ten marker) method demonstrates the companion diagnostic (EGFR-red), plus cell identification markers (CK5–green; Vimentin–blue) and immune profile markers (CD3–cyan; CD4–magenta; CD8-yellow; CD20-sepia; CD68-red hot; PD-1-grey; FoxP3-yellow hot). Squamous carcinoma, head and neck. Courtesy David Schwartz, Cell IDx. TMA from Dr. Mark Lingen, University of Chicago. (Adapted from Taylor 2018). Permission of Springer Sciences

infiltrate is never evenly distributed within or around the cancerous tissue, and the material separated for extraction may therefore over or underestimate the presence of immune cells, or by chance miss them completely.

The extent of the immune response, its constituent cells and molecular signals, together with its exact microanatomic relationship to recognizable tumor cells is best visualized *in situ* within the undisturbed tumor tissue by microscopic examination of a tissue section. However, because biomarker evaluation and assessment of the numbers and types of immune cells go hand in hand, it is necessary to employ methods that identify multiple biomarkers and phenotypic markers together in the same section, a task that at present is best accomplished by multiplex IF methods (Part II). Accordingly multiplex IF has now been added to the repertoire of methods that the cancer pathologist is required to make available. Acquiring and validating the necessary equipment, reagents, protocols and digital analytic algorithms necessary for performance and interpretation of multiplex IHC (see Chap. 14 and Part

IV) is expensive and requires new expertise, forcing the choice of establishing the method in house (preferable if volumes permit) or alternatively validating test performance at an accredited reference laboratory (Chap. 12).

3.4 FFPE Extraction Based Molecular Methods, PCR, NGS and Proteomics

Pathologists also are greatly impacted by the proliferation of molecular 'biomarker tests' that utilise extracts of FFPE tissues and which now play a major part in the companion diagnostic arena. These molecular methods include genomic analysis by PCR (polymerase chain reaction) and sequencing (Sanger or NGS—next generation sequencing), RNA expression analysis and proteomics (Gu and Taylor 2014; Yuan et al. 2016). The preparation of tissue extracts for analysis by these methods is dependent upon the availability of FFPE cancer tissue, derived from the biopsy or resection materials that are managed by the pathology laboratory, and in essence represent tissue diverted from the traditional AP tissue processing regimens designed to lead to the H&E section and the 'tissue diagnosis.' As biopsies in cancer patients become ever smaller management and prioritization of these diverse needs has become extremely difficult.

Furthermore, these methods are complex and diverse and dependent upon expensive, rapidly evolving equipment that requires the application of technical expertise not found in the traditional anatomic pathology environment. For these reasons many hospital pathologists elect not to set up some (or all) of these molecular tests in house, but instead send them out to large or specialised reference laboratories. The challenge then for the pathologist is to manage two conflicting goals: (i) to ensure the definitive tissue diagnosis is not compromised by inadvertent removal of all (or much) of the actual cancer from the submitted specimen, while (ii) also meeting the opposing goal of ensuring that the tissue selected for 'send out' has been properly fixed and processed and does in fact contain sufficient cancer to allow performance of the molecular assay.

Improper formalin fixation and processing is known to affect validity of IHC testing, an effect that is generally evident with proper controls (Part II). The effects upon molecular assays that employ extracts of FFPE tissues may be equally detrimental, but may be less evident, and again require performance of proper controls for DNA, RNA and/or protein testing. The pathologist should endeavor to submit only tissue samples that appear to have been properly fixed and processed. Critical requirements of processing of FFPE tissues for molecular methods are discussed in Chaps. 5, 6, 7, and 8.

Obviously, the pathologist should review parallel sections to those sent for extraction for the presence of cancer cells. The goal is that submitted tissue should contain a sufficient proportion of tumor cells versus normal cells (usually >20–30% for NGS), and mutated DNA versus germ line DNA among the tumor cells per se (usually >10%), in order to avoid a false negative result (Yuan et al. 2016). Even more difficult is the selection of tissue samples when the purpose is to evaluate the a 'immune cell profile', where the use of tissue extracts necessarily sacrifices morphologic information that may be critical to therapy choice. Micro-dissection and laser capture microscopy seek to enrich the cancer cells, but in so doing inevitably discard the immune cell population in whole or part.

The development of liquid biopsies, reliant upon cancer cells, of cancer derived DNA fragments in blood or other body fluids avoids the difficulties of allocation of scarce tissue materials, with attendant advantages and disadvantages discussed later in this book (Chap. 6).

3.5 Going Digital

In Chap. 1 the argument was advanced that Surgical Pathology (Histopathology) was born of technologic innovation. Following the introduction of the microscope into medical practice some 200 years ago pathologists have proven to be very adept at bringing new technologies from other disciplines into diagnostic use. The development of biomarker testing includes numerous such examples. Of the various test modalities that are commonly utilized for biomarker testing (Table 2.3), IHC and multiplex IF methods relate more or less closely to traditional histopathologic examination, and are therefore familiar to surgical pathologists, whose training is grounded in use of the microscope, such that integration of these methods is advancing, albeit not uniformly and not completely.

As mentioned above, the adoption and integration of genomics and proteomics methods into surgical pathology practice has been more difficult, because these methods are not morphology based and are more akin to clinical laboratory tests, which in most institutions are conducted in laboratories or even departments that are entirely separate from anatomic pathology, both physically and in thought process. Traditional surgical pathologists are married to their microscopes. Most have limited training or experience of the rigorous procedures that characterize a modern clinical laboratory that generates accurate quantitative results using well controlled, highly automated systems (Taylor and Becker 2011; Bogen 2019).

However, as great as these challenges are, they pale beside the demands of 'going digital,' of moving the traditional surgical pathology 'tissue diagnosis' made by light microscopy into the digital domain, thereby transmuting not only pathology but the pathologists themselves.

Yet the change may be less dramatic than it seems, a more subliminal infiltration of Pathology by AI assisted processes. Who remembers that *Siri* and *Alexa* live with us? Google, is noun, verb and a way of life. Much in the way that the smart phone has inserted itself into all aspects of our lives, from the games we play (Fig. 3.5), to finding a restaurant, a book online, a movie on TV, or simply an 'answer' on Wikipedia, so the pathologist will become integrated with the smart (intelligent) microscope, and at some point in the not so distant future will not remember when it was any other way.

Computer power and imaging (scanning) technology have advanced in leaps and bounds and are no longer major obstacles to immediate progress. In addition, novel AI assisted applications that address tissue section diagnosis (or IHC scoring) are demonstrated almost daily (as addressed in detail in Part IV). Adoption is at present greatly slowed by logistical and cost/reimbursement issues that in part are rooted in

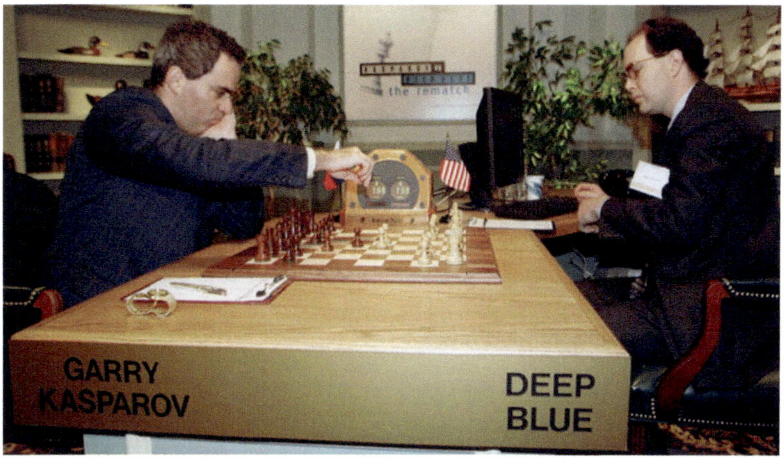

Fig. 3.5 World Champion! A landmark for AI. Garry Kasparov in 1997—*"The computer sees so deeply that it plays like God."* The World Chess Champion, losing to IBM's Deep Blue. 'Watson' and other even more recent iterations are much powerful, but we humans have not changed much. (Greenemeier 2017; Kasparov 2017). Credit Peter Morgen Reuters, Public Domain

regulatory processes that lag far behind technical capabilities. For example, digital methods and applications in surgical pathology often are measured for approval by correlation (non-inferiority) to a 'gold standard,' which usually has been microscopic interpretation of a slide by the pathologist(s), as in the study submitted for approval of primary digital diagnosis on an H&E slide (Mukhopadhyay et al. 2018), rather than absolute accuracy of diagnosis with respect to clinical outcome, surely in the near future.

The digitization of Pathology has been greatly assisted by the fact that by the turn of the millennium Radiology had "gone digital." As a result, many institutions had in place the know-how and infrastructure for moving and storing large digital files (PACs—Picture Acquisition and Communication), that was adaptable to moving digital pathology image files, although in terms of size these may be several times larger than a computed tomography (CAT) scan. Anatomic pathology, however, faced a unique and major logistical problem, namely that, at present, the generation of a digitized pathology image file still begins with a tissue section, and how that section is converted to a digital image file (Fig. 3.6).

A brief review of the process of scanning to obtain a digital image follows, as essential background to the practical discussion of biomarker tests in Parts II and III.

Part IV of this book is devoted to an in depth examination of these crucial issues and the capabilities of a fully digitized pathology environment.

In current practice the decision to generate a digital image usually is made following initial microscope examination of an IHC or H&E slide by a pathologist, for the purposes of applying a digital scoring algorithm (for IHC), or for teaching or consultation (for H&E); slides are then submitted for digital scanning (compare Fig. 3.7).

Difficulties remain. While costs are falling rapidly, high quality rapid scanners are not inexpensive, and not to be found in every pathologist's office. Thus obtaining a digital scan typically involves cost and delay as slides are conveyed to the laboratory scanner facility. Also for many of the currently approved algorithms, there are attendant additional requirements for the marking of selective FOVs (fields of view) by the pathologist. This procedure incurs further delays, unless a whole slide imaging (WSI) scanner is to be used, along with scoring or analytic algo-

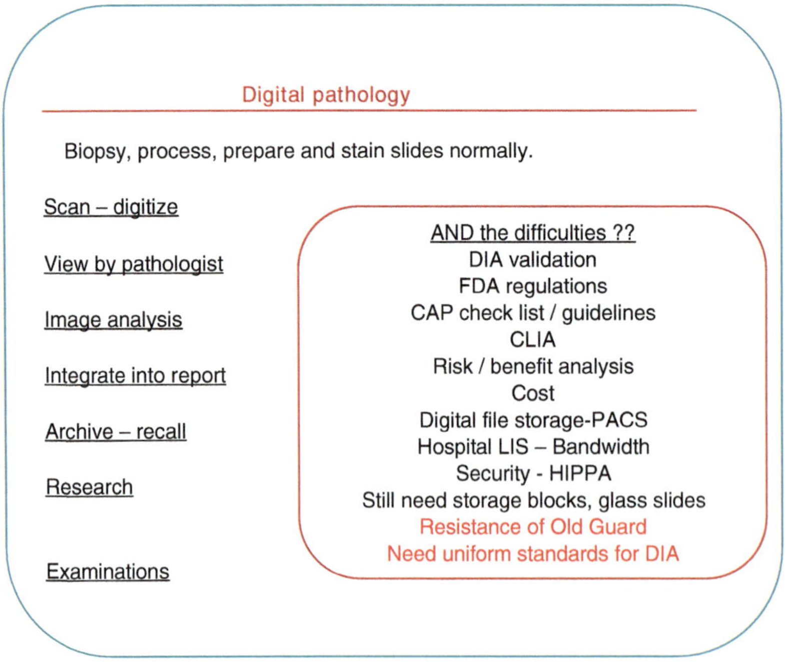

Fig. 3.6 Issues in adoption of digital pathology: difficulties remain

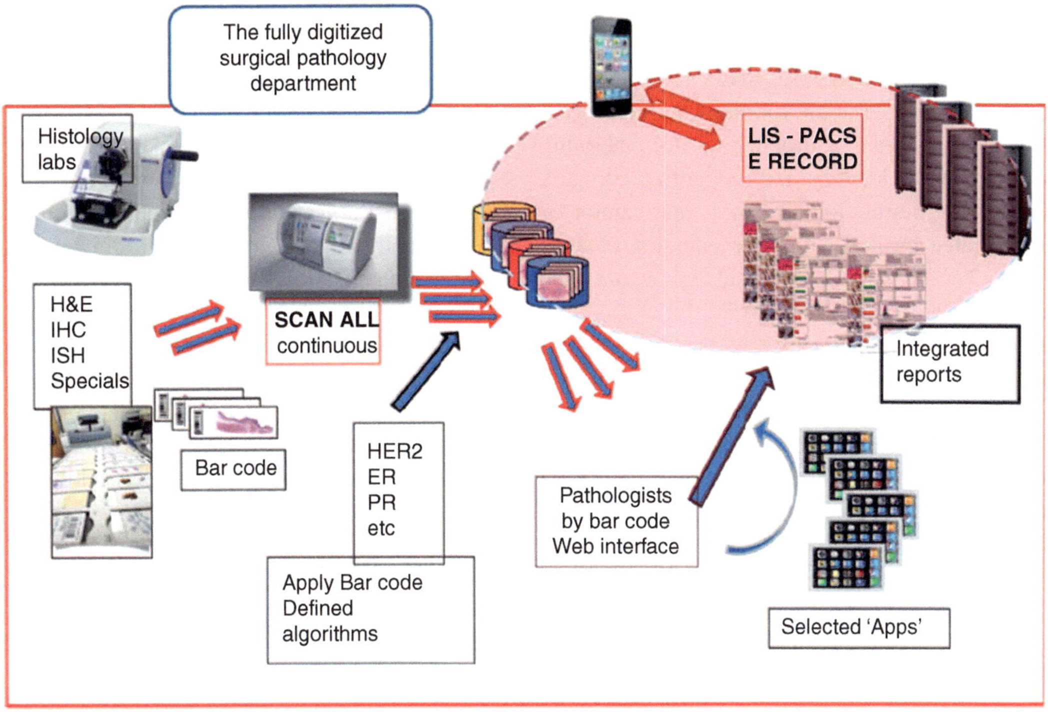

Fig. 3.7 The sequential process dependent upon ordering slide scan by pathologist is slow and cumbersome. By contrast, in a fully digitized pathology department, the glass slides are automatically scanned and subjected to AI directed analysis with the appropriate algorithms completed before distribution to the specified pathologist for review and final report. (Modified from Taylor 2011) With permission Lippincott, Williams and Wilkins

rithms that also are validated for WSI (Parts II and IV). Some multiplex IF methods are similarly encumbered by the intrinsic need for selection of FOVs, which greatly slows the process, although fluorescent scanners with WSI capabilities are gradually becoming available.

A more efficient future awaits in which processed IHC and/or H&E slides are subject to WSI scanning in the histology laboratory, immediately following preparation (Fig. 3.7). The digitized files are then automatically subject to analysis by the appropriate AI directed algorithm, and both digital files and the analytic result made available to the pathologist, along with a draft template report. The glass slides are held in reserve and submitted for examination only when the pathologist request them. A small number of anatomic pathology laboratories worldwide already operate in this totally digital mode, a glimpse into the future of AP as described fully in Part IV.

3.6 Virtual Biomarkers—Molecular Morphology in the Digital Dimension

In addition to a rapidly growing number of algorithms for scoring IHC, ISH and IF results, there are well documented examples showing that AI algorithms applied to WSI of H&E slides are able to replicate, or even exceed performance of experienced pathologists in certain tasks, such as recognizing (and counting) mitoses, identifying normal tissue types and finding micrometastases of breast cancer in lymph nodes (Van der Laak 2019) (Part IV). In most of these instances the performance of the AI algorithm is judged by comparing performance to a consensus panel of experienced pathology experts; the question being "is the AI method as good as pathologist with a light microscope?"

However, in recent years an entirely new question has merged—"is the AI method better than the pathologist with a light microscope?" (Part IV).

The very question poses that a new dimension of digital molecular morphology has emerged, founded upon the ability of AI deep learning approaches to identify and categorize complex but minute morphologic features that cannot be appreciated by the eye of the pathologist, even after 200 years of accumulated experience (Couture 2020; Jaber et al. 2020; Fu et al. 2020; Kather et al. 2020). This new capability offers promise of a new type of biomarker, the AI–Virtual Biomarker (AI–VB), which is established and validated on H&E sections through correlative studies of biomarker expression that has been detected by more conventional testing using IHC, NGS or other molecular methods.

Among the first of these reports were those relating to HER2, ER and PR status in breast cancers, where AI deep learning algorithms were developed that showed excellent correlation with actual measurement of ER, PR and HER2 levels (e.g. as determined by IHC and ISH), and also with such molecular morphologic classifications as, for example, Triple Negative Breast cancer. (Mukhopadhyay et al. 2018 and Jaber et al. 2020) (Fig. 3.8).

Studies are progressing at an astonishing pace with emerging evidence that a variety of driver gene mutations and immune related expression signatures may be detected reliably in H&E sections across more than 20 tumour types, without ever performing a formal biomarker test! (Couture 2020; Fu et al. 2020; Kather et al. 2020). This critically important topic is amplified in Part IV of this book.

If (when) the validity of this approach is substantiated for a broader range of biomarkers across the spectrum of cancer histopathology then the advantages of AID-VBs would be manifold and obvious. They include use of the existing H&E slide, obviating the need for additional (expensive) tests (such as IHC, ISH, or genomic analysis) and the incurred delays in TAT, while maximizing the use of small tissue samples. Regulatory hurdles remain, not least of which is that these new AID-VB algorithms cannot be measured by the usual approach as 'not inferior to' or equal to the usual pathologist consensus, for they are detecting features that unaided pathologists cannot detect. Validation must be against independent laboratory biomarker assays, and ultimately clinical outcome. At such a time

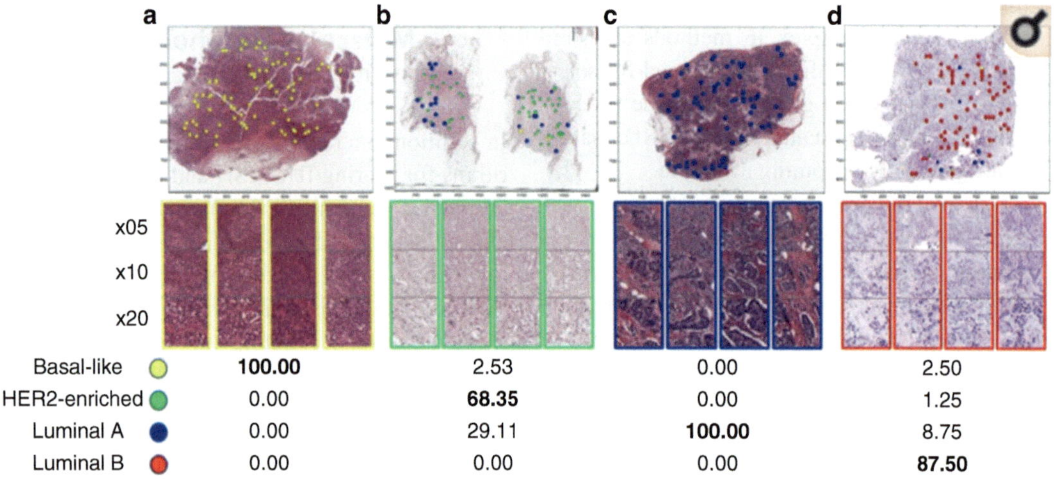

Fig. 3.8 AI Derived virtual biomarkers: Identification of breast cancer subtypes (Basal-like, HER2 enriched, Luminal A and B) by morphology without ever performing formal biomarker testing. From Jaber MI, Song B, Szeto CW, Taylor CR, et al. A deep learning approach to classifying intrinsic molecular subtypes of breast cancer from diagnostic slide images discovers significant intratumoral heterogeneity. From Breast Cancer Res 2020; 22:12, under Creative Commons 4.0 International License, with thanks to Springer Nature and the authors

that these are accomplished anatomic pathology will have changed forever. Anatomic pathology will have been re-invented for the second time in 200 years and pathologists will have undergone re-invention, or extinction.

3.7 Total Integrative Pathology; the Big Data Problem

Once upon a time, within recall of senior practicing pathologists, the pathology report described the gross and microscopic findings of the lesion, concluding with an H&E based tissue diagnosis. More than half a century past, before it became routine to add staging and grading information contingent upon criteria that evolved through international consensus among surgical pathologists as to those elements that should be represented in the report. In the 1990s the recommendations included IHC findings, and later ISH, plus other data (Table 3.2).

Pathology organizations published templates for complete pathology reports tailored to different cancer types (e.g. College of American Pathologists—CAP—Cancer Synoptic reports). https://www.cap.org/protocols-and-guidelines/cancer-reporting-tools/cancer-protocol-templates

The content and level of detail of the report had expanded enormously, but until the turn of the Millennium almost all of the essential information still was at hand to the pathologist, on the table with the microscope.

The advent of biomarker testing changed all of this. New biomarker tests extend beyond the compass of the surgical pathologist and the H&E microscopic findings. Performance requirements for the new IHC biomarker tests are beyond the capability of many laboratories and even if performed 'in-house' require extensive specific training of pathologists for scoring and interpretation. Furthermore, cancer tissues increasingly are submitted for extraction based molecular assays, such as NGS (see Table 2.3). Many of these tests are of necessity 'sent out' to reference laboratories, with the result that reams of data for each patient pour back into pathology over a period of weeks, well beyond the scope of the traditional Surgical Pathology Report. The challenge for Pathology to incorporate and integrate these diverse data sets into a comprehensive diagnostic process is just part of the Big Data problem (Gu and Taylor 2014; Parikh et al. 2019) that faces Medicine (and maybe Life) in general. How to approach this issue is a major underlying theme of Parts III and IV of this book.

Table 3.2 Growth in content of the surgical pathology report

Incorporation of IHC Data into Surgical Pathology Reports[a]
The report should include all patient demographics and tissue identifiers as for any surgical pathology report (*plus all codes for billing as required in any particular country*).
1. All IHC results should be reported, whether positive, or negative, regardless of perceived significance.
2. A 'differential diagnosis', justifying 'stain selection' should be included.
3. The report should also include:
The nature of the specimen tested (frozen, paraffin section, cytoprep. etc.)
The antibodies employed; including where appropriate the clone identifier.
The result of staining for each antibody, including cellular localization where pertinent[b]
4. An interpretation of the findings in the context of the diagnosis and with reference to associated surgical pathology report, if such is not incorporated into the same report.
5. Exact protocols, retrieval methods etc. need not be part of the report, but must be available in laboratory manuals records.

Modified from Peter Banks 1992, incorporating O'Leary 2001 and NCCLS
[a]Drawn from multiple sources as described in Chap. 13
[b]Where 'thumbnails images' are included these may fulfill this requirement
See Chap. 13 for details

3.8 Part I as an entry to Parts II, III & IV

Part II of this book addresses principles and practice and the crucial role of the pathologist to meet the increased demands of Precision Medicine.

Part III deals with how the pathologist has evolved to manage this complicated process in current day to day practice, using specific examples to illustrate the changed function and role of the pathologist with respect to current standards of diagnosis, and hence care, for the Cancer patient.

Part IV is a bridge between current approaches to biomarker analysis and a future more heavily invested in digital analysis of tissue-based results (IHC, ISH and IF), interfaced with extraction-based molecular analysis (PCR, NGS, and proteomics), and the newly developing virtual biomarkers derived from deep learning AI methods. The charge is to address the BIG data aspects of results from these multiple methods and to integrate them into a final actionable decisions for the individual cancer patient.

References

Bogen SA. A root cause analysis into the high error rate in clinical immunohistochemistry. Appl Immunohistochem Mol Morph. 2019;27:329–38.

Couture H. Deep learning-based histology biomarkers: Recent advances and challenges for clinical use. Dig Pathol Assoc. 2020. Https://Digitalpathologyassociation.Org/Blog/Deep-Learning-Based-Histology-Biomarkers-Recent-Advances-And-Challenges-For-Clinical-Use

European Parliament. Directive 98/79/EC of the European Parliament and of the Council of 27 October 1998 on in vitro diagnostic medical devices. 1998. http://eur-lex.europa.eu/LexUriServ/LexUriServ.do?uri=OJ:L:1998:331:0001:0037:EN:PDF

Fu Y, Jung AW, Viñas Torne R, Gonzalez S, Vohringer H, Shmatko A, Yates L, Jimenez-Linan N, Moore L, Gerstung M. Pan-cancer computational histopathology reveals mutations, tumor composition and prognosis. Nat Cancer. 2020;11:800–10. www.nature.com/natcancer. https://doi.org/10.1038/s43018-020-0085-8.

Greenemeier L. Scientific American. 2017. https://www.scientificamerican.com/article/20-years-after-deep-blue-how-ai-has-advanced-since-conquering-chess/ Accessed 8 Jan 2021.

Gu J, Taylor CR. Practicing pathology in the era of big data and personalized medicine. Appl Immunohistochem Mol Morph. 2014;22:1–9.

Jaber MI, Song B, Szeto CW, Taylor CR, Vaske CJ, Benz SC, Rabiizadeh S, Soon-Shiong P, Szeto CW. A deep learning approach to classifying intrinsic molecular subtypes of breast cancer from diagnostic slide images discovers significant intratumoral heterogeneity. Breast Cancer Res. 2020;22:12.

Kasparov G. Deep thinking: where machine intelligence ends and human creativity begins. New York: Public Affairs. Perseus Books; 2017.

Kather JN, Heij LR, Grabsch HI, et al. Pan-cancer image-based detection of clinically actionable genetic alterations. Nat Cancer. 2020;1:789–99. https://doi.org/10.1038/s43018-020-0087-6.

Mahoney K, Atkins MB. Prognostic and predictive markers for the new immunotherapies. Oncology. 2014;28(suppl 3):39–48. http://www.cancernetwork.com/oncology-journal/featured-resources/prognostic-and-predictive-markers-new-immunotherapies

Mukhopadhyay S, Feldman MD, Abels E, Ashfaq R, Beltaifa S, Cacciabeve G, Cathro HP, Cheng L, Cooper K, Dickey GE, Gill RM, Heaton RP Jr, Kerstens R, Lindberg GM, Malhotra RK, Mandell JW, Manlucu ED, Mills AM, Mills SE, Moskaluk CA, Nelis M, Patil DT, Przybycin CG, Reynolds JP, Rubin BR, Saboorian MH, Salicru M, Samols MA, Sturgis CD, Turner KO, Wick MR, Yoon JY, Zhao P, Taylor CR. Whole slide imaging versus microscopy for primary diagnosis in surgical pathology: a multicenter blinded randomized non-inferiority study of 1992 cases (pivotal study). Am J Surg Pathol. 2018;42:39–52. https://doi.org/10.1097/PAS.0000000000000948.

Nass SJ, Phillips J, Patlak. Policy issues in the development and adoption of biomarkers for molecularly targeted cancer therapies. National Cancer Policy Forum. Workshop Summary. The National Academies Press; 2015. NAP.edu/10766.

Parikh RB, Gdowski A, Patt DA, Hertler A, Mermel C, Bekelman JE. Using big data and predictive analytics to determine patient risk in oncology. American Society of Clinical Oncology Educational Book—published online before print May 17, 2019. https://doi.org/10.1200/EDBK_238891.

Taylor CR. From microscopy to whole slide imaging: a century and a half of image analysis. Appl Immunohistochem Mol Morphol. 2011;19:491–3.

Taylor CR. Predictive biomarkers and companion diagnostics. The future of immunohistochemistry: "in situ proteomics," or just a "stain"? Appl Immunohistochem Mol Morphol. 2014;22:555–61.

Taylor CR. Introduction to predictive biomarkers: definitions and characteristics. In Badve S, Kumar G, editors. Predictive biomarkers in oncology: applications in precision medicine. Springer Sciences; 2018.

Taylor CR, Becker KF. Liquid morphology: immunochemical analysis of proteins extracted from formalin fixed paraffin embedded tissues: combining proteomics with immunohistochemistry. Appl Immunohistochem Mol Morphol. 2011;19:1–9.

U.S. Food and Drug Administration. Guidance for industry and FDA staff. In vitro diagnostic (IVD) device studies—frequently asked questions. 2010. http://www.fda.gov/downloads/MedicalDevices/.../ucm071230.pdf.

U.S. Food and Drug Administration. List of cleared or approved companion diagnostic devices (in vitro and imaging tools). Other nucleic acid based tests are listed separately under an included link. 2021. http://www.fda.gov/MedicalDevices/ProductsandMedicalProcedures/InVitroDiagnostics/ucm301431.htm. Accessed 2 Apr 2021.

Van der Laak J. Camelyon challenges 16 and 17. 2019. www.google.com/url?sa=t&rct=j&q=&esrc=s&source=web&cd=3&ved=2ahUKEwjH5Zf9kJ_mAh-UVqZ4KHTiUDkUQFjACegQIBhAC&url=https%3A%2F%2Fdigitalpathologyassociation.org%2F_data%2Ffiles%2FAPI%2FCAMELYON_vanderlaak.pdf&usg=AOvVaw0-t5Hh5NqDMZ4e4vRFCx-p. Accessed Jan 2021.

Yaziji H, Taylor CR. PD-L1 assessment for targeted therapy testing in cancer: urgent need for realistic economic and practice expectations. Appl Immunohistochem Mol Morph. 2017;25:1–3.

Yuan J, Hegde PS, Clynes R, Foukas PG, Harari A, Kleen TO, Kvistborg P, Maccalli C, Maecker HT, Page DB, Robins H, Song W, Stack EC, Wang E, Whiteside TL, Zhao Y, Zwierzina H, Butterfield LH, Fox BA. Novel technologies and emerging biomarkers for personalized cancer immunotherapy. J ImmunoTherapy Cancer. 2016;4:3. https://doi.org/10.1186/s40425-016-0107-3.

Part II

Precision Medicine Demands Precision Pathology

4 Evolution of the Total Test Approach to Tissue Based Pathological Analysis

4.1 Introduction: The Microscope 'Invented' the Pathologist

In Part I, the historical events were reviewed whereby, almost two centuries ago, advances in manufacturing technology of microscopes and in tissue preparation methods were adopted by a number of visionary practitioners in medicine and surgery, who in effect became the first tissue pathologists (Taylor 2011, 2014, 2018; Jones and Gal 2016). 'Histopathology' or 'surgical pathology' came into being as a separate discipline and rapidly evolved to become the 'Gold Standard' for diagnosis of cancer, and a guide for subsequent therapeutic decisions.

Even today, 2021, at the time of writing this book, the essential element for initiating any form of treatment for cancer still is a "tissue diagnosis." Generally, this diagnosis is based upon a formalin fixed paraffin embedded (FFPE) H&E (hematoxylin and eosin) stained section that is interpreted by a trained (and experienced) surgical (or anatomic) pathologist by use of a light microscope or, as is increasingly the case today, by digital whole slide imaging (WSI).

Prior to the advent of biomarkers, this H&E based tissue diagnosis was sufficient for diagnosis and for choice of therapy, but not anymore.

4.1.1 Re-Invention

Technology marches on. This book will present the current diagnostic methods in Anatomic Pathology as a bridge to the introduction of two major new areas of technology:

1. analysis at a molecular level as in proteomics and genomics, and
2. advanced morphologic analysis driven by digital imaging and artificial (or augmented) (Barisoni et al. 2020) intelligence (AI).

These methods when brought together are likely to supplant the current H&E Gold Standard for cancer diagnosis in the foreseeable future, and in so doing will cause the re-invention of both anatomic pathology and the surgical pathologist.

4.1.2 Morphology Plus

Part II discusses a number of ancillary techniques currently in use in anatomic pathology, beginning with immunohistochemistry (IHC), which entered into routine surgical pathology approximately 50 years ago (review, Taylor 2020). Beginning in 1974, IHC (and related methods) gradually evolved in variety and complexity into

B. Jasani et al., *Precision Cancer Medicine*, https://doi.org/10.1007/978-3-030-84087-7_4

a range of 'special stains' that augment traditional morphologic diagnosis by means of improved cell and tissue recognition. Today IHC is embedded in the pathology literature and is part of mainstream surgical pathology diagnosis everywhere. More recently the emergence of sophisticated biomarkers, which also offer prognostic and predictive therapeutic significance, has resulted in a situation where IHC is employed for the demonstration and (attempted) quantification of these biomarkers, as will be discussed later. In this last instance the result of the IHC biomarker test serves as a necessary arbiter of therapy; in practice in an increasing proportion of cases it has therefore become a 'stand-alone' test.

During this evolving process, ever increasing requirements for greater accuracy and quality of IHC have placed great demands upon the anatomic pathology (histopathology) laboratory, technicians and pathologists alike.

4.2 IHC: A Stain 'Repurposed' as an Assay

When first used on FFPE tissues IHC was employed as a 'special stain,' the purpose of which was to impart differential staining to certain cell, tissue or tumor types, as an aid to the pathologist in diagnosis. The performance (quality and usefulness) of the IHC stain was judged in much the same way as any other histologic stain, namely by the eye of the pathologist (Taylor 2011). This evaluation was (and is) subjective, lacking any strict formal process for intra-laboratory quality control and standardization on a day to day basis, or any means of assurance of reproducibility between labs. True, controls were employed, but preparation of these controls was not standardized and their evaluation also was subjective; a situation that persists to this day (as discussed in Chap. 10). IHC was regarded a simply another tissue stain (albeit having some intrinsic specificity) that quite suddenly was pressed into use for the demonstration of biomarkers of therapeutic interest, the purpose of which is a different from the original intended use (purpose) of IHC, because it requires results that are to some degree quantitative; that is precise results having the characteristics of a quantitative assay, rather than a qualitative stain (Taylor and Levenson 2006; Taylor 2015).

In this text the term 'IHC stain' generally will be employed when the intent is to generate a tinctorial reaction that may be of value to the surgical pathologist in reaching a conventional microscopic diagnosis; that is the purpose is for the IHC result to serve as a special stain.

The term 'IHC assay' will carry the additional and vitally important connotation that the intent and purpose is to include a quantitative component as in most biomarker assays. This important distinction has far reaching implications as will be clarified in the pages that follow.

One goal of Precision Pathology, as described in this book, is effectively to convert IHC from a qualitative tissue stain into a quantitative tissue-based assay ('in situ proteomics'—ISP) (Taylor 2015). The basic requirements for a tissue based quantitative assay are summarized in the accompanying Table 4.1.

The basic approach shown in Table 4.1 was developed under the auspices of the Biologic Stain Commission in 1992, and is expanded in Table 4.3.

In order to use IHC in this mode, as a precision assay, it is necessary to improve performance standards throughout the entire set of procedures that comprise anatomic pathology. The challenge includes, but also extends beyond, technical practices and IHC protocols within the

Table 4.1 Requirements for laboratory assays of Cancer Biomarkers

Total test approach—all aspects of test system should be encompassed, including sample preparation (see Table 4.3).
Test method and analyte should have well established performance characteristics
Test should be objective for read out / interpretation
Test ideally should produce a quantitative result (objective)
Threshold and reference range should be established
Test should be 'fit for purpose'; that is designed and validated for the defined application
There should be well developed control systems that are universally available
Test should be reproducible; run to run, day to day, lab to lab
Test should be readily performed and inexpensive

Table 4.2 Performance characteristics for Enzyme Linked Immunoassay (ELISA) as compared to Immunohistochemistry (IHC)

	ELISA Quantitative 'Gold Standard' for measuring proteins in serum	IHC An 'immune based' stain; semi-quantitative scoring at best
Specimen acquisition and sample preparation	Strict standardized protocol, includes exact collection time, 'preservative,' known total time to assay. Specimen rejected if not in compliance	Absence of agreed standards other than day of collection; various fixatives; fixation times unrecorded. Minimal monitoring for compliance; no rejection
Protocol • Defined, validated reagents • Steps in protocol • Automated	Specified for the assay Closed fixed protocol Yes; reagents and protocol defined for the instrument	Wide choice of reagents; validation variable Open protocol, frequently 'tweaked' Partial; reagents and protocols vary widely
Reference standard and controls	'Universal standard' available for control and for calibration	Not available[a]; control tissues vary over time, and from lab to lab.
Interpretation; the process of measurement	Computer based readout with reference to calibration standard	Mostly manual and subjective, by the eye of the pathologist. The few approved algorithms are designed to mimic the pathologist

[a]Sections of FFPE cell line pellets in approved diagnostics kits are prepared so as to give consistent protein expression, but cannot be used to calibrate (measure) results in FFPE tissues because preparation and fixation are very different

laboratory, beyond the incorporation of AI image analysis methods, to the extent that it is necessary to change the entire mindset of anatomic pathology, pathologists included!

In this context a good starting place is for the 'IHC stain' to borrow principle and practice from a proven clinical laboratory procedures, the ELISA method (Table 4.2, see also Fig. 3.4), which is very similar in principle to IHC (it employs similar reagents), but behaves as a true quantitative assay, due to specified and more rigorous performance demands across the Total Test (Taylor 2015; Bogen 2019) (Table 4.2).

4.3 In-Situ Hybridization

In-situ hybridization (ISH) will be reviewed here briefly as a related technique, performed as the name suggests 'in-situ' on the tissue section after the manner of IHC; a more detailed description is to be found in Chap. 14.

Many of the principles of ISH on FFPE tissues are similar to IHC with a common pre-analytic phase, and similar analytic processes, except that the target in ISH is a defined nucleic acid base sequence, and the 'probe' a designed complementary sequence, in lieu of the target antigen and specific primary antibody probe employed in IHC. Sensitivity and specificity for the targeted base sequence of DNA or RNA are both high. Demonstration of the tissue bound probe may be by immunofluorescence (IF) methods, or by amplified bright field methods (here termed chromogenic ISH or CISH) that are closely analogous to those applied in IHC, with similar attendant issues of interpretation in a tissue context. Similarities between ISH and IHC extend to the post-analytic phase. Initially reading and scoring of ISH was performed by microscopy and the eye of the pathologist, but increasingly there is recourse to more accurate computerized methods (algorithms) and digital images as discussed more fully in Part IV.

4.4 Molecular Extraction Based Methods; Abandoning Morphology?

A further complication, and critical challenge, for the cancer pathologist has been the introduction and rapid expansion of a range of protein and gene based (molecular or genetic) assays, seeking to identify a variety of cancer related mutational changes. As discussed briefly in Part I and more fully in Part III, these molecular assays also take their origin from major interrelated discoveries made in the middle of the last century, the discovery of protein sequencing, DNA structure, and DNA (Sanger) sequencing. Today in the area of cancer diagnosis and therapy genomic methods are based primarily on PCR (polymerase chain reaction) and NGS (next generation sequencing) methods that are carried out on tissue extracts, which in the clinical field again perforce employ FFPE tissue, "because that is what we have."

Data as to the overall "best' method are limited, but suggest that IHC has predictive value that is comparable to gene expression profiling, and that when multiplexed (as in multiplex IF – Chap. 14) is superior because it identifies spatial relationships of the cancer and the immune response (Lu et al. 2019).

As discussed in Part I, this book maintains a focus on methods that retain the facility for morphologic evaluation in order to link current and future practice. However, it is important to emphasize that the concerns of sample preparation and pre-analytical issues that will be discussed here, also critically affect the FFPE tissues that are the primary source of extracts for molecular assays, the results of which may be compromised in ways that are not well understood or widely appreciated. A primary reason is that details of acquisition, FFPE processing and cellular composition of the tissue sample used as the source for extraction of material for analysis often are unknown, and thus very poorly controlled. Morphologic correlations are therefore tenuous, even to the extent of proportions of tumor and stromal cells in the sample.

4.5 Emerging Methods in Microscopy and Microimaging

The intent of this book is to address the emerging role of the pathologist as the key physician in the integration of biomarker data with the traditional microanatomic features that form the foundation of diagnosis in surgical pathology; namely the 'tissue diagnosis' or the H&E that still is the Gold Standard, without which treatment for cancer rarely begins.

The focus, amplified in Part III, is to assess from the perspective of the pathologist those immunologic and molecular methods that are available for precise evaluation of biomarkers in cancer, which in their application also are able to maintain the spatial relationships that are critical to making a tissue diagnosis. The microscope is the central key instrument that ties these methods to morphology, but today the microscope and indeed the whole concept of microscopy are also subject to rapid development, evolving to new formats.

The conventional optical microscope (Fig. 4.1) has a long history, reviewed briefly in Chap. 1 (Chen et al. 2011; Bock 2015; Jones and Gal 2016), where the argument was advanced that 'the microscope invented the pathologist,' by virtue of relatively sudden improvements in lens quality and manufacturing almost 200 years ago. Certainly, the first papers and texts ascribing microscopic findings to the diagnosis of cancer appeared concurrently with the widespread availability of efficient microscopes (Chap. 1, Fig. 1.2), and from 1850 onward surgical pathology evolved slowly along with the optical microscope.

Today history is repeating itself. The microscope is effectively being re-invented by the incorporation of a variety of digital imaging and machine learning (AI) methods, which in turn lend themselves to new approaches to cellular identification, down to the molecular level (Chap. 14 and Part IV). Presentation of the histopathologic features of a biopsy in digital format allows application of advanced image analysis, including accurate counting, true quantification, image segmenting methods and spectroscopic profiling. These capabilities incorporate elements of artificial intelligence (AI) somewhat resembling the smartphone 'Apps' that populate and guide our daily existence, re-inventing the conduct of our business and personal lives (Fig. 4.2).

A 're-invention of the pathologist' surely will follow as these new 'intelligent' microscopes, incorporating AI methods and Apps are assimilated into surgical pathology practice.

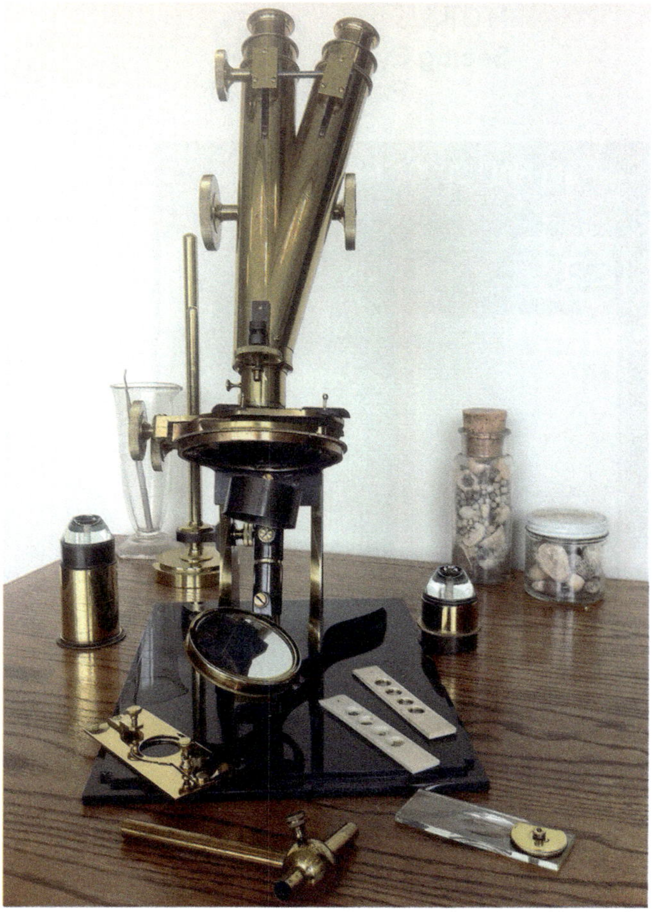

Fig. 4.1 The "Gold Standard." The 'art' of image analysis in 1870, by mind and the microscope. Henry Crouch, London; engraved n1055 with ivory mounted glass slides (Personal collection of the author, CRT)

While the primary focus of Part II of this book is on immunohistologic techniques that currently are in routine use in pathology practice (IHC, IF and ISH), some diversion into new approaches to cell and sub-cellular identification is necessary, because these methods are the future. An introduction to some of the methods that are close to clinical application follows in Chap. 14. A more detailed treatment of digital microscopy, image analysis systems and adaptations of machine learning methods follows in Part IV.

4.6 The Total Test: Pre-Analytical, Analytical and Post-Analytical Phases (Table 4.3)

The following chapters, 5 through 13, review the multiple processes and procedures that are involved in tissue based pathological analysis, integration of which is essential to proper performance of the Total Test.

The primary goal is to present principles and standards of practice for IHC that if followed will serve to improve levels of performance, quality and reproducibility of IHC (and ISH) results. It is not intended to serve as, or substitute for, a detailed laboratory IHC (or ISH) staining manual. Detailed guidelines for performance of IHC tests have been published elsewhere (Taylor and Cote 2005; Hewitt et al. 2011; Cartun and Taylor 2018).

The intent is to promote careful review of operating practices in anatomic pathology laboratories as applied to precision cancer diagnosis, leading to adjustment in procedures and manuals as warranted. The end goal of converting a qualitative IHC stain into a tissue-based assay has been addressed in several publications and provides a sound rationale for what follows here. References to recommendations for specific

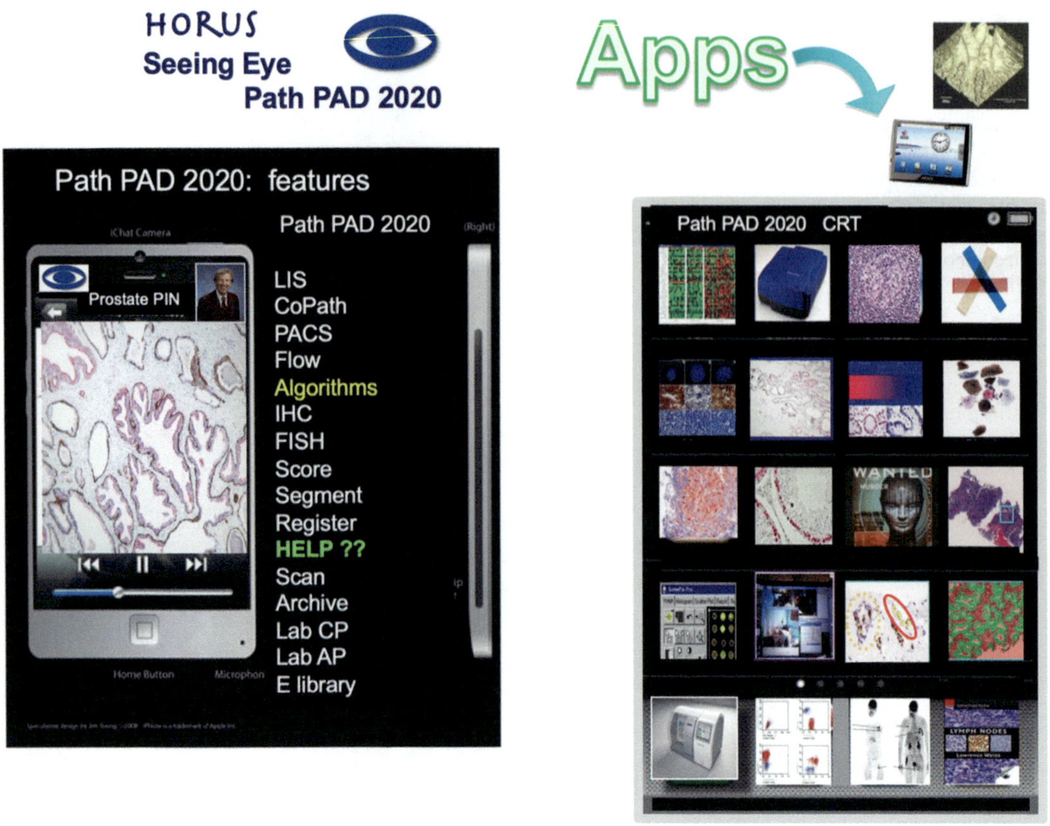

Fig. 4.2 A Vision of the digital microscope; portable and just as powerful as the latest that Microsoft of Apple can offer and evolving just as fast. (Concept is from a presentation by the author (CRT) titled 'Vision 2020, Digital Pathology.' Annual Immunohistochemistry Workshops. Vitro Molecular Laboratories. Director Hadi Yaziji 2011) Permission of Wolters Kluwer Health, Inc.

actions for improvement of IHC results will be given in context.

From the perspective of the pathologist intent upon quality assurance and elevation of IHC from a stain to an assay, each and every one of these separate steps must be scrutinized, standardized and controlled in their entirety (as far as is possible). The pathologist must assume responsibility for this 'Total Test' approach (Table 4.3 and Part III).

The focus is on methods that preserve morphologic correlations, namely advanced immunohistochemical (IHC), immunofluorescence (IF), in-situ-hybridization (ISH) and related methods that are performed directly on tissue sections. IHC and IF methods when properly performed in a Total Test environment with addition of appropriate calibration controls have the potential for combining quantitative assay of proteins with preservation of spatial and morphologic information, an assay approach that has been termed 'in situ proteomics' (ISP).

Many of the Total Test principles discussed here apply equally to proteomics and genomics methods (e.g. mass spectrometry, PCR and NGS methods), which are extraction-based assays for protein, RNA or DNA. In the clinical arena these methods also utilize extracts of FFPE tissues. The results, therefore, also may be compromised by inadequate control and quality assurance of any of the pre-analytical steps discussed below, excepting obviously those steps directly related to morphologic analysis, because all spatial correlation is lost in the extraction process.

Table 4.3 The total test: the original proposal was discussed at the US Biologic Stain Commission (Taylor 1992)

The total test
Pre-analytical: Test selection: 'fit for purpose' Specimen type Specimen acquisition—warm ischemia Specimen handling—cold ischemia, pre-fixation, transport. Fixation: type of fixative; total fixation time Processing; paraffin embedding, de-paraffinization Sectioning; thickness, storage
Analytical: Antigen retrieval (exact method) Selection of primary antibody Selection of labeling reagents (detection system) Reagent and protocol validation Selection of controls (reference standards)—fit for purpose Technologist training; laboratory certification Proficiency testing and quality assurance
Post-analytical: Assessment and recording of control performance Interpretation of result(s) / AI, computer based scoring and quantification Validation of scoring method/algorithm for prognostic/predictive significance Pathologist experience for specified biomarker test Integrated report Turn-around time Outcomes analysis/economics/reimbursement

IHC is a dynamic process with many inherent variables that may affect outcome. In recent decades, borrowing from rigorous protocols in use in hospital clinical laboratories, it has become clear that all phases of the IHC test procedure are critically important, beginning with the Pre-analytical phase (specimen handling, fixation and processing), through the Analytical phase (validation of reagents and methods) and then on to the Post-analytical phase (interpretation and reporting of the results) (Table 2.3).

Each and every step of the entire IHC Total Test process has the potential to affect performance of the succeeding steps and alter the overall result. Each step requires continuous stringent quality control and assurance against errors, in order to provide reproducible, reliable and accurate results at the individual patient level. The discussion that follows in Chaps. 5, 6, 7, 8, 9, 10, 11, 12, and 13 aims to describe established principles that, if followed, will enhance the quality and standardization of IHC, whether employed primarily for the purpose of a 'stain' or as a quantitative 'assay' for precision led evaluation of biomarkers.

References

Barisoni L, Lafata KJ, Hewitt SM, et al. Digital pathology and computational image analysis in nephropathology. Nat Rev Nephrol. 2020;16:669–85. www.nature.com/nr.neph

Bock O. A history of the development of histology up to the end of the nineteenth century. Research. 2015;2:1283. https://doi.org/10.13070/rs.en.2.1283. http://www.labome.org/research/A-history-of-the-development-of-histology-up-to-the-end-of-the-nineteenth-century.html. Accessed Sept 2020

Bogen SA. A root cause analysis into the high error rate in clinical immunohistochemistry. Appl Immunohistochem Mol Morph. 2019;27:329–38.

Cartun R, Taylor CR. Techniques of immunohistochemistry: principles, pitfalls and standardization. In: Dabbs DJ, editor. Comprehensive diagnostic immunohistochemistry. 5th ed. Amsterdam: Elsevier; 2018.

Chen X, Zheng B, Liu H. Optical and digital microscopic imaging techniques and applications in pathology. Anal Cell Pathol (Amst). 2011;34:5–18. https://doi.org/10.3233/ACP-2011-0006.

Hewitt SM, Robinowitz M, Bogen SA, Gown AM, Kalra KL, Otis CN, Spaulding B, Taylor CR. Quality assurance for design control and implementation of immunohistochemistry assays: approved guidelines, vol. 31. 2nd ed. Wayne, PA: Clinical Lab Standards Institute; 2011. p. 4.

Jones ML, Gal AA. The age of the microscope—and the "invention of the pathologist." Chapter 31. In: Van den Tweel JG, Gu J, Taylor CR, editors. From magic to molecules: an illustrated history of disease. Beijing: Beijing University Press; 2016.

Lu S, Stein JE, Rimm DL, Wang DW, Bell JM, Johnson DB, Sosman JA, Schalper DA, Anders RA, Wang H, Hoyt C, Pardoll DM, Danilova L, Taube JM. Comparison of biomarker modalities for predicting response to PD-1/PD-L1 checkpoint blockade a systematic review and meta-analysis. Jama Oncol. 2019. https://doi.org/10.1001/jamaoncol.2019.1549.

Taylor C. Quality assurance and standardization in immunohistochemistry. A proposal for the annual meeting of the biological stain commission, June, 1991. Biotech Histochem. 1992;67:110–7.

Taylor CR. From microscopy to whole slide digital images; a century and a half of image analysis. Appl Immunohistochem Mol Morph. 2011;19:491–3.

Taylor CR. Predictive biomarkers and companion diagnostics. The future of immunohistochemistry—'in situ proteomics', or just a 'stain'? Appl Immunohistochem Mol Morph. 2014;22:555–61.

Taylor CR. Quantitative in situ proteomics; a proposed pathway for quantification of immunohistochemistry at the light-microscopic level. Cell Tissue Res. 2015;360:109–20.

Taylor CR. Introduction to predictive biomarkers: definitions and characteristics. In: Badve S, Kumar G, editors. Predictive biomarkers in oncology: applications in precision medicine. Berlin: Springer Sciences; 2018.

Taylor CR, Cote RJ, editors. Immunomicroscopy: a diagnostic tool for the surgical pathologist. 3rd ed. Saunders, PA: Elsevier; 2005.

Taylor CR, Levenson RM. Quantification of immunohistochemistry—issues concerning methods, utility and semiquantitative assessment. Histopathology. 2006;49:411–24.

Taylor CR. Milestones in Immunohistochemistry and Molecular Morphology. Applied Immunohistochem Mol Morph. 2020;28:83–94

Yaziji H (2011) Pathology learning. Annual immunohistochemistry workshops. Miami, FL. https://www.vitromolecularlaboratories.com

5 Pre-Analytic Phase: Test Selection; Specimen Acquisition and Handling

5.1 The Pre-Analytical Phase Defined

The Pre-analytical phase begins the at the moment the blood supply to the tissue is interrupted in taking the biopsy or resecting the lesion. It ends with the cutting of tissue sections for subsequent examination by morphologic methods, or extraction methods for molecular or genetic methods.

The major factors in the Pre-analytic phase that are critical to test performance will be discussed in turn. The CLSI (Clinical Laboratories Standards Institute) recommendations for IHC testing are to be found in Hewitt et al. (2011). The corresponding CLSI publication for molecular testing, 'Collection, Transport, Preparation, and Storage of Specimens for Molecular Methods' is by Sheppard et al. (2020). It is important also to recognize that pre-analytic requirements also are evolving for digital imaging and AI analysis (Barisoni et al. 2020 and Part IV), and that preservation and presentation of consistent excellent morphologic detail is an absolute pre-requisite for high quality image analysis results.

5.2 Test Selection—'Fit for Purpose'

There still are limited data as to the relative effectiveness of the differing test methods for individual patients and specified biomarkers, in the context of available laboratory capabilities and clinical need (Lu et al. 2019). The discussion that follows applies primarily to methods that retain the ability to conduct morphologic analysis, either by the pathologist's eye alone, or with the aid of digital analysis. However, the principle of exercising full quality control of the total test process applies to all methods.

Ideally a test should be selected to meet the exact clinical need, and the proper specimen should be obtained to fit that purpose and the test modality to be employed. This is the usual circumstance for most Clinical Laboratory tests (e.g. blood counts, blood chemistries, serum immunoglobulin titers, blood culture, etc.). The test is ordered by the clinician and then the appropriate specimen is sought from the patient in the prescribed manner (type of specimen tube, preservative, transport conditions, strictly as per protocol).

By contrast, biomarker test selection in anatomic pathology is to a large degree an afterthought and is the type of test that can be performed then is dictated by the type of specimen that already is available. In many instances when biomarker studies are requested the specimen already has been taken (the resected tumor; lymph node biopsy etc.) and the FFPE tissue block is usually the only recourse. Test selection is then limited to whatever tests have been validated for performance on FFPE tissue. For example, the option to select a test performed by flow cytometry (e.g. of immune cell types) no longer

B. Jasani et al., *Precision Cancer Medicine*, https://doi.org/10.1007/978-3-030-84087-7_5

exists, unless a new fresh specimen is obtained, which would then be an example of test selection preceding collection, and determining the type of specimen.

As discussed in Chap. 2 and extended in Part III, the term 'biomarker' has been widely employed, prior to the current context of 'Predictive and Prognostic' biomarkers (Table 2.1). Biomarker evaluation frequently is requested only after a diagnosis of cancer (including the type) has been established following resection or biopsy, at which time usually only FFPE tissue is available for any further testing. Not only should the test that is selected have been validated in the FFPE environment, but it should be 'fit for purpose,' that is it should incorporate the notions of precision, accuracy and reliability for the intended use, in this instance of guiding the choice of a targeted therapeutic.

True, having evolved over 150 years, an FFPE H&E tissue section might be considered 'fit for purpose' being intended for the morphologic diagnosis of cancer by an experienced pathologist. However, in the context of biomarker testing the intent is different. It is to detect and measure a particular specific biomarker; the term 'fit for purpose' then has a much more precise definition. It demands that the entire test procedure is shown to be 'reliable for the intended use' with respect to one specified biomarker for a single clinical application, for which the test has been validated and approved by the appropriate regulatory authority (Cheung et al. 2017).

The specified connection of drug to biomarker may be traced back to the introduction, in about 1980, of Tamoxifen (Nolvadex; by ICI, now AstraZaneca) for treatment of breast cancer. Correlation of clinical response with ER (estrogen receptor) expression by the tumor, led to measurement of ER by cytosol extraction-based assays, which in the 1990s were replaced by IHC methods on FFPE sections (Taylor 1996; Allred et al. 1998). However, it was the FDA approval, in 1998, of the humanized HER2 antibody Trastuzumab (Herceptin: Genentech/Roche) for breast cancer, conjoined with the HerceptTest (Dako/Agilent) on FFPE sections, that gave the field its current impetus. This joint approval also set the important precedent for co-development in a clinical trial of a targeted therapeutic combined with a test to determine patient eligibility (likelihood of good clinical response). The term 'Companion Diagnostic' entered the lexicon (see Table 2.1).

Clinical applications for Herceptin/HER2, other than breast cancer (e.g. gastric and lung cancers) soon followed, as did a host of other targeted drug/biomarker combinations, led by Rituximab—CD20 (see Table 2.2).

Different assay methods (other than IHC) were advanced, particularly genomics performed on tissue extracts, as in PCR and NGS assays. All employed FFPE tissue, because that is 'what we had' available at the time of clinical need for the test. With respect to IHC the enhanced demands for reliability and accuracy plus quantification, stretched the method to (and beyond) its limits, bringing renewed attention to the necessity of improving the performance of IHC by the Total Test approach. At the same time the notion was advanced that all IHC biomarker tests should be selected and validated with the defined intended use in mind (i.e. they should be 'fit for purpose').

Examples now abound of the importance of 'fit for purpose' selection (Cheung et al. 2017); just a few serve here to illustrate the issue. More extensive discussion of this approach for assay development and implementation is reserved for Parts III and IV.

1. ALK protein (anaplastic lymphoma kinase) is dysregulated in ALCLs (anaplastic large cell lymphomas), correlating with a t(2;5) translocation. Several anti-ALK antibodies are available and when properly validated by IHC may serve as a surrogate diagnostic biomarker of ALCL. ALK is detectable in 70% of more of systemic cases of ALCL, where it has been used for many years as part of an IHC panel-(Kinney et al. 2011) to assist differential diagnosis of ALCL from other lymphomas and anaplastic tumors.

   As described in more detail in Part III, ALK has also been found to be dysregulated in a small percentage of lung cancers

(NSCLCs; less than 8%—Verma et al. 2017). ALK is a transmembrane receptor with several fusion partners leading to tyrosine activation and cell proliferation, a finding which stimulated development of targeted anti-ALK therapies and the need for a Companion Diagnostic to detect ALK expression in these cases. The same ALK IHC test that was developed for ALCL was employed initially, but was found to be very insensitive in NSCLC; the gene rearrangements differ and protein expression is much lower than in ALCL. The ALK -IHC test was therefore re-purposed for NSCLC, by increasing the detection sensitivity and conducting separate validation for clinical relevance in lung, with correlation to an independent assay (e.g. FISH). The usual positive control for ALK in ALCL is a known case of ALCL (with high ALK expression), which may not serve for an ALK IHC test also was re-purposed to NSCLC (Torlakovic et al. 2015; Cheung et al. 2017). When ordering an ALK IHC 'stain' from the laboratory it is therefore essential to select the 'fit for purpose' version, separately validated for the intended use, either ALCL diagnostic (lymphoma) or NSCLC (lung) predictive; the two are NOT interchangeable.

2. Targeted HER2 therapy was initially developed for breast cancer, but soon small percentages of other tumor types (e.g. gastric, lung) also were found to show upregulation of HER2 protein, thus offering the possibility for treatment with the antibody Herceptin and requiring new clinical trials. The original HercepTest and equivalent tests for HER2 in breast cancer from other vendors, do not serve directly for HER2 in gastric (or other) cancers, because of different expression patterns (Abrahao-Machado and Scapulatempo-Neto 2016): in breast there is a 2+ circumferential pattern; gastric adds partial, linear and basal patterns, which also means that scoring methods and algorithms are not interchangeable. Therefore while the physical assay may be the same, the scoring system is very different, requiring new clinical trials and a new 'fit for purpose' validation of the HER2 Total Test by the laboratory for gastric (or again separately, lung) cancer, once again correlating with an independent assay (e.g. FISH).

The impact of extending this approach to the use of anti-HER2 antibody drug conjugates (ADCs) is complex (Skidmore et al. 2020) and has resulted in the adaptation of HER2 IHC diagnostics to a wide variety of solid tumors, showing any level of HER2 expression (Rinnerthaler et al. 2019). Examples include ARX-788 (anti-HER2 conjugated to monomethyl auristatin F (MMAF), an auristatin analog and potent microtubule inhibitor, which is in two ongoing phase 1 trials (clinicaltrials.gov identifiers: NCT02512237 and NCT03255070). The aim in Phase 1a is to determine the recommended phase 2 dose (RP2D) in patients with HER2 positive advanced solid tumors. In the first trial, phase 1b tests safety in HER2-positive advanced breast cancer; HER2-low advanced breast cancer; and HER2 positive gastric cancer (clinicaltrials.gov identifier: NCT02512237). Phase 1b in the second trial is designed to investigate the activity and safety of the RP2D in two breast cancer cohorts: HER2 positive HER2-low (clinicaltrials.gov identifier: NCT03255070). In each of these trials there is heavy reliability on the performance of the HER2 test.

In clinical practice the issue is further complicated by the fact that several different methods exist for HER2 bioassay, providing an example of the different factors that influence selection of the optimal method of testing, whether by IHC, ISH or NGS. In lung cancer the incidence of HER2 overexpression (for potential therapy) is much lower than in breast, and is very variable in reported studies. Concordance data for the different methods are very limited and the reasoning processes that have evolved for breast cancer do not apply to lung. Factors such as cost, availability and turn-around-time become important in the decision and IHC, as a relatively inexpensive and rapid test, may be the first to be performed under conditions of very low prevalence, somewhat after the manner of a screening test, to be confirmed by a second method.

3. A third example is provided by PD-1 and PD-L1 (programmed cell death ligand-1) where the situation is even more complex. There are several different drugs (targeted antibodies to PD-1 or PD-L1 and clones thereof) from different vendors, targeted to many different tumor types, including melanoma, lung, kidney, lymphomas, with others added almost daily (see Fig. 5.1). Each targeted therapeutic has its companion or complementary test for 'predictive' evaluation of drug effectiveness (Chap. 2). Adhering to the precedent set more than 20 years ago by combined clinical trials of drug (anti-HER2 therapeutic antibody) and companion diagnostic (IHC HER2 test), each of these different PD-1, PD-L1 antibody drugs, and their corresponding tests, underwent combined trials for each new tumor type, resulting in a plethora of conjoint approvals, with each IVD (in vitro device) test approved for a defined clinical use and restricted by strict reagent and protocol requirements.

Each approved PD L-1 test is strictly fit for purpose; specifying protocol, platform, tumor type and drug, conditions that add further complexity.

The result is that the same drug (e.g. Nivolumab, antibody, clone and pharmaceutical vendor, Bristol-Myers Squibb) when intended for use in two different tumors (lung NSCLC, melanoma) engendered two distinct combined clinical trials and two distinct companion diagnostics (e.g. for NSCLC and melanoma, Phillips et al. 2015, 2018). Although both of these companion diagnostics employ the same clone, anti-PD-L1 IHC 28.8, and emanate from the same vendor

Different vendors	**FDA/CE IVDs Approved**	**Dako/Agilent**	**Dako/Agilent**	**Ventana/Roche**	**Ventana/Roche**
Different clones	Primary antibody	Rabbit monoclonal **22C3**	Rabbit monoclonal **28-8**	Rabbit monoclonal **SP263**	Rabbit monoclonal **SP142**
Different Pharma companies.	Pharma	Merck	BMS	AstraZeneca	RocheGenentech
Different drugs		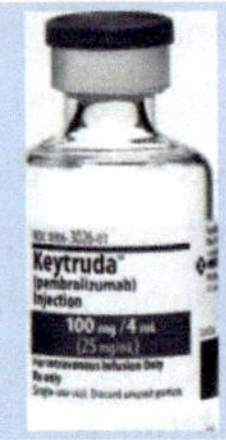	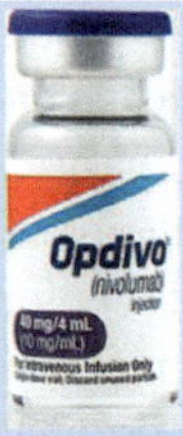	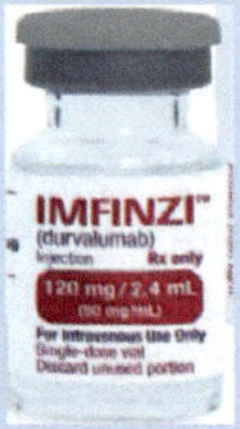	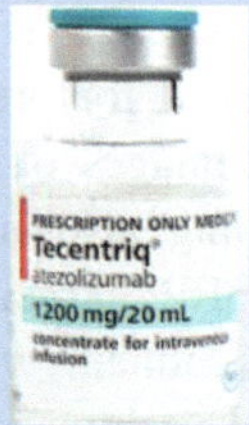
Different approvals	Biomarker teststatus	Companion Dx	Complementary Dx	Complementary Dx	Complementary Dx
Different detection	Approved configuration	RTU antibody Dako link	RTU antibody Dako link	RTU antibody Optiview Detect	RTU antibody Optiview Amp
Different platforms	Staining platform	Dako autostainer	Dako autostainer	Ventana BenchMark	Ventana BenchMark
Different thresholds for positive versus negative result, and different guidelines for counting tumor cells and / or immune cells !					

Fig. 5.1 The Diverse PD-L1 landscape. Principal approved PD-L1 tests and associated drugs. Each test must be separately established and validated by the performing laboratory and the scoring system and threshold for each is different. NordiQC and UKNEQAS data indicate that 50% of more of labs are in fact using LDT variants. Developed from discussions at NordiQC Workshop 2017 inspired by work of Suzanne Parry, UKNEQASBMS: Bristol Myers Squibb

(Dako/Agilent), the two tests were separately established and validated with distinct scoring systems. In addition to Nivolumab (anti PD-1) there are other targeted antibody drugs with similar clinical indications from other pharmaceutical companies, such as Pembrolizumab (anti-PD-1), Atezolizumab (anti-PD-L1), or Durvalumab (anti-PD-L1), each for multiple different tumor types, each of which has its corresponding diagnostic test as an approved IVD (In Vitro Device -FDA; or CE Marked test); each of which has defined intended use, specified reagents, protocol, staining platform and scoring system.

These multiple approved PD-1/PD L-1 IVD tests are not interchangeable in whole or in part, for drug or for tumor type and the need to define and select the 'fit for purpose' IHC IVD test is critical. In order to perform all of these separate IVD tests a laboratory must have in place several different staining platforms and must perform multiple in-house validations of each of these IVD tests, a prospect that is overwhelming, technically and economically (Yaziji and Taylor 2017).

Furthermore, should the user change any approved IVD test in any way (antigen retrieval method, antibody, protocol, incubation time, staining platform, intended use) then it is no longer an 'approved IVD' but is by default converted to a LDT (Laboratory Developed Test) and may show significant performance changes as shown in QC assessment surveys by NordiQC (2019) and UKNEQAS (Dodson et al. 2019). These surveys also reveal that in practice a (large) proportion of IVDs are also *de facto* LTDs, because the performing laboratories have altered some elements of the approved IVD Total Test protocol (AR, incubation time etc.), consciously, or otherwise.

In addition, a number of laboratories have responded to the near impossibility of establishing multiple different IVDs for PDL-1 by designing their own PD L-1 LDT, selecting reagents, protocol and platform of choice on the basis of experience or performance (or perhaps that most commonly demanded), and then (hopefully) performing in-house cross validation against the IVD(s) of interest, with external 'split specimen' validation as necessary. NordiQC and UKNEQAS have noted in some surveys that LTDs may account for as many as 50% of total PD-1/PD L-1 tests performed.

While this situation may evoke concern from the regulatory bodies, the same surveys show that in practice, the performance of validated LTDs in well controlled labs can be very similar to that obtained in labs using approved IVDs, when appropriate QC programs are in place.

5.3 Digital Pre-Analytic Quality

In striving to practice Precision Pathology to notion of 'fit for purpose' must now be broadened to include design of all components of the Total Test, such that the resulting tissue section, whether H&E, IHC, ISH or IF, is fit for the purposes of digital imaging and AI assisted analysis as discussed in Part IV. Published image analysis algorithms that are developed using poor quality tissues (as from tissue banks, especially if prefrozen) are likely to show poor performance in the real clinical arena, where the requirement is to preserve morphologic detail sufficient to allow the H&E Gold Standard diagnosis, and now is being further revised to meet new standards for reliable AI based image analysis. The quality of fixation and the tissue sectioning process (uniform thickness, lacking tears or artifacts (*vide infra* and Part IV), plus consistent color characteristics of the staining method are especially important (Taylor 2014; Barisoni et al. 2020).

5.4 Turn-Around Time (TAT); Cost; Reimbursement Issues

Other factors that are considered in test selection include turn-around time (TAT) and cost reimbursement issues. TAT varies widely among the different methods, and also according to whether the test is available 'in-house' or must be sent to an external reference laboratory, which inevitably delays the result. Determining the exact fully loaded cost of an 'in-house' test is not easy and is, of course, very much volume dependent for each specified test, an issue discussed above with reference to PD L-1 tests, where the large number of different approved tests effectively limits the volume of anyone of them and may render it cost prohibitive for a lab to set up all, or any of them (Yaziji and Taylor 2017). The reflex is to send such tests to an outside reference laboratory, where the cost to the patient (and the institution?) may be greater but is known, but where there is the hidden price of an extended TAT that delay treatment and extend hospitalization; these additional 'non-laboratory' costs to the patient and the health care system are usually not accounted (or even considered) in the cost analysis decision whether to set up a test in house, or to send it out.

Lastly, reimbursement procedures vary widely in different countries. In the face of rapidly growing health care costs, certain tests (and test methods) may be precluded for certain diseases, in certain patients, at some decision level, whether it be by the country, state, health care system or hospital, or by the patient's insurance (if they have it), or by the individual laboratory. Every oncologist, surgeon, and pathologist should be aware of the tests available for selection and their alternatives, the effective TAT of each, and which ones are precluded by cost (or non-reimbursement) and therefore effectively non-available.

With these factors in mind there is a growing trend in some healthcare systems (countries, hospitals, clinicians, pathologists, labs) to limit costs (and test choice) in a rationale manner by setting up test triages, with readily available, short TAT, relatively less expensive tests being performed first (often IHC), only proceeding to other assay types if the clinical situation so requires. For example, the Magee breast cancer testing algorithm allows a decision to safely avoid proceeding to expensive molecular testing (Bhargava et al. 2020) and is justified in an overall risk benefit analysis.

References

Abrahao-Machado LF, Scapulatempo-Neto C. HER2 testing in gastric cancer: an update. World J Gastroenterol. 2016;22:4619–25. https://doi.org/10.3748/wjg.v22.i19.4619.

Allred DC, Harvey JM, Berardo M, Clark GM. Prognostic and predictive factors in breast cancer by immunohistochemical analysis. Mod Pathol. 1998;11:155–68.

Barisoni L, Lafata KJ, Hewitt SM, et al. Digital pathology and computational image analysis in nephropathology. Nat Rev Nephrol. 2020;16:669–85. www.nature.com/nr.neph

Bhargava R, Clark BZ, Carter GJ, Brufsky AM, Dabbs DJ. The healthcare value of the Magee decision algorithm™: use of Magee equations™ and mitosis score to safely forgo molecular testing in breast cancer. Mod Pathol. 2020;33(8):1563–70. https://doi.org/10.1038/s41379-020-0521-4.

Cheung CC, D'Arrigo C, Dietel M, Francis GD, Fulton R, Gilks CB, Hall JA, Hornick JL, Ibrahim M, Marchetti A, Miller K, van Krieken JH, Nielsen S, Swanson PE, Taylor CR, Vyberg M, Zhou X, Torlakovic EE. Evolution of quality assurance for clinical immunohistochemistry in the era of precision medicine—part 4: tissue tools for quality assurance in immunohistochemistry. From the international society for immunohistochemistry and molecular morphology (ISIMM) and international quality network for pathology (IQN path). Appl Immunohistochem Mol Morph. 2017;25:227–30.

Dodson A, Parry S, Lissenberg-Witte B, Haragan A, Allen D, O'Grady A, McClean E, Hughes J, Miller K, Thunissen E. External quality assessment demonstrates that PD-L1 22C3 and SP263 assays are systematically different. J Pathol. 2019. https://doi.org/10.1002/cjp2.153.

Hewitt SM, Robinowitz M, Bogen SA, Gown AM, Kalra KL, Otis CN, Spaulding B, Taylor CR. Quality assurance for design control and implementation of immunohistochemistry assays: approved guidelines, vol. 31. 2nd ed. Wayne. PA: Clinical Lab Standards Institute; 2011. p. 4.

Kinney MC, Higgins RA, Am M. Anaplastic large cell lymphoma: twenty-five years of discovery. Arch Pathol Lab Med. 2011;135:19–43.

Lu S, Stein JE, Rimm DL, Wang DW, Bell JM, Johnson DB, Sosman JA, Schalper DA, Anders RA, Wang H, Hoyt C, Pardoll DM, Danilova L, Taube JM. Comparison of biomarker modalities for predicting response to PD-1/PD-L1 checkpoint blockade a systematic review and meta-analysis. Jama Oncol. 2019. https://doi.org/10.1001/jamaoncol.2019.1549.

NordiQC. Assessment run C5 2019. PD-L1 (lung). 2019. https://www.nordiqc.org/downloads/assessments/121_102.pdf

Phillips T, Simmons P, Inzunza HD, Cogswell J, Novotny J, Taylor CR, Zhang X. Development of an automated PD-L1 immunohistochemistry (IHC) assay for non small cell lung cancer. Appl Immunohistochem Mol Morph. 2015;23:541–9. https://doi.org/10.1097/PAI.0000000000000256.

Phillips T, Millett MM, Zhang X, Jansson M, Cleveland R, Simmons P, Cherryholmes G, Carnahan J, William J, Spaulding B, Satnick IR, Inzuna HD, Taylor CR, Cogswell J, Novotny J, Oroudjev E, Winther

H. Development of a diagnostic programmed cell death 1-ligand 1 immunohistochemistry assay for nivolumab therapy in melanoma. Appl Immunohistochem Mol Morph. 2018;26:6–12.

Rinnerthaler G, Gampenrieder SP, Greil R. HER2 directed antibody-drug-conjugates beyond T-DM1 in breast cancer. Int J Mol Sci. 2019;20:1115. https://doi.org/10.3390/ijms20051115.

Sheppard E, Madej RM, Alfaro MP, et al. Collection, transport, preparation, and storage of specimens for molecular methods. 2nd ed. Wayne, PA: Clinical Lab Standards Institute; 2020. MM13

Skidmore L, Sakamuri S, Knudsen KA, Hewet AG, Milutinovic S, Barkho W, Biroc SL, Kirtley J, Marsden R, Storey K, Lopez I, Yu W, Fang S-Y, Yao S, Gu Y, Tian F. ARX788, a site-specific anti-HER2 antibody–drug conjugate, demonstrates potent and selective activity in HER2-low and T-DM1–resistant breast and gastric cancers. Mol Cancer Ther. 2020;19:1833–43. https://doi.org/10.1158/1535-7163.MCT-19-1004. https://mct.aacrjournals.org/content/19/9/1833

Taylor CR. Paraffin section immunocytochemistry for estrogen receptor: the time has come. Cancer. 1996;77:2419–22.

Taylor CR. Whole slide imaging- issues for use in diagnostic pathology: 'routine;' stains, immunohistochemistry and predictive markers. Biotech Histochem. 2014;89:419–23. https://doi.org/10.3109/10520295.2013.861512.

Torlakovic EE, Francis G, Garratt J, Gilks B, Hyjek E, Ibrahim M, Miller R, Nielsen S, Petcu E, Swanson P, Taylor CR, Vyberg M. Standardization of positive controls and introduction of immunohistochemistry critical assay performance controls (iCAPCs) in diagnostic immunohistochemistry: recommendations from the international ad hoc committee. Appl Immunohistochem Mol Morph. 2015;23:1–18.

Verma S, Kumar M, Kumari M, Mehrotra R, RAS K, Goel M, Kumar A, Kant S. An immunohistochemical study of anaplastic lymphoma kinase and epidermal growth factor receptor mutation in non-small cell lung carcinoma. J Clin Diagn Res. 2017;11:EC22–5. https://doi.org/10.7860/JCDR/2017/27941.10279.

Yaziji H, Taylor CR. PD-L1 assessment for targeted therapy testing in cancer: urgent need for realistic economic and practice expectations. Appl Immunohistochem Mol Morph. 2017;25:1–3.

6 Pre-Analytic Phase: Specimen Type and Acquisition

6.1 The Specimen

The type of specimen, how and where it is obtained, is in many cases outside the direct control of the pathologist. This state of affairs, albeit inevitable for reasons of cost and logistics, contributes to many of the problems that follow and may from the very beginning preclude the possibility of reliable assay results. Specimens derive from diverse sources in each health care system, from multiple clinics and operating rooms manned by various clinical and surgical departments, which makes it difficult, or impossible, to establish and adhere to a rigorous protocol for fixation and processing. In most cases total duration of exposure to fixative(s) is at best an estimate, and indeed in large specimens may vary to an unknown degree, from periphery to center, due to differences in tissue size, density and rate of penetration of fixative.

Yet, for many analytes, fixation matters.

In the Hospital Clinical Laboratory if a specimen is received that is inappropriate for the assay that has been requested (e.g. wrong specimen tube, extended or unknown transport time), then the standard protocol response is to reject the specimen (knowing that the result may be unreliable, but is readily repeatable) and request a new one.

In anatomic pathology obtaining a new specimen is less easy; at the minimum it involves a new (invasive) biopsy procedure for the patient, but often it is not possible at all, because the lesion of interest may have been entirely removed while obtaining the initial biopsy, or in the course of surgical resection of the tumor.

Depending upon the tumor type and accessibility, the major categories of specimen that are most commonly resourced for biomarker assay are Excision Biopsies and Surgical Resections, followed by Fine Needle Aspiration (FNA) and Core Needle biopsies (American Cancer Society 2015).

Cytologic preparations obtained by smear techniques or FNA are used less often for biomarker assays, because of small number of available cancer cells, lack of intact tumour associated stromal tissue and loss of architecture. However, in developing nations FNA remains the mainstay biopsy procedure because of affordability, plus lack of resources and expertise for performance of other types of biopsy.

More recently a fourth type of specimen has found increasing application, namely Liquid Biopsy, which is a blood or body fluid sample, leading to special sample preparation and assay procedures.

In every instance the rules apply of attaching physician and patient information, clinical information including site and reason for biopsy, and collection time. The requisition form should allow (or better, require) entry of key time points as the specimen moves forward (see below).

B. Jasani et al., *Precision Cancer Medicine*, https://doi.org/10.1007/978-3-030-84087-7_6

6.2 Excision Biopsy and Surgical Resection

For excision biopsies the primary purpose is to establish a tissue diagnosis. Biopsy is initiated by the oncologists, surgeon or other clinician. The resultant specimen is usually placed in formalin fixative and submitted to the laboratory to 'fit the purpose' of allowing an H&E diagnosis. Formalin (see below) is a good fixative for morphologic preservation, and very forgiving in terms of process scheduling, but with significant disadvantages in relation to preservation and/or accessibility of tissue molecules for their subsequent detection and measurement.

For surgical resections the primary purpose is clinical, intrinsic to the course of surgical treatment, and specimen handling is geared to morphologic diagnosis and further assessment by H&E (grading, staging). Similar processing constraints exist to those discussed above for excision biopsies, but with some additional concerns. In large, difficult cancer resections interruption of blood supply to areas of the resected tissue is not uniform, which affects onset of autolysis as described below. Once removed it is placed in a container where the amount of fixative often is inadequate for the size of the tissue, and formalin penetration, hence fixation, in large tissue masses is not uniform. In central areas fixation may not even begin until the specimen reaches the lab where it is dissected into small blocks ("grossing") and placed in fresh fixative; the timing and duration of this phase are widely variable, and often entirely unknown. In this context, the commonly used term, 'standard' formalin fixation, does not at all exist.

Does this lack of a standard formalin solution matter? When judged by morphology alone, often not very much, but it is known that for biomarker studies results are compromised by many of the same factors that cause molecular degradation in IHC in general (Chaps. 7 and 8).

6.3 FNA, Core Needle Biopsy

FNA and core needle biopsies mostly are ordered to meet a defined clinical need, namely a relatively non-invasive method for diagnosis of a nodule or mass. These types of biopsies yield small tissue specimens but typically follow a strict sample handling protocol, with immediate fixation and standard FFPE processing. Many of the pre-analytic issues discussed below are thereby avoided. In one sense these biopsies are ideal for biomarker evaluation, but at the cost of obtaining only a small amount of one of the key tissues of interest (i.e. the tumor and associated stroma). The small size and lack of stromal cells may critically limit the number and types of biomarker assays that can be performed, after the initial H&E evaluation has confirmed the presence of tumor, thereby generating a need for biomarker testing.

For IHC, most of the approved IVD biomarker tests have a minimum threshold requirement of at least 100 tumor cells in the cut-stained section for a valid test score. Extraction based methods (NGS or PCR) also have an effective minimum threshold number of tumor cells for performance, plus requirements for minimum proportion of tumor cells versus wild type cells (usually requiring 20% or more of cells that may harbor mutations and genes of interest). Selecting part(s) of a thick tissue section (FOVs—fields of view) for extraction is therefore often necessary to enrich for tumor cells, but is time consuming and technically difficult, demanding both expertise and experience of a qualified pathologist. Areas of interest may be removed manually, and crudely, by scalpel tip, or more precisely by laser microdissection. The latter method requires special equipment, and experience.

With either approach cell selection should be performed by an experienced surgical pathologist, able to identify with some certainty the areas (cells) of interest. Even then, selection on a cell to cell basis is highly subjective, and involves compromise. For example, in order to enrich for cancer cells, the stroma and immune cells are typically discarded, although their presence is essential for some assays. Also, in microinvasive cancers the distinction and separation of individual invading tumor cells is impossible by any method. In small biopsies, following H&E evaluation there may be insufficient tumor remaining for extraction assays, and the use of multiple methods for cross confirmation or further study is usually is not possible.

6.4 Cytologic Preparations

In many ways cytologic preparations form a separate category in terms of obtaining the specimen and subsequent processing and evaluation. The goal often is screening rather than definitive final diagnosis, and cells are obtained in smaller numbers, often insufficient for extraction based genomic studies. However, with the advent of extensive biomarker testing in tumors of lung and gastric origin, diagnosis and evaluation increasingly is by small biopsies and necessity has forced adaption of methods to include cytologic or 'cell block' preparations.

Cytologic 'cytospin' preparations generally are not formalin fixed and are processed in a manner distinct from FFPE. While IHC reagents may be in common and the principles of the Total Test certainly apply, specific details of the assay do not. There is no cross validation of cytologic IHC and FFPE IHC methods and usually no cross validation of controls; a separate process is required. In cytologic 'cell block' procedures, where aspirated cells are pelleted and then formalin fixed and embedded in paraffin, the material may be treated in a fashion analogous to a small FFPE biopsy.

6.5 Liquid Biopsy

It is a sign of rapidly changing times and technology, that this book, although its primary focus is on methods that retain morphologic features, cannot pass without some brief discussion of 'Liquid Biopsies.' In most instances the term Liquid Biopsy has been applied to blood (plasma) or other fluid specimens (CSF, urine, effusions, saliva, stool etc.) (Sisson et al. 2019), although some authors have included 'liquid tissue extracts' prepared from regular tissue biopsies.

In the present context, a liquid biopsy is most often obtained primarily for the purpose of molecular or genomic assays. In this sense a liquid biopsy may be considered a 'fit for purpose' test—namely the performance of a molecular or genomic assay on isolated cell free DNA (cfDNA) or circulating tumor DNA fragments (ctDNA) in blood or other body fluids. Some assays target methylated tumor DNA (ctmDNA). Blood specimens may of course be evaluated for intact circulating tumor cells and immune cell profiles, as well as for free cancer associated proteins (biomarkers) such as PSA, but these latter tests have traditionally not fallen under the rubric of liquid biopsy.

With respect to genomic biomarkers in cancer the intent of a liquid biopsy is to sample ctDNA fragments in blood regardless of tumor type and site, and whether tumor is primary or metastatic. The proportion of advanced cancer patients with detectable ctDNA may be as high as 80% in certain tumor types, but is considerably less in others, especially early stage.

Liquid biopsy differs from the preceding types of biopsies in providing no morphologic information (that is not the intent or purpose). It has advantages in ease of obtaining the specimen; a blood draw is straightforward and is less invasive and less expensive. It may also be used when a tumor mass is not identifiable or accessible for tissue biopsy. For these reasons liquid biopsy may more readily be repeated to monitor the progress and course of disease.

Most of the pre-analytic issues discussed below with respect to tissue biopsy (e.g. cold ischemia, fixation) are avoided. However, issues of specimen collection, handling and transport remain and require standardization and conformance to protocol. Plasma is usually preferred to serum because the latter may contain more cfDNA from leucocytes, a concern that increases if separation is delayed, leading to false assay results. Separation and cfDNA extraction are therefore critical, specifically the centrifugation step(s) and the method of DNA extraction and isolation, which affect integrity and yield of the DNA and thus test outcome. Choice and handling of control materials (identical to that for test DNA) is paramount and quality control (QC) of the entire analytic process (Total Test) is critical, but is still evolving as to what is the best approach (Sisson et al. 2019). Verification and validation requirements for Liquid Biopsy results, whatever the analytic method employed (the Total Test), are no less severe than anything discussed in these pages with respect to tissue-based methods.

The assays employed in 'liquid biopsies' are rapidly evolving and detailed discussion is beyond the design of the current text, which retains a primary morphologic connection. However, in principle the isolated DNA may be subjected to various types of molecular assays, either searching for targeted mutations, or aimed at a more generic search for mutations of possible interest. Commonly employed methods include variants of PCR and deep sequencing, such as CAPP-Seq and SafeSeq, which usually are employed for known specified mutations that serve as biomarkers in the mode of a companion diagnostics: e.g. Roche's EGFR Mutation PCR Test v2 with Tarceva in NSCLC was the first to be FDA approved (in 2018). NGS methods are usually employed for genome wide testing using panels of genes. Several well established commercial vendors exist and currently offer panels up to about 80 'cancer genes,' about to expand to more than 300.

Recent reports describe a variant of NGS that examines DNA methylation haplotype patterns that are indicative of cancer and are claimed to be more readily separable from normal DNA patterns (Chen et al. 2020), and thus (potentially) both highly sensitive and highly specific. The data generated by these methods are so extensive that AI and machine learning methods are necessary for their interpretation; all must be part of a Total Test validation process.

Comparative studies of different molecular assays on identical case materials reinforce the concern for independent validation with complete concordance for detecting the 'same cancer genes' falling below 10% in one study, and 20% in another when normal genes were excluded. (Chae et al. 2017; Torga and Pienta 2018; Sisson et al. 2019). There are several possible reasons for low concordance in these studies, not least the lack of maturity and experience with these methods. Performance is likely to improve across the board with time and with more rigorous QC. Commercial vendors report higher concordance on matched samples, but with some selective bias.

For the next several years liquid biopsy and traditional biopsies evaluated by morphologic methods clearly will exist side by side; oncologists and pathologists will need to learn how to use the full repertoire of methods in a complimentary 'fit for purpose' approach.

References

American Cancer Society. Types of biopsies used to look for cancer. 2015. https://www.cancer.org/treatment/understanding-your-diagnosis/tests/testing-biopsy-and-cytology-specimens-for-cancer/biopsy-types.html. Accessed 30 July 2015.

Chae YK, Davis AD, Jain S, Santa-Maria C, Flaum L, Beaubier N, Platanias LC, Gradishar W, Giles FC, Cristofanilli M. Concordance of genomic alterations by next-generation sequencing in tumor tissue versus circulating tumor DNA in breast cancer. Mol Cancer Ther. 2017;16:1412–20.

Chen X, Gole J, Gore A, et al. Non-invasive early detection of cancer four years before conventional diagnosis using a blood test. Nat Commun. 2020;11:3475. https://doi.org/10.1038/s41467-020-17316-z.

Sisson BA, Uvalic J, Kelly K, Selvam P, Hesse AN, Ananda G, Chandok H, Bergeron D, Holinka L, Reddi HV. Technical and regulatory considerations for taking liquid biopsy to the clinic. Validation of JAX PlasmaMonitor™ Assay. Biomark Insights. 2019; 14. https://doi.org/10.1177/1177271919826545.

Torga G, Pienta KJ. Patient-paired sample congruence between 2 commercial liquid biopsy tests. JAMA Oncol. 2018;4:868–70.

7 Pre-Analytical Phase: Biopsy/Tissue Handling and Processing

7.1 Pre-Analytical Variables (Table 7.1)

The critical importance of careful control to all steps in acquiring and processing tissues for biomarker studies (Taylor 2015) has only quite recently been given the public attention it warrants, at an NCI-NIST Workshop (NCI 2011; Taylor 2011).

7.2 Transport, Warm and Cold Ischemia

Specimen Acquisition involves removal of the specimen, with possible phases of Warm Ischemia and Cold Ischemia (Delay to formalin fixation) during transport to the laboratory and onset of processing. The pathologist should assume oversight of this entire process (Part III).

When blood supply to a tissue is interrupted, as in an excision biopsy or a resection procedure, autolysis begins in minutes and only is halted when fixation is complete.

Warm ischemia is that period extending from the interruption of blood supply until removal of the tissue from the body. It is an inevitable part of the surgical process. For excision biopsies this period may be short, minutes only, but with extensive resections it may be considerable depending upon the complexities of the surgical procedure. As already noted for needle and core biopsies the time between interruption of blood

Table 7.1 The major Pre-analytic variables that affect the results of IHC "staining" and all extraction-based methods that use FFPE material

Process effects represent general 'truths': Detailed impact is mostly unknown for individual analytes (proteins)
Autolysis
Anoxic damage; proteins, RNA, DNA degraded to unknown extent.
Warm ischemia vessels clamped at surgery.
Cold ischemia time prior to fixation; transport time and conditions.
Grossing (further cutting of tissue in pathology laboratory as necessary)
Time elapsed to 'grossing' of specimen; block size/thickness: 2–3 mm maximum
Fixation
Placement of specimen in fixative (usually 'formalin solution (see text).
Variable penetration and fixation within large specimen or block; varies with tissue type of fixative; total time in fixative; state of fixative, freshness; pH; degree of cross linking of proteins leading to "loss of antigenicity" IHC, and decreased ability to detect analytes by other methods including extraction.
Parts of tissue block that are poorly fixed in formalin will be alcohol-fixed
Processing: dehydration, clearing, impregnation in paraffin wax
Variable times in alcohols, xylol, and paraffin. Temperature of wax
Storage as FFPE block time and conditions of block storage effects unknown
Cutting thickness of section; avoidance of tears; time from cutting to staining
Thick sections may show apparent increase in intensity; tears may give artifacts; loss of antigenicity for some protein
Blocks used for frozen sections might show diffusion of protein(s) and ischemic change, prior to being fixed. Of these factors, variable fixation is likely to be the most important

B. Jasani et al., *Precision Cancer Medicine*, https://doi.org/10.1007/978-3-030-84087-7_7

supply and exposure to fixative may be close to zero. While warm ischemia is not considered a major factor affecting the demonstration of most proteins (antigens; epitopes) by IHC, metabolically labile proteins, including phosphorylated proteins of clinical interest, may behave differently (Lerch et al. 2020) reflecting the fact that hypoxic cellular degenerative changes begin within minutes. Similarly, the action of RNAases may cause rapid and significant break down of RNA if fixation is delayed. DNA is considered relatively stable.

Cold ischemia is that period extending from the time that tissue is removed from the body, until it is placed in fixative. Ideally, if specimen is small and is placed in formalin immediately, this period can be very short. The term Delay to Formalin Fixation (DFF) has been used synonymously for cold ischemia. It is vital to recognize that placement in fixative is neither synonymous nor synchronous with actual fixation, because the fixative must penetrate the tissue before fixation can begin, and with formalin the fixation process is itself not instantaneous (referred to as a 'clock reaction' by Shi et al. 2011, 2019).

For resected large tissue specimens there is a variable delay in penetration (and thus fixation) that is both unknown and unequal throughout the tissue, and can only be mitigated by immediate transport to the lab for 'grossing' (i.e. dissection into small blocks) that promotes rapid and even fixation as described below. Cooling (refrigeration) of the tissue following removal from the body does slow the autolytic process, but is uneven and less effective in larger tissue masses. Also, it should be noted that tissue blocks that have been employed for frozen section examination and are then processed to FFPE blocks, have undergone prolonged cold ischemia, in addition to suffering cellular change due to freezing artifacts and diffusion of free proteins.

There is general consensus that cold ischemia has adverse impact on detection of some biomarkers, regardless of method employed for their detection (Fig. 7.1). Much of the published biomarker data relates to ER, PR and HER2. Results across several different studies are not uniform (not surprisingly!), but some data specific to IHC on FFPE tissues are available (Yildiz-Aktas et al. 2012; Khoury 2018). HER2 showed a progressive decrease in score values when cold ischemia exceeded 1 h, most evident in lower intensity staining cases (2+ and 1+). ER and PR were affected in some studies, but not others. In one study variation was dependent upon which antibody was used for detection; SP1 was better than 1D5 and 6F11 for ER; and 1E2 better than PgR636 and 16 for PR (Qiu et al. 2018). Both intensity and percentage scores were affected. Refrigerated specimens were less impacted than those undergoing cold ischemia at room temperature (Isil et al. 2012). This obvious intrinsic variability speaks to the importance of controlling, and instituting controls for, the cold ischemic phase as a routine part of Total Test validation.

For newer biomarkers data are even more limited. Ventana did report that for their PD-L1 approved test, using antibody SP263, cold ischemia up to 24 h had no detectable deleterious effect under experimental conditions (Zajac et al. 2019). However, in view of the diversity of tests (antibodies, platforms and scoring systems) it is unlikely that this conclusion holds true in broad application across other antibodies and biomarkers.

Not only does cold ischemia allow an ongoing slow rate of autolysis, it also permits diffusion within the tissue of molecules that are not structurally bound, including partially autolyzed products that may confuse IHC (or IF) staining in their dislocated position. Molecular degradation and diffusion occurring in the cold ischemic phase is irreversible, that is, it is not affected by AR (antigen retrieval). Problems of loss of intensity of staining and diffusion artefacts are well known, having been observed in conventional IHC studies of frozen section blocks that subsequently are processed by FFPE. An unfortunate corollary is that many commercial IVD and pharmaceutical companies perforce rely in their R&D process upon purchased tumor (and normal) tissues, mostly in the form of FFPE blocks. On examination of sections from such TMAs freeze artefacts frequently are apparent, showing that the source blocks were derived from previously frozen tissues, or in other instances from

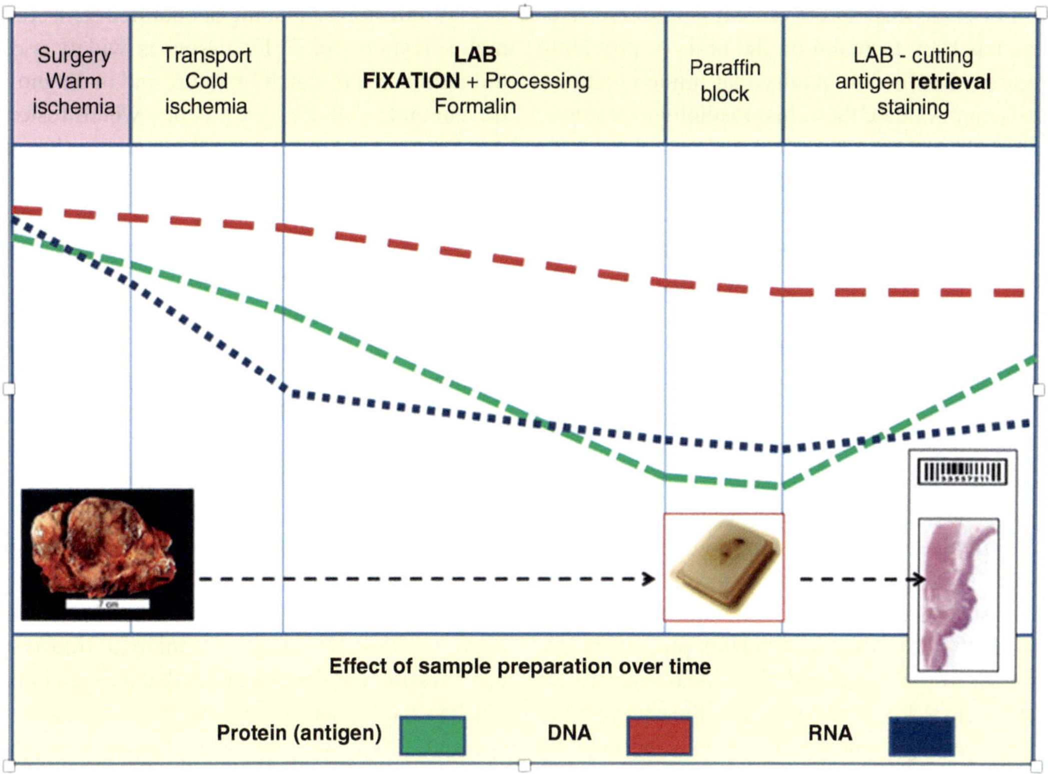

Fig. 7.1 During the pre-analytic phase there is a variable decrease in ability to detect proteins, DNA and RNA in tissue sections (by IHC, ISH, or IF) and in tissue extracts (by NGS, PCR etc.). The proportionate loss during ischemia and fixation, or extent of possible recovery following AR, is largely unknown for any specific analyte. Fresh tissue is on the left, with the paraffin block and the H&E tissue section on the right (Taylor 2015; Permission Springer Nature)

tissues fixed in unknown ways for unknown times. In almost all cases the extent of cold ischemia is unknown. For these reasons the development and validation of commercial tests, including tests employed in clinical trials, that employed commercially sourced TMAs of uncertain provenance in the development phase, may be compromised.

Together these potentially adverse effects are reason enough to urge rapid placement of the specimen in fixative and rapid transfer to the laboratory for processing immediately upon arrival if biomarker studies are anticipated. In this context, as already noted, FNA and core needle biopsies are in many respects ideal specimens as they are placed in fixative solution almost immediately upon taking the sample. Being small they are rapidly and evenly fixed, in which instance the start time for fixation may be reliably recorded. Conversely their small size may limit morphologic assessment and restricts the types and numbers of tests that may be performed.

7.3 Fixation and Paraffin Embedding (FFPE)

Type of fixative, amount, freshness (pH), penetration of tissue and total fixation time. Throughout this book the unspoken assumption is that the tissue being tested has been fixed in formalin and embedded in paraffin (FFPE) in a 'standard' or 'routine' manner. What this means in practice is discussed in detail below, with the caveat, as mentioned earlier, that there is no such thing as 'standard formalin fixation.' For any other fixation conditions consensus data are almost non-existent.

For more than a 100 years the preferred fixative has been formalin on the basis of providing tissues of sufficient quality that trained pathologists can evaluate those histopathologic features, which have been described and established for disease entities over the last 200 years (namely, the H&E 'Gold Standard'—Chap. 1). In this context, unless otherwise specified, 'formalin' means 10% neutral buffered formalin (NBF) effectively a 4% solution of 37–40% paraformaldehyde, at pH 7.0 to 7.4 (Grizzle 2009), including, unfortunately, numerous unspecified local variants thereof.

When morphology alone is the end goal, the exact fixation time is not critical, extending from 6 h to days or even months with little compromise in histologic appearance. While formalin is generally forgiving in this respect, the variable rate of penetration of tissues does remain an issue. If the blocks destined for processing are not cut to recommended size (ideally not larger than 1 cm × 1 cm × 0.5 cm) then the central areas may undergo more advanced degenerative changes, or may be primarily alcohol fixed, due to delayed penetration of the formalin, and hence inadequate fixation by formalin, a process which, as already noted, is not instantaneous, but is a 'clock reaction' requiring of time (up to 24 h Shi et al. 2011, 2019).

The morphology in partially fixed areas may be compromised and IHC often shows variable quality of staining extending from the peripheral part of the block (well fixed) to the center (partially fixed). Furthermore, not all proteins behave in identical manner, depending upon their relative degree of preservation upon exposure to alcohol and formalin, and the extent to which prolonged formalin fixation may mask epitopes. The smaller the tissue block, the more uniform and more rapid is the exposure to formalin, and the less these issues are a problem. During this phase of processing care should be taken to ensure that the specimen does not dry out, as subsequent staining will be compromised by additional staining artifacts, which may be especially evident at the tissue edges (so called edge-artifact).

It is unfortunate that the unqualified term 'formalin fixation' (or FFPE tissue) is widely used throughout the research literature and in diagnostic anatomic pathology, a practice which fosters the long standing, and often unquestioned, assumption that formalin fixation is a single uniform process, which it is not. All FFPE tissues are, therefore, not the same with respect to preservation of protein, DNA or RNA.

In surgical pathology practice there is no precise control over the amount of fixative present in specimen containers distributed around the institution, in relation to the bulk of the tissue placed therein (should be at least a ten-fold volume of fixative in relation to tissue), or the freshness of the fixative and hence its pH. Once placed in fixative the time of transport up to the point of initiation of tissue processing in the laboratory (grossing) is highly variable, being dependent upon location, the facility's internal transport mechanisms and the exact time that the specimen reaches the lab and is placed in the queue for grossing (dissection) into small blocks. Notably, the single quality assurance measure (QA criterion) for this entire diaspora is limited to whether the resultant morphology is judged by the pathologist to be satisfactory on examination of the H&E! (see also Part III).

Therefore, although this process often is termed 'routine' or 'standard' formalin fixation, there is in reality no such thing as 'standard' and the precise total fixation time for any particular tissue specimen usually is unknown, even within a single laboratory. With the advent of biomarker evaluation more rigorous protocols are required and have been introduced in some centers, requiring as a minimum the recording of key time points as the specimen moves through the system (see below). An approximation of total fixation time may thus be made more widely available.

While generalizations may be made about the overall impact of these variables on outcome (Fig. 7.1), the ability to demonstrate any particular analyte in any particular laboratory can only be determined by experimental evidence (hence, validation). These complications are now well recognized in IHC methods, and control processes exist to compensate to some degree (Chaps. 11 and 12).

It is equally important, but much less appreciated, to recognize that proteomics and genomics (mass spectrometry, PCR and NGS), and other methods that rely upon extraction from FFPE tissue are equally, or more, vulnerable to variations in sample preparation, because in these methods adequacy of fixation of the tissue (cells) that are the source of the extract is rarely assessed, even by such a crude measure as morphology. In addition, the internal 'house keeper' proteins and nucleic acids that are used as internal controls are impacted by all of these same factors, including the fixation status of the various cell, and the differing subtypes and proportions thereof that are present in the sample. These aspects of tissue handling will be discussed in more detail for specified analytes in Parts III and IV.

There is no fixative that is ideal for all antigens and no antigen that perfectly survives all fixatives (Taylor and Cote 2005). Fixatives other than 4% neutral buffered formalin have been sometimes employed in the belief of superior morphology or better preservation of antigenicity. Torlakovic et al. (2010) reviewed the topic with respect to IHC. Data for specific biomarker testing are very limited, yet (almost) all approved or certified biomarker tests to date have used FFPE tissues. All are thus subject to the inherent and unknown intrinsic variability of the pre-analytic process.

For these reasons discussion in this book is largely restricted to FFPE tissue. The pre-analytic concerns apply both to studies of intact sections and to extracts made for molecular or protein analysis.

7.3.1 Total Fixation Time

Under controlled experimental conditions and by inference in anatomic pathology practice, fixation times in NBF from 6 h upwards to 72 h (and in some instances longer) are satisfactory for the subsequent demonstration of many, but not all, antigens (including protein biomarkers). ASCO/CAP guidelines for ER extend up to 72 h and HER2 up to 48 h, but in all cases the lower limit is 6 h (noting that even for needle biopsies formalin fixation ideally requires 24 h to complete) (Hammond et al. 2010). The fixation times of many (most) biomarkers are not known in detail, but are assumed to fall within these parameters. As a matter of practice any fixation regimen outside of these guidelines requires laboratory validation of its effectiveness for ER and HER2, and for all new biomarkers where specific information is not available. With approved IVD tests the manufacturer's package insert should be consulted and may contain information to the extent that it is known.

There is a consensus that 'under-fixation' is more damaging than 'over-fixation.' With respect to under-fixation, 'stat' or same day turn-around-time (TAT) tests necessarily employ fixation times of less than the minimum 6 h, sometimes accompanied by methods to accelerate fixation (as by microwave or ultrasound exposure). Results obtained by any of these rapid approaches should be regarded with suspicion unless extensively validated within the laboratory for the biomarker in question. With respect to over-fixation, there is extensive literature attesting to the fact the prolonged formalin fixation does render it more difficult to detect many antigens by IHC methods. Just how difficult, or whether it is possible at all, depends upon several factors, principal among which are the nature of the antigen (protein and its epitopes), the type of fixative and total time of exposure, the exact type and duration of the antigen retrieval (AR) protocol, the antibody employed for detection, and the technical sensitivity of the IHC labeling or detection system (Shi et al. 2011, 2019; Hewitt et al. 2011).

In an approach to standardization, and better to understand how all of these variables affect test results, some institutions have begun routinely to record on the specimen request form key time points in the specimen handling process; time of removal from body, time of placement in fixative, time of grossing into small blocks in formalin in the lab, time of placement in the auto-processor, and total formalin exposure in processor cycle (Hammond et al. 2010; Khoury 2018). Given the standard auto-processor cycle the total exposure to formalin can easily be calculated, with the caveat that at times the cycle may be adjusted to accommodate lab schedules (weekends, and holidays), this also may alter total time of formalin exposure. This approach is to be recommended and may in practice reduce variations in fixation, so limiting the adverse effects that are discussed below; at a minimum it will allow retrospective investigation of disparate results in relation to fixation time etc. Specific details (fixation type and time) should be included in the final pathology report, because the information may influence the selection and protocol (e.g. AR method) of any subsequent tests that may be performed on the FFPE block.

7.3.2 Nature of the Antigen

Different antigens (proteins, epitopes) are affected differently by the complex cross-linking reactions occurring during formalin fixation. While there is an extensive literature on the subject, information is mostly lacking with respect to individual proteins, and is very limited for the more recent novel biomarkers. There is the added complication that the ability to detect any particular biomarker protein in FFPE tissues by IHC not only is impacted by the variables already described, but also is critically dependent upon the exact antibody/detection system selected for its detection (Chap. 9).

In essence, the only definitive statement that can be made is that the ability for detecting each individual biomarker by IHC in FFPE tissues must be demonstrated and validated de novo in each laboratory (or research bench experiment) for every step of the specified Total Test (Chaps. 9, 10, 11, and 12). The use of an approved IVD (FDA or CE Marked) has the practical advantage that intra-laboratory validation is less demanding, because components of the IVD kits (reagents, protocol) will have been extensively validated by the vendor. However, it is important to note that performance validation by the vendor, does not guarantee that the test will perform to required standards on tissues processed in the user's laboratory, because fixation and processing of tissue will not be the same.

7.3.3 Fixation Time in Relation to Effectiveness of Different Antibodies

Today most of the antibodies used in IHC and IF are monoclonal, as opposed to the use of antisera (polyclonal antibodies). The implications for practical performance of IHC and IF stains or assays are significant, but often not appreciated. The key factors are outlined below.

In the early IHC (and IF) studies on FFPE tissues the primary and secondary antibodies used were in fact antisera, which are in fact mixtures of many different antibodies (polyclonal) (Fig. 7.2), some of which have specificity (with varying affinity) to the target protein (used as the immunogen), and others which have low or irrelevant specificity with respect to the target, reflecting the prior immune history of the animal in which the antiserum was generated.

The fact that the immunogen (antigen) used to make an antiserum induces several different antibody clones against different epitopes was an advantage in early experiments trying to effect IHC on FFE tissue, because some of these epitopes survived formalin masking better than others, contributing to the success of the initial studies for immunoglobulins, lysozyme, transferrin etc. (Taylor and Burns 1974; Mason et al. 1975). On the other hand, with antisera the presence of subsets of antibodies of irrelevant specificity, may give unexpected false positive (spurious) staining, as well as increased background due to non-specific non-immunologic binding.

In this context the discovery and application of monoclonal antibodies was huge step forward, because antibodies could be developed or selected or, more recently, engineered to have reactivity against defined formalin fixed target epitopes (Fig. 7.3). The antibodies used in biomarker detection are for this reason monoclonal antibodies that have been developed, selected and validated as fit for purpose for detection of the

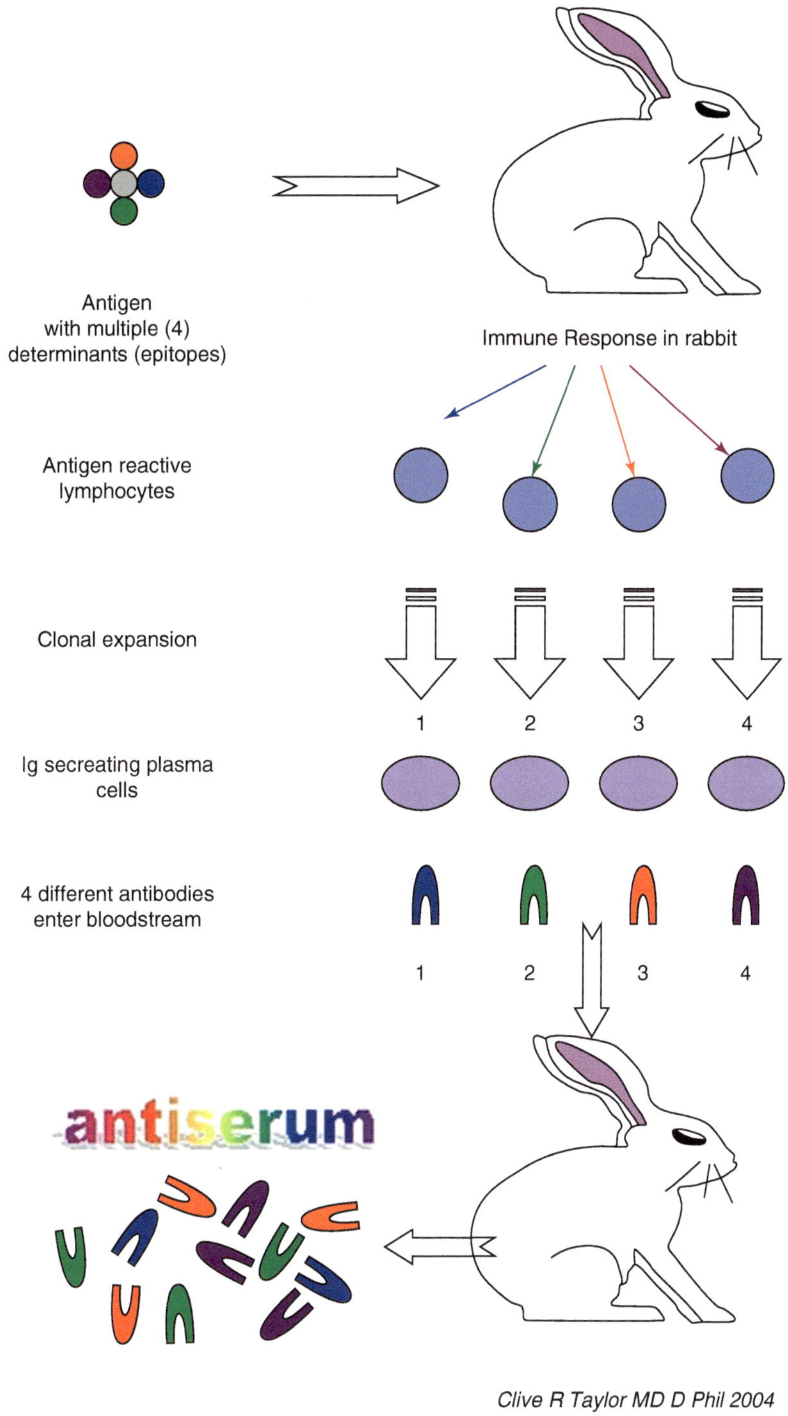

Fig. 7.2 Simplified depiction of antiserum (polyclonal antibody) production in rabbit. The resulting antiserum contains many different antibodies having differing specificity and affinity for the immunogen, which itself may display multiple epitopes; in this illustration the immunogen is shown as having just 4 epitopes, generating 4 distinct antibodies in the serum—in reality there are many more (This figure was published in Immunomicroscopy, A Diagnostic Tool for the Surgical Pathologist. Eds. Taylor and Cote (2005); by permissions Elsevier)

targeted epitope in FFPE tissues. The utility of each primary monoclonal antibody in any other condition, with any other fixative, cannot be assumed, but must be separately validated.

A further advantage is that in theory, once established, a monoclonal antibody can be produced indefinitely, with basic performance validation; this is not true of an antiserum, where

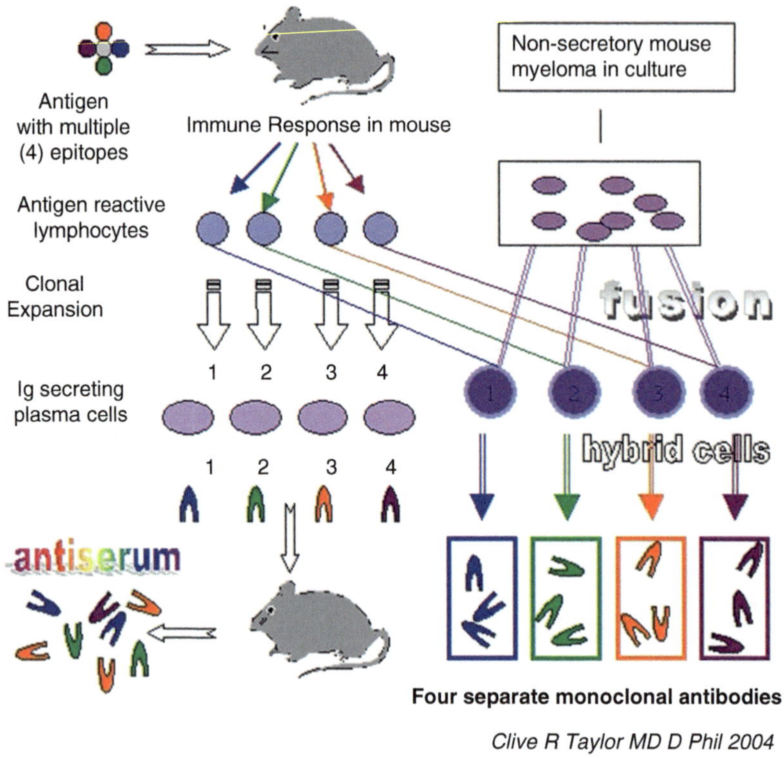

Fig. 7.3 Antiserum production in the mouse (L side) mirrors that in rabbit (Fig. 7.2). A simplified depiction of monoclonal antibody production is shown on the right. The immunologically reacting lymphocytes are removed and separately hybridized with a murine plasma cell line, following which selection occurs for the clone(s) that produce antibody with the required characteristics. For illustrative purposes the immunogen is shown as having 4 epitopes resulting in 4 uniquely specific monoclonal antibodies (This figure was published in Immunomicroscopy, A Diagnostic Tool for the Surgical Pathologist. Eds. Taylor and Cote (2005); by permissions Elsevier)

each batch (drawn from the immunized animal) is different, and validation complex, plus when the animal is extinguished, so is the antiserum.

7.3.4 Antigen Retrieval (in Analytic Phase)

Antigen retrieval (AR) or epitope retrieval is discussed by some authors as part of the pre-analytic phase. In this book AR will be considered as part of the analytic process, principally because changes in the AR method may radically impact test outcome and because for FDA and CE marked tests the exact AR method usually is described as an intrinsic part of the approved test protocol. Heat induced retrieval AR will be addressed in Chap. 8, under 'Analytic Phase' as the preferred retrieval method for most purposes and that most commonly used. Enzymatic digestion may be required occasionally in addition to, or in lieu of, AR and will be discussed as appropriate.

7.3.5 Fixation of Tissues Employed for Validation and Controls

(discussed more fully in Chaps. 10 and 11, and in Part III with respect to the crucial role of the pathologist).

Tissues to be used for controls, subject to verification and validation, should be obtained from within the performing laboratory. In practice the usual source is from archival FFPE blocks, an approach that allows some uniformity of overall

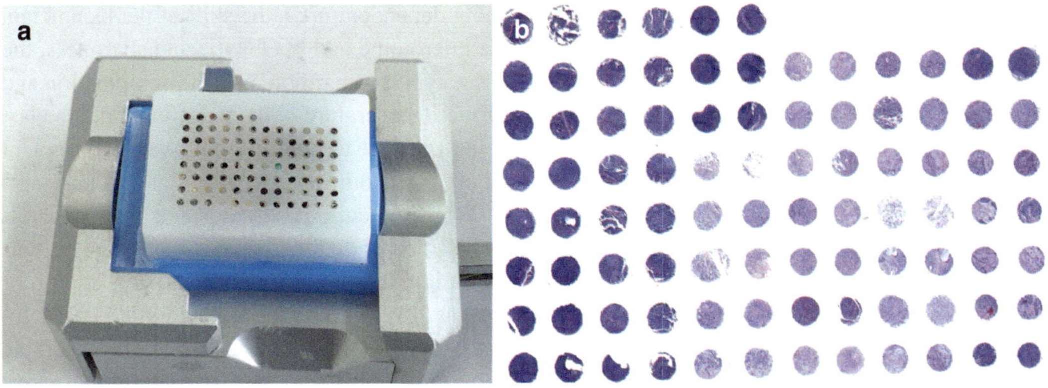

Fig. 7.4 (**a**) shows a 96 × 1 mm core paraffin block Tissue Micro-Array (TMA). (**b**) shows cut section of the 96 FFPE cores with H&E stain. These are duplicate cores of ovarian cancer, representing an excellent way for testing antibody reactivity on multiple tumor specimens (48 in this instance) using only one slide. Courtesy of Dr. Regan Fulton, Array Science, Sausalito, CA

tissue preparation because the 'in-house' fixation method and processing protocol is then broadly similar for controls and tissues being tested. Selection of normal FFPE tissues as method control materials should follow the same approach. However, just as detailed total fixation time may not always be recorded for the test tissue, the same may also be true of the archival blocks used as controls. For these reasons planned collection of specimens for controls is preferable, by setting up protocols in which most of the recommendations discussed herein are incorporated.

In order to evaluate large numbers of normal or tumor tissues with a particular primary antibody, multi-tissue blocks or tissue microarrays (TMAs) often may be used for convenience and economy (Fig. 7.4).

TMAs prepared from tissue processed under closely controlled protocols for this defined purpose represent the optimal choice. Preparation from existing in-house archival tissue is the second, and most commonly used, option and is preferred over purchased TMAs. The reason previously alluded to is that by definition TMAs contain tissue cores taken from several or many different tissue blocks, which in the commercial setting may be of unknown provenance: almost by definition these blocks will not have been subjected to the same (or even similar) tissue preparation protocols and fixation may be unknown, beyond simple categorization as 'formalin fixed.' Thus if using TMAs attention should be given to how the source tissues have been fixed and processed, which will have been documented for good 'in house' protocols as well as by the better commercial suppliers.

The preparation, verification and validation of optimal control tissues is a key part of establishing a successful biomarker test, and is discussed in more detail in the Analytic phase (Chaps. 10 and 11).

7.4 Processing

To produce a FFPE tissue block requires that the fixed tissue be impregnated with paraffin wax (or similar material) prior to sectioning. This is termed 'processing' and has general features in common across most laboratories. It involves first displacing water by exposing the tissue to increasing concentrations of alcohol up to 100%, and then replacing the alcohol with a solvent that is miscible with heated liquid paraffin, usually xylene.

Many service laboratories employ tissue autoprocessors to perform these sequential steps according to a pre-set timed cycle, using reagents supplied by the manufacturer, which does introduce some degree of uniformity across laboratories using common instruments. However, it falls far short of standardization. There is the ability to change schedule times over weekends and holidays, when tissues may be paused for longer periods in formalin solution or alcohol. Also, there are several commercial auto-processors available, and likewise different reagents and paraffin waxes of different melting points (or substitutes—generally the lower the melting point the better).

Manual processing of tissues in smaller labs and in research labs is subject to even greater variation particularly with regard to total time in fixative, an important factor that is rarely mentioned in research papers, though it often is critical to the results reported and to whether or not findings are repeatable by others.

Small excision and core needle biopsies frequently require special handling in order to preserve the limited amounts of tissue present. Usually there are established protocols that are more closely standardized because of the extra care required in handling. Drying of tissue surfaces is a particular threat and requires extra precautions. The IHC results obtained in such tissues compare well with those obtained in optimally processed tissue blocks.

As with the term 'standard formalin fixation' there is in reality no standard for the remaining stages of tissue processing to achieve a paraffin block. This wide intrinsic variability from lab to lab (and even tissue to tissue within a lab) merely underlines how vital it is that the Total Test must be validated for performance within each and every laboratory for each specified biomarker—that is proven 'fit for purpose.'

7.5 Tissue Sectioning and Storage

7.5.1 Sectioning: Thickness

The usual recommended FFPE section thickness for IHC (and routine H&E) is 4 μm. Any histology technologist or technician can attest to how difficult it is consistently to cut sections from different tissue blocks to uniform 4 μm thickness, being dependent upon the skill of the technician, the microtome and blade type and sharpness, the tissue type and fixation, and the composition and surface temperature of the paraffin block, the last being difficult to control under varying ambient laboratory conditions.

With conventional tissue stains such as H&E and also basic qualitative IHC stains such as keratin, minor changes in thickness, of a micron or less, are likely not to be detected by the pathologist's eye. More major changes, for example between 4 μm and 8 μm, might not affect interpretation of qualitative staining of slides when they are viewed separately, but in the authors' experience usually are readily apparent when slides of different thickness are viewed side by side, as by split screen microscopy, or by digital imaging. Indeed, decades ago Tony Leong (see editorial review, Leong 2009) (Fig. 7.5) among his many major contributions showed that section thickness impacted ER scores, both the observed intensity and percentage score, with the potential for false positive and false negative results.

Thick sections may also pose difficulties in penetration of antibody and large molecule labeling reagents, and impair the effectiveness of wash

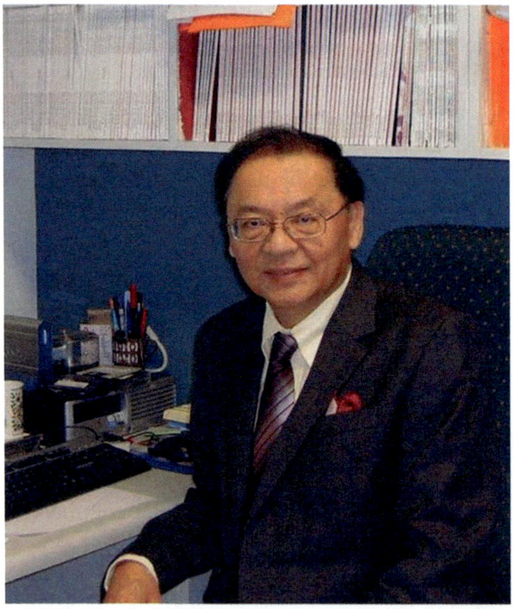

Fig. 7.5 A Leong. Professor Anthony Siew-Yin Leong (1945–2011). (Personal collection of author—CRT)

stages, which have been set by the manufacturers as optimal for 4 µm sections. Thicker sections also impact on the intensity of haematoxylin counterstaining, which can indirectly affect, by contrast, the relative intensity of the biomarker related staining, or may entirely obscure low intensity IHC nuclear staining (Dunstan et al. 2011).

As noted, by default 4 µm has become the standard, because with the microtome set at 4 it is possible under careful conditions to produce evenly cut sections that consistently are close to 4 µm, which is fine for H&E examination and thus is the default norm for IHC.

There are relatively few recent reports that address this issue, and the findings are in conflict. As already noted, Leong (2009) pointed out that when comparing section of 4 µm versus 7 µm, subcellular elements of membrane, cytoplasm and nucleus may be represented very differently, which clearly impacts assessment by IHC of proteins represented in each of these compartments. More recently, McCampbell et al. (2019) provided elegant confirmation using 2 µm, 4 µm, 6 µm and 8 µm thickness sections (confirmed by interferometry) in a study of representative nuclear (Ki-67, BCL6), membranous (CD7) and cytoplasmic (keratin) markers. When assessed by eye and, more accurately, by an algorithmically defined pixel score, the results were clear. The thickness of the section had significant impact on any attempt at scoring of cells (proportion of positive versus negative). In a subsequent study, Libard et al. (2019) demonstrated that differences in thickness (4–7 µm) significantly affected IHC 'scoring' of several microglial marker proteins, (synaptophysin, GFAP and neurofilament H), whether assessed by eye (greater intensity), or by digital imaging and basic morphometric analysis (pixel count); scores increased by as much as 72% in 7 µm versus 4 µm sections. CD68 and HLA DR were similarly affected. Libard's interest was primarily in quantitative evaluation in Age Related Tauopathy, but the principles relate directly to quantification of biomarkers in cancer.

As part of a biomarker immune profile study, Zajac et al. (2019) described conflicting results using sections that were cut at 1 µm intervals, from 2 to 7 µm. They evaluated PD-L1 staining with SP263 antibody in urothelial cancer and reported that the differences in thickness "maintained the same PD-L1 expression status." While this finding is encouraging in a practical sense, it also is very surprising because there is a greater than three-fold variation in thickness and in tissue volume, and thus potentially in the real amount of analyte present on the slide (PD-L1 protein in this instance). In view of earlier accepted data that thickness does matter it is likely that the complex nature of the visual PD L-1 scoring system used in this study is simply not sufficiently sensitive to detect a three-fold change (in intensity), in part because the human eye is unable to detect even major changes in intensity of high intensity IHC signals. Other confounding factors include the fact that in IHC (for several reasons) intensity is not directly proportional to the amount of targeted analyte present. In addition, penetration of the antibody and labeling system (large molecules) will be very different in a 2 µm section versus a 7 µm section at fixed incubation times; decreased penetration may counteract any increase in stain intensity in thick sections.

QC and QA studies also support the contention that section thickness is an important part of overall standardization (Nielsen 2015; Vyberg and Nielsen 2016; NordiQC 2019). Furthermore, as digital algorithms and objective quantification increasingly become available for 'reading' IHC biomarker slides, the assessment of intensity and percentage against reference standards shows that thickness does matter (Matenaers et al. 2018; McCampbell et al. 2019; Matsuda et al. 2021).

In the study by Masuda and colleagues it is of particular note that HER2 scoring was markedly affected the authors introduced an interesting approach to measure and compensate for thickness variation. While they used a polyclonal antibody which, as discussed earlier in this chapter is not recommended for widescale biomarker assays, the principles still apply.

Absent a body of evidence to the contrary, strict adherence and QA measures are recommended to achieve a consistent 4 µm thickness. Digital imaging systems are able to monitor that cut sections are within acceptable limits. Obviously, control sections must be cut to the same thickness as the test tissue section, whether or not they are mounted on separate slides or, as preferred, on the same slide (discussed in Chaps. 10 and 11).

7.5.2 Glass Slides

The glass slides typically are coated with some form of adhesive or are positively charged to promote adhesion of the tissue section (which has a net negative charge). If using an automated staining platform, it is recommended to use glass slides exactly as listed by the manufacturer, because the instrument will have been calibrated and quality controlled for these specific slides in terms of adhesion, effectiveness of wash stages and overall quality.

7.5.3 Section Storage Time: Cut Slide Stability

It has long been recognized that IHC stains may yield poor results on FFPE sections that have been cut and stored for long periods. There is no universal guide as to exactly how long a cut section may be stored before the quality of staining is affected. It is likely to vary for different antigens and of course according to storage conditions. There are data, however, that for some (many?) antigens storage for up to 6 months does not noticeably affect outcome, that is within the limits of qualitative assessment by eye (Zajac et al. 2019). Exact storage conditions also matter; airtight storage at 4 °C being preferred to room temperature, whatever that may be. It is generally accepted that dipping cut slides in melted paraffin prior to storage provides a protective surface coating and prolongs utility.

In light of the above observations, there is general consensus that cut FFPE sections should be submitted for IHC staining as soon as possible, ideally within 7 days. This standard is usually achieved in routine anatomic pathology practice. Cut sections that are to be used as controls, including on-slide controls, should be handled in like manner. Resorting to sections that have longer storage times is often an issue for research studies that seek to collect and aggregate archival FFPE sections in the many instances when original blocks are not made available. If FFPE blocks are collected for study, it is wise to defer sectioning of all blocks until such a time as staining can be performed. Degradation of proteins in FFPE blocks is thought to be a much slower process, provided, again, that the blocks are stored at consistent cool temperatures.

It is important to recognize that while it is known that storage time of cut slides may affect outcome for IHC, the same potential adverse effects apply to ISH studies. It is generally not recognized that storage degradation applies equally to genomic methods that employ extracts made from FFPE sections, although few data are available as to RNA and DNA degradation under these conditions. It is difficult to gather meta-data on this issue from the literature, because unfortunately most research publications do not reference whether extracts were taken from archival blocks or from stored pre-cut slides or from sections freshly cut from archival blocks: the last is to be preferred.

References

Dunstan RW, Wharton KA, Quigley C, Lowe A. The use of immunohistochemistry for biomarker assessment—can it compete with other technologies? Toxicol Pathol. 2011;39:988–1002. http://tpx.sagepub.com/content/39/6/988

Grizzle WE. Models of fixation and tissue processing. Biotech Histochem. 2009;84:185–93.

Hammond ME, Hayes DF, Dowsett M, et al. American Society of Clinical Oncology/College Of American Pathologists guideline recommendations for immunohistochemical testing of estrogen and progesterone receptors in breast cancer. J Clin Oncol. 2010;28:2784–95. https://doi.org/10.1200/JCO.2009.25.6529.

Hewitt SM, Robinowitz M, Bogen SA, Gown AM, Kalra KL, Otis CN, Spaulding B, Taylor CR. Quality assurance for design control and implementation of immunohistochemistry assays: approved guidelines, vol. 31.

2nd ed. Wayne, PA: Clinical Lab Standards Institute; 2011. p. 4.

Khoury T. Delay to formalin fixation (cold ischemia time) effect on breast cancer molecules. Am J Clin Pathol. 2018;149:275–92. https://doi.org/10.1093/ajcp/aqx164.

Leong AS-Y. Quantitative immunohistology: tissue section thickness, another glitch in the path to standardization. Appl Immunohistochem Mol Morph. 2009;17:465–9. https://doi.org/10.1097/PAI.0b013e3181a60898.

Lerch ML, Kenerson HL, Chafin D, Westerhoff M, Theiss A, Otter M, Yeung RS, Baid GS. Effect of immediate cold formalin fixation on phosphoprotein IHC tumor biomarker signal in liver tumors using a cold transport device. Sci Rep. 2020;10:2147. https://doi.org/10.1038/s41598-020-58257-3. https://www.nature.com/articles/s41598-020-58257-3

Libard S, Cerjan D, Alafuzoff I. Characteristics of the tissue section that influence the staining outcome in immunohistochemistry. Histochem Cell Biol. 2019;151:91–6. https://doi.org/10.1007/s00418-018-1742-1

Mason DY, Farrell C, Taylor CR. The detection of intracellular antigens in human leucocytes by immunoperoxidase staining. Br J Haematol. 1975;31:361–70.

Matenaers C, Popper B, Rieger A, Wanke R, Blutke A. Practicable methods for histological section thickness measurement in quantitative stereological analyses. PLoS One. 2018;e0192879:13. https://doi.org/10.1371/journal.pone.0192879.

Matsuda S, Susuki R, Kitano Y, Nishimaki H, Kobayishi H, Nakanishi Y, Yokoi H. Tissue thickness interferes with the estimation of immunohistochmeical intensity: introduction of a control system for managing tissue thickness. Appl Immunohistochem Mol Morphol. 2021;29:118–26.

McCampbell AS, Raghunathan V, Tom-Moy M, Workman RK, Haven R, Ben-Dor A, Rasmussen OF, Jacobsen L, Lindberg M, Yamada NA, Schembri C. Tissue thickness effects on immunohistochemical staining intensity of markers of cancer. Appl Immunohistochem Mol Morphol. 2019;27:345–55. https://doi.org/10.1097/PAI.0000000000000593.

National Cancer Institute Best Practices for Biospecimens. Report of the NCI-NIST biospecimen quality assessment & standards development workshop. 2011. Washington DC. https://biospecimens.cancer.gov/bestpractices/2011-NCIBestPractices.pdf. Accessed 20–22 Oct 2010.

Nielsen S. External quality assessment for immunohistochemistry: experiences from NordiQC. Biotech Histochem. 2015;9:1–10. https://doi.org/10.3109/10520295.2015.1033462.

NordiQC Assessment Run C5. PD-L1 (lung). 2019. 2019. https://www.nordiqc.org/downloads/assessments/121_102.pdf

Qiu J, Kulkarni S, Chandrasekhar R, Rees M, Hyde K, Wilding G, Tan D, Khoury T. Effect of delayed formalin fixation on estrogen and progesterone receptors in breast cancer: a study of three different clones. Am J Clin Pathol. 2018;134:813–9.

Shi SR, Shi Y, Taylor CR. Antigen retrieval immunohistochemistry: review of research and diagnostic applications over two decades. J Histochem Cytochem. 2011;59:13–32.

Shi SR, Shi Y, Taylor CR, Gu J. New dimensions of antigen retrieval technique: 28 years of development, practice and expansion. Appl Immunohistochem Mol Morph. 2019;27:715–21.

Taylor CR. Focus on biospecimens: the issue is the tissue. Observations on the "NCI-NIST fitness for purpose quality assessment and standards workshop". October 2010. Appl Histochem Mol Morph. 2011;19:95–8.

Taylor CR. Quantitative in situ proteomics; a proposed pathway for quantification of immunohistochemistry at the light-microscopic level. Cell Tissue Res. 2015;360:109–20.

Taylor CR, Burns J. The demonstration of plasma cells and other immunoglobulin- containing cells in formalin-fixed, paraffin-embedded tissues using peroxidase-labelled antibody. J Clin Pathol. 1974;27:14–20.

Taylor CR, Cote RJ, editors. Immunomicroscopy: a diagnostic tool for the surgical pathologist. 3rd ed. Saunders, PA: Elsevier; 2005. (1st edition, Taylor was 1986; 2nd edition, Taylor and Cote was 1994)

Torlakovic EE, Riddell R, Banerjee D, et al. Canadian Association of Pathologists-Association canadienne des pathologistes National Standards Committee. Canadian Association of Pathologists- Association canadienne des pathologists National Standards Committee / immunohistochemistry: best practice recommendations for standardization of immunohistochemistry tests. Am J Clin Pathol. 2010;133:354–65.

Vyberg M, Nielsen S. Proficiency testing in immunohistochemistry—experiences from Nordic immunohistochemical quality control (NordiQC). Virchows Arch. 2016;468:19–29. https://doi.org/10.1007/s00428-015-1829-1.

Yildiz-Aktas IZ, Dabbs DJ, Bhargava R. The effect of cold ischemic time on the immunohistochemical evaluation of estrogen receptor, progesterone receptor, and HER2 expression in invasive breast carcinoma. Mod Pathol. 2012;25:1098–105.

Zajac M, Boothman A-M, Yong B, et al. Analytic validation and clinical utility of an immunohistochemical programmed death ligand-1 diagnostic assay and combined tumor and immne cell scoring algorithm for Durvalumab in urothelial cancer. Arch Path Lab Med. 2019;143:722–31.

8 Analytical Phase: Protocol and Antigen Retrieval

8.1 The Analytical Phase Defined

A few general comments with respect to methods will be followed by review of the key individual steps in the Analytic Phase. The following is designed primarily to highlight those parts of the process that may impact results; it is not intended to substitute for a required laboratory staining manual, guidance for which may be found elsewhere (Hewitt et al. 2011; Taylor and Cote 2005; Cartun and Taylor 2018).

In terms of laboratory procedures, the Analytic Phase begins with 'deparaffinization' of the cut FFPE tissue section in xylene, followed by passage through graduated alcohols to reduce the tissue to aqueous medium. Next comes antigen retrieval, and optional blocking steps to reduce non-specific antibody binding or to block endogenous peroxidase activity and or biotin. Primary antibody incubation is then followed by application of the labeling system with multiple washes. The chromogen (enzyme substrate) then is added, before dehydration in reverse graduated alcohols and finally permanent mounting under a coverslip.

The entire procedure involves more than 20 separate steps (manipulations of the slides, Fig. 8.1), with the exact timing of several steps being critical to the outcome. Details may be found in the above cited guidelines. With so many disconnected variables, and considering only the major categories, well over 1,000,000 different protocol variations are possible! In this context the importance of developing and validating strict protocols with proven quality control systems, and then adhering to them, should be obvious. The role of the pathologist in assuring quality is detailed in Part III.

If this is not variation enough, then the accompanying table (Table 8.1) shows the astonishing variation in reagents and protocols among a sample of 365 laboratories. This table also illustrates the critical value of external QC programs in providing feedback across participating laboratories, which can lead to overall improved results, as discussed more fully in Taylor 2015 and in Chaps. 12 and 13.

External QC programs (such as NordiQC, UKNEQAS, CPQA and CBQA [formerly CiQC)]) have shown repeatedly that laboratories that are experienced in the use of IHC methods, and have well validated protocols with established control systems, show excellent reproducibility of IHC results, both internally and among similar laboratories. Most of these laboratories use automated. IHC staining platforms.

Unfortunately, the methods used in many research papers, and in clinical laboratories having limited experience in IHC methods, frequently neglect proper validation and control procedures, which is one of the main reasons for reportedly poor performance of IHC. A principal reason for the perception of poor performance of IHC by research investigators is that, judging from the 'Methods' sections of many research publications, they do not follow or adhere to

B. Jasani et al., *Precision Cancer Medicine*, https://doi.org/10.1007/978-3-030-84087-7_8

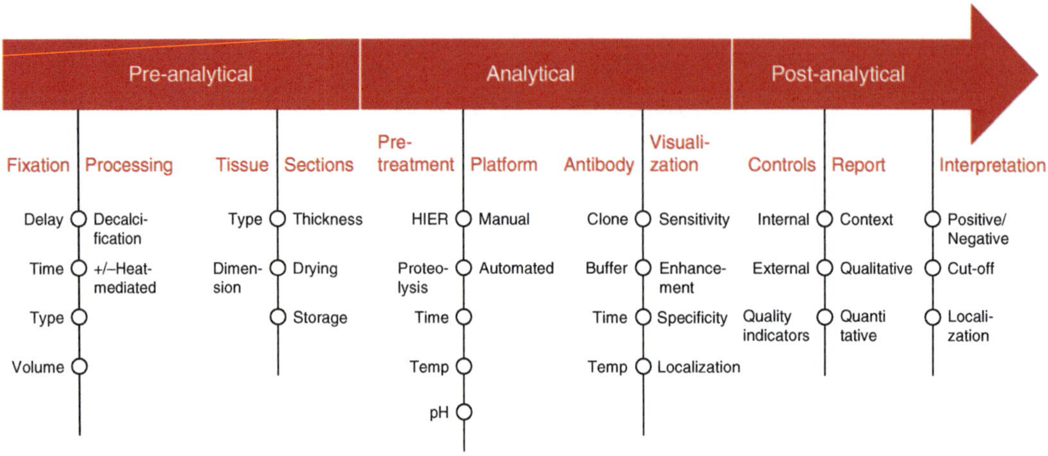

Fig. 8.1 Summary of the many variables that must be controlled in the total IHC test; pre-analytical (Chaps. 5, 6, and 7), analytical (Chaps. 8, 9, 10, and 11) and post analytical (Chaps. 12 and 13). (From Nielsen S 2013). Note that many of these factors also adversely affect genomic and molecular assays that use FFPE tissues, a circumstance not obvious to the performing laboratory, which may receive assay materials that were extracted elsewhere. Reproduced with Permission, Courtesy of Agilent Technologies, Inc. © Agilent Technologies, Inc. 2013

standardized procedures for IHC as described briefly here, and given in more detail in the CLSI guidelines (Hewitt et al. 2011). Apart from the Analytic phase issues described here, the other main reasons for inferior results are variability in the Pre-Analytic Phase (especially fixation) and inconsistent interpretation of results and scores (Fig. 8.1).

IHC, when used in the traditional Anatomic Pathology mode as a 'special stain,' is a very forgiving stain in terms of reagents and performance requirements. The fact that the IHC method allows so much variability in reagents and protocol, but still is able to yield a 'brown (or red) positive stain' can mislead the user into a false confidence, which leads in turn to a lax approach to overall control of the method. Indeed, IHC is often treated in the pathology laboratory in much the same manner in terms of lack of stringency as an H&E stain. Typically in an H&E, the hematoxylin stain reaction can be adjusted by the technologists in terms of intensity and color, deep blue to purple to red, more or less to please the observer (the pathologist), and there is much variation from lab to lab and even within a single lab catering for the preferences of different pathologists. In this mode of performance, the IHC stain also is often adjusted in a similar manner and repeated upon demand until a result (more or less intense) is obtained that 'pleases the pathologist.' Provided that all adjustments are made in accordance with satisfactory performance as judged by external (and internal) positive and negative controls (as will be discussed in Chap. 10), this modus operandi for IHC has served for four decades, as a qualitative 'special stain.' In the hands of experienced pathologists this open, somewhat flexible approach is (just) sufficient for the purpose of a stain, but not for IHC repurposed as an assay, and unfortunately this flexible approach has permeated the entire anatomic pathology literature establishing a mind-set that is difficult to change.

If any form of quantified measurement (or scoring) is intended, which is a requirement of most biomarker tests (i.e. the purpose is not just a stain, but an assay), then we must abandon past and the established practice and accept that more standardization of the IHC method is required, with strictly validated protocols and rigorous control of performance, outcome and interpretation (Chaps. 10, 11, 12, 13, and Part III).

The IHC tests that most nearly approach to this goal are those IHC biomarker tests that are

Table 8.1 External quality control (QC) survey illustrative of the great range of Analytic Phase variables among laboratories performing the 'same' IHC test as a stain

	Markers SMA, CK	Markers SMA, CD34/CD31
Retrieval method		
Heat - Enzymatic - Retrieval reagents	297 labs; 76% acceptable results 146 labs; 32% acceptable Varied; mostly pH6 or 9	336 labs; 83% acceptable results 32 labs; 29% acceptable Varied; mostly pH6 or 9
Primary antibodies		
SMA – CK – CD34/CD31 –	18 antibodies from 10 suppliers 26 antibodies from 16 suppliers	20 antibodies from 9 suppliers 25 antibodies,11 suppliers
Detection reagents	26 different from 13 suppliers	23 different from 11 suppliers
Autostainers	17 instruments from 7 suppliers	17 instruments from 7 suppliers
Chromogen+	Mostly DAB from 19 suppliers	Mostly DAB from 11 suppliers

UKNEQAS data show the enormous variation in practice among 365 participating laboratories in for QC Runs 97 and 97 available online at https://ukneqasiccish.org/. In these studies UKNEQAS distributed paired slides and requested that the performing lab 'stain' them with the designated antibodies, reporting the results and returning one slide for central review. SMA—smooth muscle actin; CK, cytokeratin

FDA approved or CE Marked. These tests are in essence RTU kits (Ready to Use) that have been developed by the vendor to very high levels of verification and validation with respect to reagents and protocol, but which also include clinical correlation with respect to predicting response to the drug for which the test was designed.

As described in Part I, an FDA approved biomarker test, exemplified by the several PD-L1 IVDs that are available (see Fig. 5.1), is developed in a planned conjoint clinical trial along with its companion drug, and is approved within strict specifications, including the intended use (drug, tumor type), reagents, protocol, automated platform and scoring system. Any deviation from the approved specifications (as slight as a change in incubation time or in the AR method) voids the entire validation process; the approved test in these circumstances becomes, by default, an LDT, requiring of a separate new and extensive validation process (Chaps. 2 and 3).

The detailed Analytic Phase discussion that follows here is largely redundant for approved IVDs, where the single and absolute instruction is to follow exactly the manufacturer's FDA (or CE Mark) approved protocol, using the specified reagents, platform and scoring methodology. Performance still must be validated for the FFPE tissues and conditions in the performing laboratory, either by comparison with an established independent method, or with the same assay performed and already validated in a separate laboratory. Generally, correlation over 30 cases is required; it is recommended to include a minimum of 10 cases close to the threshold value selected for a clinical positive or negative result; but these vary in different countries and should be checked locally.

The discussion of the Analytic Phase that follows also recognizes that increasing numbers of laboratories are using automated platforms, of which several excellent and well proven versions exist. When using an automated platform, reagents and protocols are available that have been validated for performance by the vendor for that specified platform, which should be followed, according to the degree to which the system is closed (i.e. reagents and protocol cannot be changed), or open. It may be possible (in open systems) to use protocols and reagents, other than those provided by the instrument vendor, which sometimes is tempting for perceived economic reasons. However, to do so requires new verification and much more extensive performance validation, as vendors usually do not cross validate to competitors' platforms. Reagent manufacturers who do not market their own automated platform may include data in package inserts with respect to performance on selected platforms, but again these must be validated in house. In every instance it is critical to note that validation by the vendor, however extensive, will not have included validation with the laboratory's own 'in-house' pre-analytic and FFPE (fixation) processes (Chaps. 4, 5, 6, and Part III).

The reduced emphasis in this book on manual methods for IHC is also due in large part to the fact that there are no approved Companion Diagnostics with manual protocols. The additional variability inherent in trying to reproduce a 20–30 step IHC procedure (Fig. 8.1) by manual methods has rendered the manual method approach undesirable, indeed untenable for biomarker testing. A specified automated platform is an absolute requirement for approved IHC biomarker IVDs; if an LTD approach is chosen for reagents and protocol, the use of proven automated platform is essential to the total validation process in order to establish a test that is reproducible, day to day, week to week.

8.2 Deparaffinization and Optional Blocking Procedures

As already described, prior to performing AR, the first analytic step is deparaffinization of the FFPE section.

Various blocking steps may then be employed and usually follow AR in sequence within the overall procedure. These may include blocking for (i) endogenous enzyme activity, (ii) nonspecific protein (antibody) binding, or (iii) endogenous biotin. These methods are well described in AP laboratory manuals and in IHC manuals (Hewitt et al. 2011); only a brief outline is given here.

Deparaffinization classically uses xylene (xylol, or equivalent) to solubilize the paraffin, and then successive exposure to graduated alcohols to remove the xylene, ending with the section in aqueous medium (ideally buffer solution). This essentially reverses the paraffin embedment process described in Chap. 7. Several commercial products and protocols also are available for this process, including proprietary 'all in one' aqueous based products. Whatever the method of choice, it must be validated as part of the Total Test result. When using an automated platform, or an RTU kit, then the manufacturer's recommendations should be employed; if not any substitutions must be separately validated. If performed correctly, deparaffinization yields tissue sections in an aqueous environment suitable for IHC (and for ISH, and for first step of most extraction methods).

Deparaffinization is not known to have major effect upon IHC outcome, providing that the process is performed completely, and all traces of solvent and paraffin (wax) are removed when the tissue is returned to the aqueous phase. However, if the process is incomplete, for example because of exhausted reagents, results are compromised because immiscible water, solvent and paraffin droplets may remain in the tissue section and interfere with staining and with visualization of the result. Existence of this problem usually will be apparent on microscopy as the section will appear unclear, or hazy, sometimes with refractile paraffin remaining. Extraction methods similarly are impacted, though not obviously because there is no visual cue to show that the extract still contains paraffin or solvents, which interfere with assay results.

8.2.1 Blocking Steps

1. There are several 'blocking' procedures (including commercial products) that involve treating the section with dilute hydrogen peroxide with the goal of reducing endogenous peroxidase (and related) enzyme activity that might be confused with a true positive test signal, when using DAB, diaminobenzidine, or similar 'chromogens'. With alkaline phosphatase labels levamisole is used instead of hydrogen peroxide. Blocking is, in a sense, optional, being necessary only for tissues where this problem may be anticipated. However, in routine practice this blocking step is generally performed for all cases as it is not known to have adverse effects, and it allows for a uniform procedure on all slides, particularly in automated laboratories, where the recommendations of the vendor should be followed.

2. A second 'blocking step', consisting of application of protein solution is designed to reduce background staining caused by non-specific (non-immunological) charge-based binding of proteins (specifically the primary antibody). Initially albumin solution was used, but today non-immune immunoglobulin (or serum) is preferred. This procedure does not affect test outcome if the blocking immunoglobulin is properly chosen so as not to interfere with, or bind with, either primary or secondary antibodies (usually it is non-immune immunoglobulin of same species as the secondary link or labeling antibody). For kits and RTU reagents the package insert will usually include recommendations for reagents and methods; again, for approved tests the manufacturer's protocol must be followed exactly.
3. Blocking for endogenous biotin is advised when using streptavidin or ABC (avidin biotin complex) labeling methods, to obviate the possibility of false positive reactions due to direct binding of avidin (in the labeling reagent) with biotin present in cells in the tissues. The occurrence of this type of false positive binding will be detected in the appropriate negative controls. Because endogenous biotin varies in amount from tissue to tissue and in tumors it is usual in biotin labeled methods routinely to include a biotin blocking step. Traditionally egg white was used for this purpose, but many good commercial products are available and are to be preferred for reasons of standardization. Avidin biotin labeling has largely been superseded by polymer based labeling methods, which avoid this problem and in addition have higher levels of sensitivity in detection (Chap. 9).

8.3 Antigen Retrieval (AR) or Heat Induced Epitope Retrieval (HIER)

When the feasibility of use of labeled antibody methods with FFPE tissues was first established (Chaps. 1 and 4) the range of antigens that could be detected was limited by several factors; the quality and number of antisera (polyclonal antibodies) available; the poor detection sensitivity of the labeling methods; and the recognized loss (really decrease in detectability) of antigens following formalin fixation. Subsequently antibodies that were more effective in FFPE tissues were developed (including monoclonal antibodies) and the sensitivity of labeling methods improved dramatically. However, the adverse effects of formalin 'masking' of antigenic sites (or epitopes) remained a significant issue.

The first method to show improved IHC staining, or recovery of antigenicity, involved enzymatic (proteolytic) digestion. The detection of a limited number of antigens in FFPE sections was improved. Several different digestion methods and enzymes were trialed, but the methods were fickle and results difficult to reproduce across different laboratories and working conditions. Today enzyme-based retrieval is used only in very limited circumstances for 'antigens that are difficult to demonstrate' in FFPE sections and, even then, often together with other methods.

The breakthrough, when it came, was unexpected, but not entirely without precedent (reviews Shi et al. 1997, 2011, 2019). Shan-Rong Shi developed the idea for a process that he was to call 'Antigen Retrieval' from an exhaustive review of the old literature, specifically the work of Fraenkel-Conrat and Olcott (1948), who showed that it was possible to restore the immunogenicity of tetanus toxoid preparations that had been 'detoxified' by formalin treatment prior to injection into horses for producing antitoxin, by heating the formalin treated toxoid in water. One of the authors (CRT) recalls Dr. Shi describing that his idea was to transfer this heating approach to FFPE tissue sections and confesses to a response along the lines that 'heat treatment of protein antigens was likely make things worse, not better! After lengthy discussion it was clear that the only resolution was to test the hypothesis by performing the experiment. It worked! The rest is history (reviews Shi et al. 1997). Shi and colleagues in the Cancer Diagnostic program at USC went on to further develop and apply the AR method (Shi et al. 2011, 2019), which incidentally also became the basic underlying method for FFPE extraction procedures for protein and molecular analysis (Shi et al. 2002, 2006). Just as the detailed mechanism of formalin fixation remains unclear, so exactly how AR exerts its effect is not fully understood, but is discussed in detail in the reviews cited above and in related texts (Shi et al. 2000; Shi and Taylor 2010).

What is clear is that AR was dramatically successful in practice, making it possible to demonstrate numerous antigens, hitherto hidden or masked in FFPE sections, by the simple process of boiling the deparaffinized sections in buffer solution. The success of AR was rapidly confirmed by numerous other investigators, some of whom have suggested alternative nomenclatures (heat induced epitope retrieval—HIER, 'unmasking,' 'uncloaking,' or 'decloaking'). Throughout this book the term AR will be used in recognition of Dr. Shi's original proposal, carrying the meaning of Heat Induced Antigen (or Epitope) Retrieval; any other method having the goal of restoring antigenicity will be described directly, as in the example of enzymatic retrieval briefly described above. All biomarker assays beginning with FFPE tissue may be assumed to include a defined, validated form of AR, unless otherwise specified.

There are several important points to be made with respect to AR and testing for biomarkers in FFPE tissues, most important among which is that not all AR is the same.

1. AR is part of the Analytic Phase of the Total Test and thus must be part of the overall test validation. When using an approved Companion (or Complementary) Diagnostic IHC test (FDA or CE marked), the exact AR method is to be found in the protocol and should not be changed in any respect. Changing it simply invalidates the test. The same mandate applies to an LDT test; once established and validated in the laboratory the exact AR method is defined and cannot be changed.

   There is historical precedent. Soon after the FDA approved the HercepTest IVD and released it for sale (1998) a number of laboratories changed the prescribed AR conditions in order to produce more intense staining with HercepTest on their FFPE tissues, which they deemed desirable (easier to see and to score). The result, however, was that HER2 scores from those laboratories were no longer comparable to scores from other labs. In attempting to 'improve' the test interlaboratory reproducibility fell by the wayside.

   If the intensity or pattern of staining obtained for HER2 (or any other biomarker) is judged to be less than that expected in test sections and 'in-house' controls, the first recourse should be to go back and review carefully all steps in the Pre-Analytic Phase, and bring all steps within recommended procedures, before re-evaluating the Total Test, with AR and protocol unchanged. Reaching out and obtaining examples of FFPE tissues (sections or blocks) with known scores from other labs that are using the same validated assay is of value in identifying pre-analytic (fixation) issues as the root cause of deficient staining.
2. AR is to be preferred to enzymatic digestion in terms of efficacy and reproducibility for IHC in general, a recommendation clearly supported by external QC studies of multiple laboratories performing IHC stains, including testing for biomarkers (Table 8.1). Laboratories using enzyme-based retrieval reveal a much higher failure rate in achieving 'sufficient staining' than labs using AR and switching those labs to optimized AR improves outcomes immediately. In seeking to establish a biomarker test (for research or for clinical practice) an essential pre-requisite is to identify the optimal AR method as an intrinsic part of the Total Test procedure as described below (iv).
3. The efficiency of AR is affected by several factors, particularly the nature and pH of the buffer solution and the heating conditions, temperature and time (refs). While

numerous antigens benefit from AR there is variation of effectiveness under differing conditions. The two most commonly employed buffers are citrate pH 6.0 and Tris pH 9.0. The most common temperature is 100C (usually 98C, to avoid vigorous boiling which may disrupt the tissue), and the most frequent used heating time 20 minutes (2 × 10 min. exposures in a microwave).

4. Because of variation in the effectiveness of different AR procedures, it is necessary to select the 'optimized AR' conditions for each antigen (protein/biomarker) that is to be demonstrated by IHC. In practice, if starting from scratch with a new antibody, a laboratory may best find the optimized AR method by a 'Test Battery' approach, as recommended by Shi and colleagues (Shi et al. 1996, reviews Shi et al. 2011, 2019). Guidance as to the optimal AR method may also be found in the package insert provided by the vendor of the reagent (primary antibody) or kit. Such guidance is useful as a start point in determining the optimized AR, but must be validated for performance on 'in-house' test and control FFPE tissues.
5. AR is generally included as a routine part of IHC staining on automated staining platforms. The vendors of auto-stainers often offer proprietary trademarked AR solutions, usually one of pH6 and one of pH9. The performance of these proprietary solutions (including heating conditions) will have been validated extensively by the manufacturer across a broad range of IHC stains and will be programmed into the auto-stainer protocol. As a general rule it is simplest to use these proprietary AR solutions exactly as recommended; any change in an attempt to obtain improved results on in-house FFPE tissues, must be validated; as noted above in paragraph (i). When using an approved test (FDA IVD) changes in AR are not allowed; if made they invalidate the approval.
6. In addition to the manufacturers of staining platforms, many other IHC vendors offer proprietary AR solutions, kits or methods; sometimes withholding the exact composition and nature (even the pH) of the products. Some of these commercial products are effective, but if incorporated into the analytic phase again must be validated for Total Test performance for each biomarker (antigen) under study. The use of a proprietary 'secret sauce' handicaps attempts to achieve standardization.
7. While the success of AR provided great impetus to IHC in diagnostic pathology and in research, there have been some unanticipated downside effects (Table 8.2). The widespread adoption of this simple and inexpensive method of improving IHC results led inevitably to many attempts to adapt or improve upon the method. Within a short time period, a range of different buffer solutions, different heating methods and different times and temperatures was described, none of which were cross validated. Not only were different AR solutions tried and promoted, but also several different methods of heating (microwave, autoclave, water bath). As a simple guide, the lower the temperature (e.g. 80C) the longer the time period necessary for heating to achieve near equivalent results ('temperature x time'—Shi et al. 2011, 2019), and the more fierce the heating (e.g. autoclave) the shorter the period, at the possible cost of more disruption of tissue architecture.
8. The end result of all of this experimentation has been to introduce yet another variable into the IHC Total Test, namely AR (Table 8.2)(see also Shi et al. 2011, 2019); another variable that must be optimized and validated in the context of the Total Test procedure, any change in which may impact overall outcome. In short just as there is no standard 'formalin fixation' so there is no standard AR, meaning that whatever method is employed it must be given in detail, and then followed exactly.

Table 8.2 Caveats in the use of antigen retrieval methods

1. While most antigens are enhanced, this is not true for all.
2. Some antibodies outperform others post-AR; just as they did pre-AR. Polyclonal antibodies (anti-sera) may continue to detect antigens that monoclonal reagents 'miss', but attendant specificity issues remain
3. Different antibody/antigen pairs may require different AR approaches, both heating and AR solutions
4. Because more antigen is 'available' post-AR IHC stains appear to be more 'sensitive' and antibodies may need to be diluted and re-optimized (see 3.0 Methods)
5. A case that was previously 'negative' for an antigen, may be 'positive' post-AR
6. Semi-quantitative stains (such as ER and PR) will give higher values post-AR: cases judged 'negative' may be revealed as 'positive'
7. The 'pre-AR' literature (before about 1996) is obsolete and irrelevant with regard to which lesions express which antigens (in formalin paraffin sections).
8. Many different AR methods/protocols exist in different labs, and different AR solutions are available commercially, adding yet another variable to the IHC method.

References

Canadian Biomarker Quality Assurance—Programme canadien d'assurance de la qualité des biomarqueurs. https://www.cbqa.ca/

Canadian Pathology Quality Assurance—Programme Assurance qualité Canadienne en pathologie. http://www.cpqa.ca/

Cartun R, Taylor CR. Techniques of immunohistochemistry: principles, pitfalls and standardization. In: Dabbs DJ, editor. Comprehensive diagnostic immunohistochemistry. 5th ed. Amsterdam: Elsevier; 2018.

Fraenkel-Conrat H, Olcott HS. The reaction of formaldehyde with proteins. V. Cross-linking between amino and primary amide or guanidyl groups. J Am Chem Soc. 1948;70:2673–84.

Hewitt SM, Robinowitz M, Bogen SA, Gown AM, Kalra KL, Otis CN, Spaulding B, Taylor CR. Quality assurance for design control and implementation of immunohistochemistry assays: approved guidelines, vol. 31. 2nd ed. Wayne, PA: Clinical Lab Standards Institute; 2011. p. 4.

Nielsen S. In: Taylor CR, editor. Selection of primary antibody. Chapter 4 in immunohistochemistry staining methods. Copenhagen: Dako Publications; 2013.

NordiQC. https://www.nordiqc.org/

Shi SR, Taylor CR, editors. Immunohistochemistry and antigen retrieval based research and diagnosis. Hoboken, NJ: Wiley; 2010.

Shi SR, Cote RJ, Wu L, Liu C, Datar R, Shi Y, Liu D, Lim H, Taylor CR. Development of an optimal protocol for antigen retrieval: a 'test battery' approach exemplified with reference to the staining of retinoblastoma protein (pRB) in formalin fixed paraffin sections. J Pathol. 1996;179:347–52.

Shi SR, Cote RJ, Taylor CR. Antigen retrieval immunohistochemistry: past, present and future. J Histochem Cytochem. 1997;45:327–43.

Shi SR, Gu J, Taylor CR, editors. Antigen retrieval techniques: immunohistochemistry and molecular morphology. BioTechniques books. Natick, MA: Eaton Publishing; 2000.

Shi SR, Cote RJ, Wu L, et al. DNA extraction from archival formalin-fixed, paraffin embedded tissue sections based on the antigen retrieval principle: heating under the influence of pH. J Histochem Cytochem. 2002;50:1005–11.

Shi S-R, Liu C, Balgley BM, Lee C, Taylor CR. Protein extraction from formalin fixed, paraffin embedded tissue sections: quality evaluation by mass spectrometry. J Histochem Cytochem. 2006;54:739–43.

Shi SR, Shi Y, Taylor CR. Antigen retrieval immunohistochemistry: review of research and diagnostic applications over two decades following introduction of the method to The Journal of Histochemistry and Cytochemistry. J Histochem Cytochem. 2011;59:13–32.

Shi SR, Shi Y, Taylor CR, Gu J. New dimensions of antigen retrieval technique: 28 years of development, practice and expansion. Appl Immunohistochem Mol Morph. 2019;27:715–21.

Taylor CR. Quantitative in situ proteomics; a proposed pathway for quantification of immunohistochemistry at the light-microscopic level. Cell Tissue Res. 2015;360:109–20.

Taylor CR, Cote RJ, editors. Immunomicroscopy: A diagnostic tool for the surgical pathologist. 3rd ed. Saunders, PA: Elsevier; 2005. (1st edition, Taylor was 1986; 2nd edition, Taylor and Cote was 1994)

UKNEQAS. Immunocytochemistry and in situ hybridization. https://ukneqasiccish.org/

Analytical Phase: Principles for Immunohistochemistry (IHC) 9

9.1 Reagents and Protocol for Biomarker Labelling; Selection and Validation

The major steps of the Analytic Phase will be described for IHC specifically, but in most cases the principles apply equally to ISH and IF methods that will be discussed in Chap. 14.

Among the many variables that affect the outcome of an IHC test, selection of the primary antibody remains the single most important factor, in addition to which it must be shown to perform to the required level in the context of the Total Test. For all IHC biomarker tests other than approved tests, whether developed by a clinical service lab for diagnostic practice (LDT), or by a research group (research test), all parts of the test protocol must be established and validated separately, and then finally validated again by the result of the Total Test, that is against the performance with respect to the intended use. Again this vital step is the responsibility of the pathologist (Part III).

9.2 Lab Developed Tests (LDTs)—Manual and Automated

There are two broad approaches to setting up an IHC test in the laboratory, whether for manual use or on an automated platform, either to develop the test 'de novo' or to utilize a purchased kit containing prepackaged reagents.

In the first approach the entire test is set up 'de novo' in the performing laboratory, selecting all reagents and developing the protocol to meet laboratory requirements and intended use for its clinical application. The same requirements exist for a research project, although in research the common practice is to follow a previous published paper, in which the methods often are not explicit and are much less well defined than the guidelines used by clinical diagnostic laboratories (e.g. CSLI guidelines, Hewitt et al. 2011). Results often therefore are suspect.

These are in fact the traditional approaches to setting up IHC stains, which were of course performed manually from 1974, until automated platforms became generally available in the 1990s.

The setting up of an IHC stain, that is properly controlled and validated and will thus provide reproducible results, is far more complicated than most potential users realize (vide infra and Tables 9.1 and 9.2). Simply to buy the necessary reagents from vendors, read some prior research papers or package inserts, and then expect the test to perform perfectly (or at all) is a serious, but common, mistake.

The most common shortfall is lack of 'fit for purpose' controls (Chaps. 10 and 11), coupled with absence of proper validation of the assay in the context of the tissues being tested, including how the result is to be read and reported (see also Part III). In many respects, when primary antibody is made within the research laboratory, or is

B. Jasani et al., *Precision Cancer Medicine*, https://doi.org/10.1007/978-3-030-84087-7_9

Table 9.1 Comparison of manual methods versus automated platforms

Manual platform	Automated platform
More rapid, less expensive initial set up	Automated platforms available from several vendors, with variable cost according to sophistication.
Often used in research labs having no access to automated platforms	All service and large throughput labs use automated platforms
Development and validation of protocol is more complex requires experience and technical expertise	Recommended protocol is frequently part of vendor package
While set up is less expensive, manual staining cost more in technician time	
Little standardization across labs, as difficult to reproduce exact protocol and reagents vary widely	Often forces uniform use of recommended protocols and reagents having initial vendor validation
Necessary to develop controls from basic principles	

Table 9.2 Features of lab developed tests (LDTs) and ready to use tests (RTUs)

LDT (Home brew)	RTU kit (Ready-to-Use): includes approved tests (FDA or CE marked)
Determine intent or goal of test Identify protocol 'fit for purpose' from literature (or from manufacturer). Select primary antibody, purchase Select labeling (link) antibody, purchase Select appropriate chromogen, purchase Identify, purchase, prepare necessary buffers Perform checker-board titration to identify optimal dilution and incubation times for primary and labeling antibody Make solution of chromogen to appropriate concentration (and incubation time) Identify and obtain appropriate control tissue Test complete protocol on controls. Establish interpretation or scoring method; either manual of computer assisted. Validate performance on in-house tissues	Determine intent or goal of test Select RTU kit 'fit for purpose', purchase; includes protocol, often designed for a specified auto-stainer platform. Primary antibody and labeling antibody included. Buffers may be included or recommended. Primary and labeling antibodies are pe-diluted with recommended incubation times. Chromogen may be included or recommended Recommendations for controls included Test kit on controls Recommended interpretation/scoring included Validate performance on in-house tissues Side benefit of improving standardization within and across labs using the same kit. Any change in reagents or protocol, voids all manufacturer's validation (and 'warranty') on test performance.

obtained from other investigators, the situation is still worse, because validation of the antibody is usually far less rigorous than for the best commercial reagents. In developing reagents for biomarker testing, which requires the most exacting levels of performance, manufacturers go to great lengths to carry out complete characterization, verification and validation of the primary antibody, a process beyond the capabilities of all but a few research or service laboratories. In addition, for biomarker testing validation must encompass its performance in the context of the final Total Test, including documented results, which also includes the scoring protocols. For examples of just how extensive is the process see Phillips et al. (2015, 2018).

Details of how to set up an IHC test (stain) using manual protocols are available in several excellent IHC texts and practice guidelines (Taylor and Cote 2005; Hewitt et al. 2011; Cartun and Taylor 2018; Taylor 2018). Again it must be emphasized, however, that manual protocols are not suitable for biomarker assays.

The second approach is to purchase the principal test components in a ready to use (RTU) format. Intrinsic to this decision is to determine whether reagents are validated to the available automated staining platform(s).

When developed in-house, a process which includes assembling the reagents and establishing a protocol, it is termed a lab developed test (LDT); sometimes referred to colloquially as 'home brew.' When using a vendor supplied kit containing optimized reagents and protocol then it is termed 'ready to use' (RTU) (see Table 3.1).

9.2.1 Manual IHC Stains

Manual methods have been replaced by use of automated platforms (auto-stainers) in most service laboratories for many reasons (Table 9.1). This is less true in the research environment, in part because of lack of access to automated platforms, and in part due to lack of experience in their use. Many research publications neglect to state whether or not the protocol was performed manually or by an automated method, or designate which instrument.

9.2.2 Automated IHC Stains

Automated platforms usually are accompanied by recommended reagents and protocols from the same vendor. However, most of these platforms technically are 'open' to the extent that they allow the users some choice of primary antibodies and labeling systems, including selecting the dilutions and incubation times. When operating in the open mode the user may select primary antibody and labeling reagents from other vendors, in which case the user must perform the steps summarized in Tables 3.1 and 9.2, under the LDT column, including checker-board titrations to determine optimal dilutions and incubation times. The instrument then serves simply to conduct the manipulations of the slides, the incubations and washes etc.

Today most platforms are set up and validated by the manufacturer with recommended protocol(s) using of course antibodies and other reagents (such as AR solutions) prepared, validated and sold by the manufacturer in kit form as RTUs (vide infra). Alternatively, these reagents may be purchased individually (e.g. concentrated primary antibody) from the vendor, usually with guidelines for usage included in the package insert. In this instance incubation times and dilutions for optimal performance must be established in the performing laboratory, again requiring checker board titrations.

9.3 Ready to Use IHC Tests (RTUs)

A second increasingly popular alternative approach is to purchase all of the principal reagents in a Ready to Use (RTU) kit, which includes a defined protocol, usually for a specified staining platform produced by the manufacturer of the RTU kit. RTUs generally have been developed by vendors for specified automated platforms. As such they represent the most straightforward approach to establishing an IHC lab service, obviating the need to perform many of the more complex steps in Tables 9.1 and 9.2. The RTU kit is run as shown in the righthand column and tested (validated) on in-house control tissues. If performance is satisfactory then the RTU assay is ready for further in-house validation in the actual test environment, and can be placed in service.

If performance of the RTU in a given laboratory is not satisfactory (negative or too weak) then one recourse is to adjust (increase) incubation times, but in so doing it must be remembered that the manufacturer's validation is thereby voided (and the test become a defacto LDT). A better approach is to go back and optimize all of the pre-analytic processes (e.g. fixation) and then rerun the test. If performance still is unsatisfactory then it is useful to obtain FFPE sections (or TMAs) of tissues shown to be positive for the analyte in question having been tested by validated methods in other accredited laboratories. Reliance upon TMAs from commercial sources carries the caveat that each tissue core in the TMA may have undergone unknown and different pre-analytic conditions; usually a TMA is simply designated as FFPE, encumbering all of the attendant variables discussed previously (Chaps. 7 and 8).

The pros and cons of these two approaches are summarized in Table 9.2.

- The vendor package insert should be regarded as a start point only. At a minimum the primary antibody should separately be tested for appropriate specificity (detects the target antigen), plus validated for high specificity, that is there should be no false positive staining in the context of the labeling method employed. Also, it should show the desired level of sensitivity with the test protocol, that is absence of false negative staining in the intended use.

9.4 Approved IHC Biomarker Assays (FDA, CE Marked)

When an FDA (or CE marked) approved test is utilized then the decision as to which primary antibody will be used already has been made by the vendor of the test, in conjunction with the manufacturer of the associated drug (targeted antibody, as discussed Chaps. 2 and 3). In this context issues of sensitivity and specificity, both technical and clinical, have been addressed and validated in a planned clinical trial as part of the GMP (Good Manufacturing Practice) development and approval process. The primary antibody may not then be changed by the user in any way, neither in dilution nor incubation time, and cannot be substituted by a different antibody (source or clone, even if purported to have the same or better performance characteristics). Similarly, the protocol and all other test reagents have been pre-selected and validated by the manufacturer and cannot be changed without voiding the validation.

In establishing an IHC stain or assay as described above, not only is the selection or the primary antibody critical, but also the selection of the detection system. Detection or labeling systems show enormous variation in ability to detect primary antibody (so called detection sensitivity as discussed below), and both primary antibody and detection system must be optimized in concert, essentially optimization of the entire analytic protocol, including all steps that are intended to amplify or increase the visible stain reaction. It is not generally appreciated that when using highly sensitive detection systems (polymer labels and tyramine amplification), even what would seem to be slight changes in incubation times (as little as from 20 seconds and 30 seconds) can produce intensity changes that are visible even to the naked eye, and thus may impact biomarker scoring.

In RTU kits, and in all approved certified biomarker tests, the detection and optimization of the detection system will have been performed by the vendor, and should be regarded as 'locked.' Any change in reagent, or dilution, or incubation conditions negates any implied warranty or approval and requires revalidation of the entire test.

9.5 Detection Systems and Amplification

In the beginning when IHC was applied to FFPE tissues, one approach to the recognized loss of antigenicity (masking) of antigens was to increase the technical sensitivity of the detection method (Taylor 1978; reviewed by Taylor and Cote 2005). In brief, the indirect conjugate method was replaced by PAP methods and then by ABC systems which allowed for detection of some antigens hitherto not visualized in FFPE sections (Fig. 9.1a–c).

The advent of AR, described above in Chap. 8, restored (to some degree) the antigenicity of many molecules, and detection was further enhanced by still more sensitive labeling methods, based on tyramine amplification and polymer labels (Fig. 9.2a and b), both of which are effective methods of assembling multiple active enzyme labeling molecules ate the site of the antigen.

Today several approaches to maximizing the technical sensitivity of detection of antigens by IHC are in general use in LDTs, RTUs, and Approved Biomarker assays. The major approaches to amplification (or increased technical sensitivity) are summarized in the accompa-

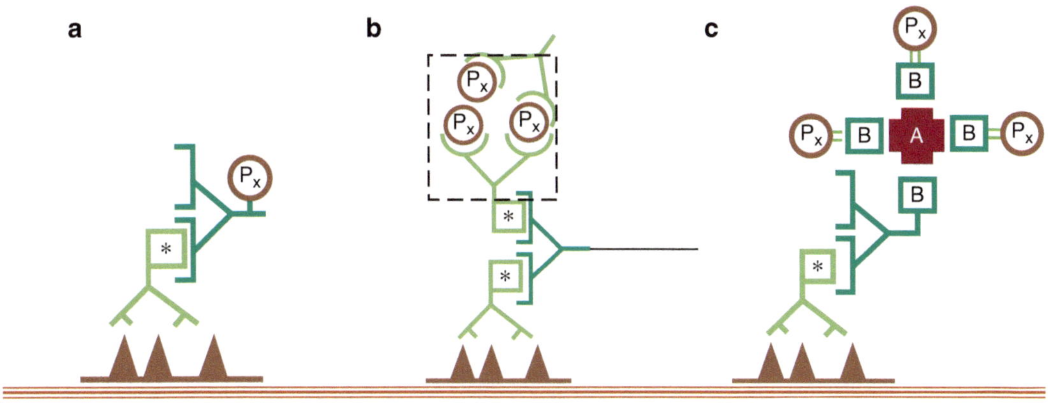

Fig. 9.1 (**a**, **b** and **c**) Basic methods for increasing detection sensitivity. The Direct conjugate (**a**), and PAP (Peroxidase-Anti-Peroxidase) (**b**) and ABC (Avidin Biotin Conjugate) (**c**) methods. PAP and ABC methods increase detection sensitivity by enabling more peroxidase enzyme molecules at the antigen site. In this diagram the primary rabbit antibody (light green) bears an epitope [*] that is bound by the secondary or labeling antibody (dark green). (Px) signifies peroxidase enzyme (This figure was published in Immunomicroscopy, A Diagnostic Tool for the Surgical Pathologist. Eds. Taylor and Cote (2005); by permissions Elsevier)

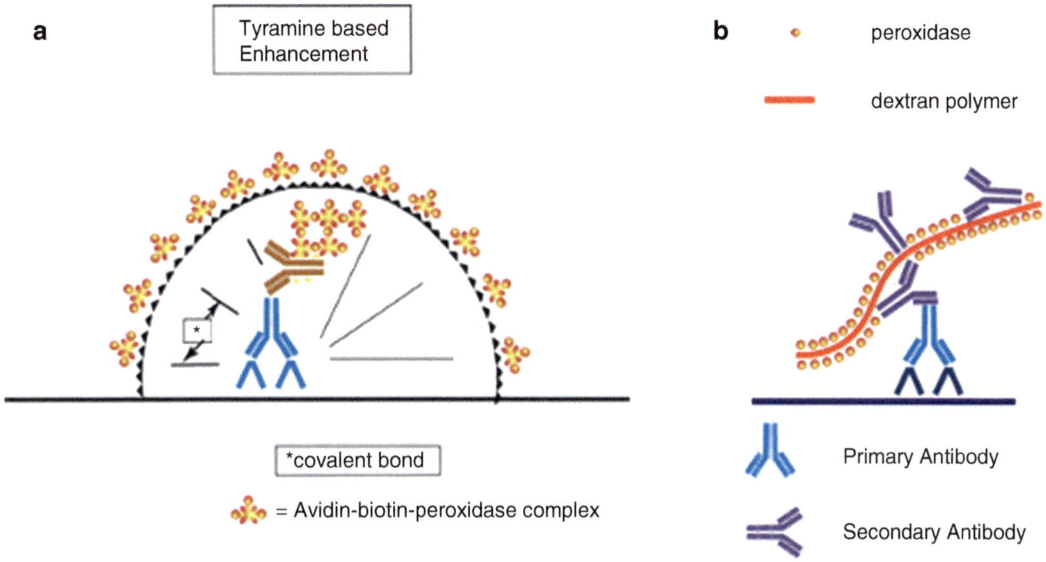

Fig. 9.2 (**a** and **b**). Highly sensitive detection methods assemble numerous enzyme molecules at the antigen site. (**a**) Tyramine amplification relies upon the catalyzed deposition of multiple biotin-tyramine molecules (depicted as a halo) at the site of an initial immunoperoxidase reaction, giving the method great sensitivity. Control of the intensity at the 'end-point' is challenging. (**b**) Polymer carrier methods rely upon linkage of multiple molecules of enzyme to one or more molecules of secondary antibody, resulting in high sensitivity. Major advantages are that reagents are stable and endogenous biotin is not a concern. (This figure was published in Immunomicroscopy, A Diagnostic Tool for the Surgical Pathologist. Eds. Taylor and Cote (2005); by permissions Elsevier)

nying table (Table 9.3). Some approaches may be combined. Whichever approaches are adopted, they must be incorporated into the verification-validation process. Details of principles and practice may be found in the relevant package inserts from vendors and in IHC manuals and methods texts (Hewitt et al. 2011; Cartun and Taylor 2018).

Table 9.3 Summary of methods employed to increase IHC signal

Stage at which effect occurs	Principles of action	Pros and cons
Pre-detection amplification		
(antigen recovery) Enzyme digestion methods Antigen (epitope) retrieval	Attempts to 'unfix' tissue, restoring antigens or epitopes masked or lost due to formalin fixation effects.	Simple and inexpensive. Improves staining for most, but not all, antigens
Detection phase amplification		
Use of highly 'sensitive' detection systems, such as ABC, polymeric and tyramine based methods.	Increases number of molecules of enzymatic label that are deposited at the reaction site.	Controls must be extended to include assessment of sensitivity. May detect antigens that basic methods miss.
Post-detection amplification		
DAB enhancement (imidazole) Gold-silver enhancement	Intensifies DAB color. Intensifies DAM-brown/ black.	Intensifying the end signal tends also to increase the background, and contrast may be impaired.

Any such steps must also be applied to control materials and must be part of Total Test validation

9.6 Introduction to Fit for Purpose Controls: Required Characteristics

In 2004 NIST (The National Institute of Standards and Technology) convened a meeting in Washington DC, in large part responding to widely discrepant HER2 results from different clinical laboratories, even when using 'approved' versions of the HER2 test. There was extensive debate as to causes and consequences, and possible course of action.

In retrospect three main concerns held sway;

Table 9.4 Summary of required characteristics for controls (reference standards) for IHC on FFPE tissues, including increased requirements for quantitative bioassays by IHC

Immunohistochemical control (reference standard): Requirements
1. Identical pre-analytic phase • The control must be subjected to all of the same rigors of sample preparation (ischemia, transport, fixation) as the "test" tissue.
2. Identical analytic and post-analytic phases • The control must be integrated into all steps of the test (assay) protocol, including evaluation of the result.
3. The control should contain a **known amount and dynamic range of the reference standard** protein.
4. The control tissues should be **universally available** to all laboratories performing the assay.
5. It should be **inexhaustible and inexpensive**.
6. The control material should be **fit for purpose.**

1. the variable and unknown impact of differences in fixation (since expanded to the wider concept of all Pre-Analytic issues);
2. the lack of a standard universal control (to augment the cell line controls in the approved kit);
3. the relatively poor reproducibility of scores rendered by pathologists (a factor in the introduction in the USA of additional reimbursement for computer assisted scoring).

The recommendations with respect to controls (Table 9.4) were quite obvious to those pathologists familiar with testing procedures in hospital chemistry laboratories, but less so to colleagues in anatomic pathology laboratories just down the hallway, or to researchers across campus. Fifteen years later considerable progress has been made with respect to meeting the first and second requirements (1 and 2, Table 9.4). A sixth requirement that controls should be 'fit for purpose' has since been added. In addressing the remaining characteristics (3, 4 and 5, Table 9.2), a beginning has been made, but no more.

From the very beginning of use of IHC with routine FFPE tissues (Taylor and Burns 1974) pathology laboratories have used tissue based controls (positive and negative and internal controls as a minimum, *vide infra*) in performing IHC for the purpose of a special stain. Use of the term reference standard (in lieu of control) carries the additional connotation of meeting all of the requirements in Table 9.4, which conventional IHC controls do only in part.

9.6.1 The Six Required Characteristics of Controls—Reference Standards

1. The control tissues must be subjected to all of the same rigors of sample preparation (ischemia, transport, fixation) as the "test" tissue (Identical Pre-Analytic Phase).

   The requirement that control tissues should have undergone an identical pre-analytic phase dawned gradually but is today generally accepted. Even so it not always achievable. For example, the FDA approved HER2 tests include control materials provided by the vendor in the form of cell line preparations, which cannot be considered to have identical pre-analytic phase to the test tissue. Cell line controls are validated and standardized but can serve only as a control signal that the reagents and protocol yield the expected levels of staining intensity in the control. They do not provide assurance that the test will perform on FFPE tissues accessioned into the service laboratory. In the event that the test fails to perform well in FFPE tissues it is vital to recognize that the fault is likely not in the 'kit' but in the pre-analytic process; tweaking the components of the kit is NOT the answer.

   Among the many pre-analytic variables, fixation was the first to be addressed in practical terms. Historically it is of interest that attempts to improve IHC staining in FFPE tissues focused first on improving detection, and next on recovery of lost antigenicity by using enzymatic digestion, then AR, prior to any real effort to introduce and maintain standard fixation methods. That is, the philosophy of pathologists and vendors alike was to manipulate reagents and protocol, not to 'fix the fixation' problem. This precept held true within individual institutions, and even more across different laboratories or countries. In many ways it reflected a pragmatic approach, tacit recognition of the huge logistical issues of obtaining any agreement as to what the standard FFPE fixation should be, and then, if agreed, bringing it into uniform large scale practice.

   There are real practical consequences stemming from lack of a standardized FFPE method. In the selection of controls 'in-house' archival tissues are preferred to FFPE blocks obtained from other sources, or to purchased 'control' blocks or sections. The presumption is that in-house archival tissues will have undergone a pre-analytic process that is similar, although not identical, to the test tissue. As already noted, no such assumption can be made for purchased blocks or slides or TMAs. In fact, the issue is compounded when using commercial TMAs in which each core set will have undergone a different pre-analytic phase (cold ischemia and fixation time), details unknown! It can scarcely be over emphasized that the common practice of employing such TMAs for initial antibody verification and subsequent validation potentially is a significant source of error.

   In order to optimize selection of control material the preferred approach within a laboratory is to set up a schedule specifically for collection of control tissues (normal and pathologic) by harvesting those tissues not essential to the diagnostic process (that otherwise would be discarded), with careful control and documentation of ischemic time, fixation time and processing. Over a short period a 'bank' FFPE control tissues can be developed that conforms with existing guidelines for biomarker testing, and may be used for TMA production internally. The NCI (2016) has published extensive guidelines, that if universally followed would help resolve the issues described here. NordiQC (https://www.nordiqc.org/) has used this approach to develop standard in house TMAs, which by careful selection of normal tissue types are able to serve as controls for a surprisingly broad range of IHC stains (Nielsen 2015). In general, the use of normal tissues as controls is preferable, for practical reasons of availability, and also because expression of many antigens will be more consistent from specimen to specimen in. normal tissues than in pathologic specimens (see Chap. 10). Successive normal tissue blocks selected as controls will be relatively more similar to the exhausted block that they replace, requiring less validation, thereby promoting consistency within the laboratory, and also by inference across different laboratories that utilize the same approach.

For antigens not usually expressed in normal tissues then pathologic tissues are used as control sources and should be banked under controlled pre-analytic conditions as indicated for normal tissues. Validation of these control blocks, and their replacement by 'new' blocks when exhausted must be more extensive in order to maintain consistency of the Total Test result.

Newer control materials are becoming available in the form of cell line preparations (as in HER 2 tests), xenograft tumors (Hasan et al. 2015) and faux-tissue blocks (or 3D 'histoids') (Kaur et al. 2011) all of which are considered in detail in Chap. 11. These control preparations also do not have identical pre-analytic phase to the test specimen, but xenografts and histoids can be processed by FFPE, yielding sections whose preparation and appearances closely resembles regular FFPE tissue sections. Protein deposits (spots) have also been developed (review, Bogen 2019, see Chap. 11). These 'spots' also have not undergone a similar pre-analytic phase, or the usual FFPE process, and they have no morphologic resemblance to tissues. However, they do have the singular advantage that they can be engineered to contain known amounts of the target protein, for calibration and quantification. It is probable that some combination of these newer controls may come close to meeting the advanced control requirements given in Table 9.4 and discussed in more detail in Chap. 11.

These and other important factors that influence the overall quality of the control process are discussed in greater depth in 'The Control Series' of six papers published in Appled Immunohistochemistry and Molecular Morphology by the International Ad Hoc Expert Panel for QC in IHC (Chap. 10). Selection criteria for negative and positive controls are described at length with the attendant rationale and practical approach. This series of papers (Torlakovic et al. 2014, 2015; Cheung et al. 2017a, b; Torlakovic et al. 2017a, b) is strongly recommended for all IHC labs, whether their prime intent is to perform basic IHC stains, or the goal is to meet the more rigorous demands of performing IHC to the level of a biomarker assay. Equally many research investigators using IHC in a more limited and focused approach would almost certainly benefit from knowledge of these guidelines.

2. The control tissues must be integrated into all steps of the test (assay) protocol, including evaluation of the result (Identical Analytic and Post-analytic Phases).

   In meeting the requirement of identical Analytic Phase it is most important to ensure that all control materials undergo an identical AR process to the test tissue, a fact often overlooked if AR is considered as part of the pre-analytic process. The best way to ensure this condition is by the use on 'on-slide' controls (Fig. 9.3 and Chap. 10), which (almost) guarantees that control and test tissues are subjected to identical analytic conditions, inclusive of AR, reagents, and incubation times. Note that internal controls (Chaps. 10 and 11), by definition, are integrated into all phases of the test protocol.

3. The control should contain a known amount and dynamic range of the reference standard protein.

   The development of a universal external reference standard that contains a known amount and ideally dynamic range of the target analyte (protein), and also meets all of the

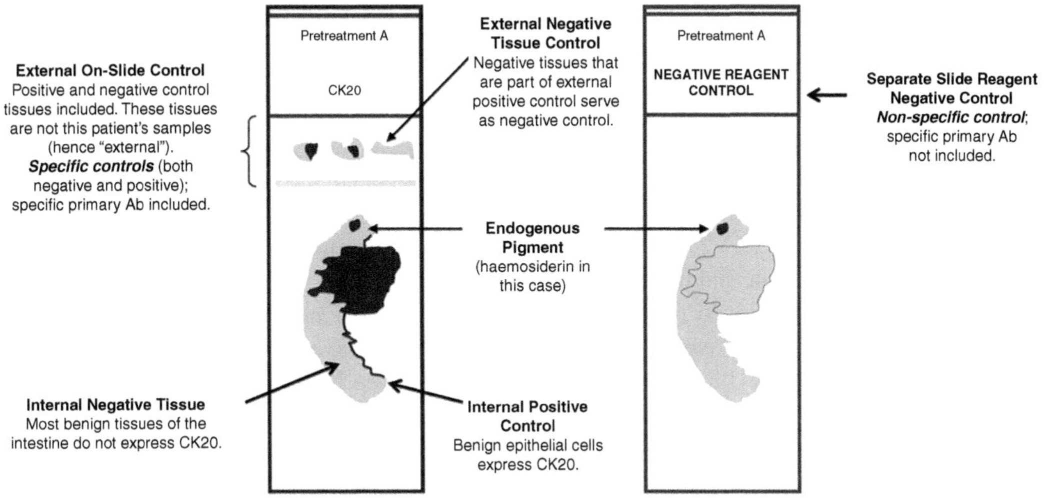

Fig. 9.3 On-slide controls. "On-slide" external tissue provide best assurance that analytic protocol is identical to test section. Pre-analytic phase should be as similar as possible. Internal controls will have identical pre-analytic and analytic phases (see Chap. 10 and Figs. 10.7 for further discussion). (From Torlakovic et al. 2014, by permission of Wolters Kluwer Health Inc.)

other desired characteristics expressed in Table 9.4 has proven to be difficult for manifold reasons, scientific, practical and economic. A universal reference control should share the characteristics of calibration standards employed in clinical pathology (Taylor and Levenson 2006; Taylor 2015), very well summarized in the recent review by Bogen (2019).

Currently the ultimate quality of IHC tests is limited by the types of available control materials. Positive control sections, even when selected rigorously using normal tissue samples, can at best provide comparable patterns of staining and similar levels of intensity, day to day, month to month, lab to lab. In no case is the actual amount of target analyte (protein) known in quantitative terms on a per cell basis, nor can it be known in absolute terms, because control sections are prepared from blocks, which are regularly exhausted and replaced within the laboratory, and are drawn from different tissues in different laboratories. In short positive controls are all different; selected to be as similar as possible, but in fact different. At present the only approach that provides defined measured levels of the analyte is the 'protein spot method, considered in Chap. 11 (review, Bogen 2019).

4. The control tissues should be universally available to all laboratories performing the assay.

As alluded to previously, current tissue controls, both positive and negative, are local in nature, in fact unique to the lab that develops them from in house archival tissues. Each control block yields only a finite number of sections and when exhausted must be replaced by a new block, often from a different specimen. Use of control blocks to generate cores for TMAs can extend the lifetime use of a block, but only serves to delay the time when the block (and TMA) must be replaced. In seeking to resolve this problem different investigators (and companies) have proposed several approaches, alluded to above, and described in more detail in Chap. 11: cell line preparations, xenograft tumors (Hasan et al. 2015) and faux-tissue blocks (or 3D 'histoids') (Kaur et al. 2011) and quantifiable internal reference standards, all of which are considered in detail in Chap. 11.

Positive control sections and TMAs are available for purchase and are marketed for use as controls. However, as already noted, these suffer from the major disadvantage that the pre-analytic conditions vary widely or are often entirely unknown, beyond the claim of being 'FFPE processed.' Finally purchased controls fall foul of desired characteristic #5 discussed below, in that they are often expensive for routine use.

5. It should be inexhaustible and inexpensive.

   Tissue controls developed from in house archival blocks are inexpensive in terms of materials (the archival blocks are freely available in house), but do require technical effort and time in procurement and preparation. And time is money! Also as described above in-house archival controls are not inexhaustible. Possible solutions will be discussed in the section below dealing in detail with controls, following a similar approach to that described for #3 and #4: namely cell lines, 'faux' tissues, and protein 'spots.'
6. The control material should be fit for purpose.

   In current diagnostic practice pathologists use IHC tests for different purposes.

(a) As noted, historically IHC was first used on FFPE as a kind of special stain, a practice that continues.

(b) In addition, today IHC is increasingly being adapted to a higher level of use, as a biomarker assay.

In this second category the selection and validation of controls is more rigorous to meet this different purpose.

It is a theme throughout this text that the Total IHC test must be developed, both in performance and interpretation, in a fit for purpose manner, because radically different weighting is given to the IHC findings, according to the intended use (or purpose). These differences are reflected in the classification of IHC tests developed by regulatory and QC organizations.

9.7 FDA Classification of IHC Tests: Classes I, II and III

In the United States, the FDA lists IHC tests under the category of diagnostic devices (Code of Federal Regulations. Title 21). The FDA subclassifies IHC test/devices on the basis of risk to the patient into three classes (classes I to III) (US FDA 2010, 2021; Nass et al. 2015; Yuan et al. 2016). Europe in the CE Mark (European Parliament 1998) and other countries follow principles that are both similar and different, all of which for the specified region should be referenced directly as needed, because these are apt to undergo regular revision.

1. Class I IHC test results include the traditional IHC 'special stains' and are interpreted by the pathologist much as any other stain, in the context of morphology and other relevant clinical information. Class I IHC tests (stains) generally are ordered by the pathologist as part of working up the case. They are used as an adjunct to traditional histopathology (H&E) and may contribute to primary and differential diagnosis, and assessment of grade and or invasion. The results are entered into the pathologist's report as part of the final diagnosis or as an addended final diagnosis (see Chap. 13, Table 13.1).
2. Class II IHC tests are intended for the detection/ measurement of well established biomarkers that provide prognostic or predictive information that cannot be derived directly by routine histopathologic methods. A Class II test may be ordered by the pathologist or the clinician and may be reported as independent diagnostic information, or within the final complete pathology report, or both. The biomarkers included under Class II IHC tests have a sufficient history of clinical used accompanied by valid scientific evidence (e.g. ER. PR).
3. The FDA defines Class IHC III (biomarker) tests as any IHC test not falling under classes I or II. Under this definition they are of higher

risk and have less extensive history of use with less supporting evidence. Typically they produce 'stand alone' results that are not confirmed by other histopathologic criteria that the pathologist uses in rendering a report. The FDA requires that Class III devices go through a Pre-Market Approval (PMA) approach, including the development of defined guidelines for test reagents, protocols, controls, and interpretation, usually developed in conjoint clinical trials as discussed in Part I.

The HercepTest (Dako, Agilent) with the corresponding drug Herceptin (Genentech, Roche) serves as the first historical example of this class.

The FDA classification relates to the IHC devices (and reagents), but it is the pathologist (and the clinician) who determine the actual effective use within the regulatory environment of each separate country. This practical consideration is reflected in a slightly different classification of IHC test usage promulgated by the Canadian CIQC (now the Canadian Biomarker Quality Assurance Program (https://www.cbqa.ca/) into Levels I and II only—the gist of which is it is up to the end user (usually pathologist) to determine how and for what purpose various IHC tests are used. For example, ALK-1 in lung cancer is a "predictive" IHC test and differs in purpose from ALK-1 for lymphoma, which is a diagnostic IHC test). As already discussed in Chap. 5, these two different usages must be reflected in the development of the ALK IHC test so as to be fit for two different purposes (in reality this means two different and separate tests, albeit that the basic reagents are identical).

References

Bogen SA. A root cause analysis into the high error rate in clinical immunohistochemistry. Appl Immunohistochem Mol Morph. 2019;27:329–38.

Canadian Biomarker Quality Assurance. Programme canadien d'assurance de la qualité des biomarqueurs. (n.d.). https://www.cbqa.ca/

Cartun R, Taylor CR. Techniques of immunohistochemistry: principles, pitfalls and standardization. In: Dabbs DJ, editor. Comprehensive diagnostic immunohistochemistry. 5th ed. Amsterdam: Elsevier; 2018.

Cheung CC, D'Arrigo C, Dietel M, et al. Evolution of quality assurance of clinical immunohistochemistry in the era of precision medicine—part 1: fit-for-purpose approach to classification of clinical immunohistochemistry tests. From the International Society for Immunohistochemistry and Molecular Morphology (ISIMM) and international quality network for pathology (IQN path). Appl Immunohistochem Mol Morph. 2017a;25:4–11.

Cheung CC, D'Arrigo C, Dietel M, et al. Evolution of quality assurance for clinical immunohistochemistry in the era of precision medicine—part 4: tissue tools for quality assurance in immunohistochemistry. From the international society for immunohistochemistry and molecular morphology (ISIMM) and international quality network for pathology (IQN path). Appl Immunohistochem Mol Morph. 2017b;25:227–30.

European Parliament. Directive 98/79/EC of the European Parliament and of the Council of 27 October 1998 on in vitro diagnostic medical devices. 1998. http://eurlex.europa.eu/LexUriServ/LexUriServ.do?uri=OJ:L:1998:331:0001:0037:EN:PDF.

Hasan T, Carter B, Denic N, Gai L, Power J, Volsey K, Kao KR. Evaluation of cell-line-derived xenograft tumours as controls for immunohistochemical testing for ER and PR. J Clin Pathol. 2015;68:746–51. https://doi.org/10.1136/jclinpath-2015-203066.

Hewitt SM, Robinowitz M, Bogen SA, Gown AM, Kalra KL, Otis CN, Spaulding B, Taylor CR. Quality assurance for design control and implementation of immunohistochemistry assays: approved guidelines, vol. 31. 2nd ed. Wayne, PA: Clinical Lab Standards Institute; 2011. p. 4.

Kaur P, Ward B, Saha B, Young L, Groshen S, Techy G, Lu Y, Atkinson R, Taylor CR, Ingram M, Imam A. Human breast cancer Histioid: an in vitro 3D co-culture model that mimics breast tumor tissue. J Histochem Cytochem. 2011;59:1087–100.

Nass SJ, Phillips J, Patlak. Policy issues in the development and adoption of biomarkers for molecularly targeted cancer therapies. National Cancer Policy Forum. Workshop Summary. The National Academies Press; 2015. NAP.edu/10766.

National Cancer Institute. NCI best practices for biospecimen resources. National Cancer Institute; 2016. https://biospecimens.cancer.gov/bestpractices/2016-NCIBestPractices.pdf

Nielsen S. External quality assessment for immunohistochemistry: experiences from NordiQC. Biotech Histochem. 2015;90:1–10. https://doi.org/10.3109/10520295.2015.1033462.

Phillips T, Simmons P, Inzunza HD, Cogswell J, Novotny J, Taylor CR, Zhang X. Development of an automated PD-L1 immunohistochemistry (IHC) assay for non small cell lung cancer. Appl Immunohistochem Mol Morph. 2015;23:541–9. https://doi.org/10.1097/PAI.0000000000000256.

Phillips T, Millett MM, Zhang X, Jansson M, Cleveland R, Simmons P, Cherryholmes G, Carnahan J, William J, Spaulding B, Satnick IR, Inzuna HD, Taylor CR, Cogswell J, Novotny J, Oroudjev E, Winther H. Development of a diagnostic programmed cell death 1-ligand 1 immunohistochemistry assay for Nivolumab therapy in melanoma. Appl Immunohistochem Mol Morph. 2018;26:6–12.

Taylor CR. Immunoperoxidase techniques: practical and theoretical aspects. Arch Pathol Lab Med. 1978;102:113–21.

Taylor CR. Quantitative in situ proteomics; a proposed pathway for quantification of immunohistochemistry at the light-microscopic level. Cell Tissue Res. 2015;360:109–20.

Taylor CR. Introduction to predictive biomarkers: definitions and characteristics. In: Badve S, Kumar G, editors. Predictive biomarkers in oncology: applications in precision medicine. Berlin: Springer Sciences; 2018.

Taylor CR, Burns J. The demonstration of plasma cells and other immunoglobulin- containing cells in formalin-fixed, paraffin-embedded tissues using peroxidase-labelled antibody. J Clin Pathol. 1974;27:14–20.

Taylor CR, Cote RJ, editors. Immunomicroscopy: a diagnostic tool for the surgical pathologist. 3rd ed. Saunders, Philadelphia: Elsevier; 2005. (1st edition, Taylor was 1986; 2nd edition, Taylor and Cote was 1994)

Taylor CR, Levenson RM. Quantification of immunohistochemistry—issues concerning methods, utility and semiquantitative assessment. Histopathology. 2006;49:411–24.

Torlakovic EE, Francis G, Garratt J, Gilks B, Hyjek E, Ibrahim M, Miller R, Nielsen S, Petcu E, Swanson P, Taylor CR, Vyberg M. Standardization of negative controls in diagnostic immunohistochemistry: recommendations from the international ad hoc committee. Appl Immunohistochem Mol Morph. 2014;22:241–52.

Torlakovic EE, Francis G, Garratt J, Gilks B, Hyjek E, Ibrahim M, Miller R, Nielsen S, Petcu E, Swanson P, Taylor CR, Vyberg M. Standardization of positive controls and introduction of immunohistochemistry critical assay performance controls (iCAPCs) in diagnostic immunohistochemistry: recommendations from the international ad hoc committee. Appl Immunohistochem Mol Morph. 2015;23:1–18.

Torlakovic EE, Cheung CC, D'Arrigo C, et al. Evolution of quality assurance of clinical immunohistochemistry in the era of precision medicine—part 2: immunohistochemistry test performance characteristics. From the international society for immunohistochemistry and molecular morphology (ISIMM) and international quality network for pathology (IQN path). Appl Immunohistochem Mol Morph. 2017a;25:79–85.

Torlakovic EE, Cheung CC, D'Arrigo C, et al. Evolution of quality assurance for clinical immunohistochemistry in the era of precision medicine—part 3: technical validation of immunohistochemistry (IHC) assays in clinical IHC laboratories. From the international society for immunohistochemistry and molecular morphology (ISIMM) and international quality network for pathology (IQN path). Appl Immunohistochem Mol Morph. 2017b;25:151–9.

U.S. Food and Drug Administration. Guidance for industry and FDA staff. In vitro diagnostic (IVD) device studies—frequently asked questions. 2010. http://www.fda.gov/downloads/MedicalDevices/.../ucm071230.pdf.

U.S. Food and Drug Administration. List of cleared or approved companion diagnostic devices (in vitro and imaging tools). 2021. Other nucleic acid based tests are listed separately under an included link. http://www.fda.gov/MedicalDevices/ProductsandMedicalProcedures/InVitroDiagnostics/ucm301431.htm. Accessed 2 Apr 2021.

Yuan J, Hegde PS, Clynes R, et al. Novel technologies and emerging biomarkers for personalized cancer immunotherapy. J Immunol Ther Cancer. 2016;4:3.

10 Analytical Phase: Current Controls; Fit for Purpose Selection and Validation

10.1 Guides for Selection of Control Materials

In the preceding discussion of required characteristics of controls, reference was made to the types of materials (including archival tissues) that are available today and may be adapted to fill the range of necessary IHC controls. Reference also was made to the AIMM Control Series of papers that represent the most complete published survey of how to establish optimal control systems. The current text is focused upon principles and limitations that may affect outcome of biomarker testing; for practical recommendations on how to establish optimal control systems the original AIMM control series should be consulted. These papers are listed in Table 10.1 for convenience; their content underlies much of the basis of this chapter.

A complete panel of negative and positive controls should be employed in initial set up and validation of every new IHC test or assay, but once validated the controls may be more streamlined in day-to-day practice. At the very minimum, negative and positive controls are essential for IHC when used as a stain, but controls are more extensive and more rigorous when IHC is re-purposed to serve as a quantitative biomarker assay (Torlakovic et al. 2015).

10.2 Negative Controls

The principal types of negative controls for IHC are summarized in Table 10.2, followed by discussion of the major issues relevant for biomarker assays. “Best Practice” recommendations may be found in the original papers in the AIMM Control Series (Table 10.1), in the CSLI Guidelines (Hewitt et al. 2011), in practical IHC texts (Taylor and Cote 2005; Cartun and Taylor 2018) and in recommendations from leading QC organisations (e.g. NordiQC, UKNEQAS, CBQA, CAP Accreditation Checklist, which covers all aspects of pathology laboratory practice including IHC and molecular studies).

10.2.1 Negative Reagent Controls (See Table 10.2)

The negative reagent control omits the primary antibody. Replacement with buffer may suffice in some circumstances, but the use of an identical concentration of non-immune Ig of same species and immunoglobulin isotype is preferred, in order to detect any non-specific non-immune binding of Ig of that species to the test section.

The desired result is absence of staining.

The presumption then is that any observed staining reaction in the test section is due directly

B. Jasani et al., *Precision Cancer Medicine*, https://doi.org/10.1007/978-3-030-84087-7_10

Table 10.1 The AIMM control series of papers—applied immunohistochemistry and molecular morphology

Standardization of negative controls in diagnostic immunohistochemistry: Recommendations from the international ad hoc committee.	Torlakovic et al. (2014)	Appl Immunohistochem Mol Morph 22:241–252.
Standardization of positive controls and introduction of immunohistochemistry critical assay performance controls (iCAPCs) in diagnostic immunohistochemistry: Recommendations from the international ad hoc committee.	Torlakovic et al. (2015)	Appl Immunohistochem Mol Morph 23:1–18.
Evolution of quality Assurance of Clinical Immunohistochemistry in the era of precision medicine—Part 1: Fit-for-purpose approach to classification of clinical immunohistochemistry tests.	Cheung et al. (2017a)	Appl Immunohistochem Mol Morph 25: 4–11.
Evolution of quality Assurance of Clinical Immunohistochemistry in the era of precision medicine—Part 2: Immunohistochemistry test performance characteristics.	Torlakovic et al. (2017a)	Appl Immunohistochem Mol Morph 25:79–85.
Evolution of quality Assurance of Clinical Immunohistochemistry in the era of precision medicine—Part 3: Technical validation of immunohistochemistry (IHC) assays in clinical IHC Laboratories.	Torlakovic et al. (2017b)	Appl Immunohistochem Mol Morph 25:151–159.
Evolution of quality Assurance for Clinical Immunohistochemistry in the era of precision medicine—Part 4: Tissue tools for quality assurance immunohistochemistry.	Cheung et al. (2017b)	Appl Immunohistochem Mol Morph 25:227–230.

Table lists a series of 'Control publications' emanating from the Ad Hoc Committee: International Society for Immunohistochemistry and Molecular Morphology (ISIMM) and International Quality Network for Pathology (IQN Path). (Cheung et al. 2017a, b; Torlakovic et al. 2014, 2015, 2017a, b)

Table 10.2 Summary of principal negative controls for IHC staining and IHC biomarker assays

Control material	Control process	Interpretation	Fit for purpose
Negative reagent control.	Use test tissue: Replace primary Ab with same concentration of non-immune Ig of same species.	Desired result is complete absence of stain reaction	Purpose is to detect false positive staining in test tissue
Negative internal tissue control (cells in test tissue known not to contain the target Ag)	Control cells are in test tissue and have identical pre-analytic and analytic phase.	Desired result is absence of stain reaction in negative control cells	Purpose is to detect false positive staining (non-specific) within test tissue
Negative external tissue control: a. Archival tissue; b. Cell line prep, pseudo-tissue, or protein spot (all known not to contain target Ag)	Treat control with identical protocol as test section—Optimally using on-slide control.	Desired result is complete absence of stain reaction	Purpose is to detect false positive staining in control tissue, cell line or protein spot (non-specific). Option b. often used in biomarker assays

Summary based on data from Torlakovic et al. (2014)

to specific binding by the primary antibody, and not to non-specific binding of the detection steps or intrinsic false positivity, as by endogenous peroxidase or endogenous biotin (if a biotin labeled method is employed). This presumption is of itself not absolute proof of the specificity of the primary antibody for the desired target. For example, an antibody to PSAP (prostate specific acid phosphatase), mislabeled as anti-PSA (prostate specific antigen), would give a qualitative staining reaction similar to that expected for PSA; the stain reaction would be absent when the primary antibody is omitted, but the mislabeling (false specificity) would not be detected.

As noted above, verification and validation of the specificity of the primary antibody to meet the intended purpose must be included in the initial test set up, but complete validation extends beyond the capabilities of most service and research laboratories. Information from the manufacturer (package labeling) is valuable but should not be relied upon exclusively. The primary antibody should give tissue staining patterns in conformation with experience and with the literature for the target in question. Anomalous patterns may be (mis) interpreted as novel findings and require additional validation of the specificity of the primary antibody and validity of the Total Test before reaching such a conclusion. For 'new' and research antibodies, having no established prior literature, the onus of proof of specificity is extremely high. The controls listed in Table 10.2 together with a full range of positive controls are then essential, but still of themselves not sufficient. Independent methods for verification of primary antibody specificity (including of course any primary polyclonal antibody or antiserum) are then required as described elsewhere (Hewitt et al. 2011; NordiQC; CAP checklist 2020).

Biotin (avidin) detection systems are not recommended for biomarker assays and in practice have largely been replaced by polymer-based labeling reagents. Most authorities accept that if not using a biotin labeling method then, after initial validation studies, the negative reagent control is no longer routinely necessary, providing a considerable savings in effort, tissue and cost. If a biotin avidin detection system is employed, it must also be noted that AR methods may increase false staining due to endogenous biotin.

When a panel of stains are performed on parallel sections of the same tissue using the same detection process, the different primary antibodies employed may to a degree serve as negative reagent controls, each for the others.

10.2.2 Negative Tissue Controls: External and Internal

Some clarification of nomenclature may be necessary. The term 'internal (or intrinsic) control' refers to a cell or tissue element that is to be found within the actual tissue section being tested. It is not to be confused with an 'in house control', generated from archival blocks within the performing laboratory. Such a section is in fact an 'external control' in that the control elements are NOT part of the tissue section being tested. That such external controls are generated from tissues available 'in house' (i.e. internally within the lab) as opposed to being purchased has led to confusion. As described later controls prepared in house usually are preferable to purchased controls.

Negative external tissue controls are tissues (sections thereof) that are selected for known absence of the test antigen or biomarker. Tissues that are selected for use as negative controls should have undergone a pre-analytic phase identical to the test tissue section (as far as possible). Negative (and positive) tissue controls should preferably be 'on slide' (Fig. 9.3) to maximize exposure to an identical analytic phase, including AR and all reagents and incubation times.

Negative control sections mounted on separate slides, serve as batch controls for a number of test sections treated with the same primary antibody. They are more economical in use of tissue, but cannot ensure that analytic steps are identical across the entire batch of slides in manual methods, due to delays in reagent application from slide to slide or inadvertent missed steps. This concern exists also for automated methods, which provide higher fidelity, but still cannot guarantee that each section in a run is treated identically; as already mentioned with highly sensitive detection of modern methods, even a few seconds difference in incubation time may affect the observed intensity.

Negative control tissues are designed to detect non-specific reaction due to the primary antibody, the detection system or any other factor, including for example brown material within cells due to melanin, that might otherwise be confused with specific positive staining (e.g. for S100 or PD L-1 when applied to a melanoma: see Fig. 9.3).

The detection of a spurious (unexpected) staining reaction in negative controls, internal or external, requires detailed study as to cause, and may include testing of an additional range of control materials, and new verification and validation of all steps of the Total Test process.

Alternative control materials mentioned in Table 9.2 are discussed more fully in the context of positive controls and in Chap. 11.

Negative internal tissue controls signify the use of cells that are known not to contain the target antigen but are located within test tissue. They serve as the ideal negative control, having experienced identical pre-analytic and analytic conditions and being situated in close adjacency to the positively stained elements. The utility of internal negative control elements is limited only by the extent of existing data that assures absence of the antigen (biomarker) in question, or at least absence of expression at levels that are detectable by the established purposed assay.

10.3 Positive Controls: External and Internal

All IHC tests, whether employed as stains or as assays for biomarkers must include the appropriate positive controls.

The principal types of positive controls for IHC are summarized in Table 10.3, which is followed by discussion of the major issues relevant for biomarker assays. "Best Practice" recommendations may be found in the original papers in the AIMM Control Series (Table 10.1), in the CSLI Guidelines (Hewitt et al. 2011), in practical IHC texts (Taylor and Cote 2005; Cartun and Taylor 2018) and in recommendations from leading QC organisations (e.g. NordiQC, UKNEQAS, CBQA, CAP Accreditation Checklist, which covers all aspects of pathology laboratory practice including IHC and molecular studies).

10.3.1 Positive External Tissue Controls

Historically, when IHC is used for the purpose of a special stain, the positive control most commonly employed is a tissue section made from an archival block within the laboratory, on the presumption, as with negative controls, that the pre-analytic phase (including fixation) will be similar to that of the test tissue.

Table 10.3 Summary of Principal positive controls for IHC staining and IHC biomarker assays

Control material	Control process	Interpretation	Fit for purpose
Positive internal tissue control (cells within test known to contain the target Ag)	Control cells/tissues are in test tissue and have identical pre-analytic and analytic phase.	Desired result is presence of expected stain reaction in positive control cells. When present this is the optimal control.	Purpose is to demonstrate expected positive staining in test tissue. An internal positive control may not always be present.
Quantitative internal reference standard; a form of positive internal tissue control in which the amount of analyte of interest is known.	The control is within test tissue; has identical pre-analytic and analytic phase.	The intensity of stain reaction is correlated with amount of antigen present.	Purpose is to provide calibration point(s) for quantification
Positive external tissue control: a. Archival tissue b. iCAP: Characterized archival tissue c. Low/high expressor qualitative control d. Cell line prep, pseudo-tissue, or protein spot (all known to contain target Ag) e. Quantitative external control (subset of d. above in which amount of analyte is known).	Treat the control with identical protocol as test section—Optimally using on-slide control	Desired result is expected positive stain reaction. Does not control for the pre-analytic phase.	Purpose is to demonstrate expected intensity and pattern of positive staining in control tissue. Options b and d. often used in biomarker assays. Purpose of option c. is to match level of expression of control to that anticipated in test section. Cell lines and protein spots cannot match tissue stain patterns

All IHC tests, whether employed as stains or as assays must include appropriate positive controls
iCAP: immunohistochemistry critical assay performance controls
Table drawn from data in Torlakovic et al. (2015), which should be consulted for complete information

The positive control tissue block is selected also on the basis of a second presumption, namely that it contains the antigen in question, based upon independent evidence, or upon knowledge and experience of the tissue type (e.g. skin, contains high molecular weight keratin, and prostate contains PSA, and so forth). As discussed for negative controls, normal tissues are preferred over diseased tissues because expression of most proteins (antigens) in normal tissues may be expected to be similar from sample to sample. Successive selected control blocks may thus be expected to show similarity within a lab and across labs, giving some rudimentary basis for standardization of results. This practice, however, falls short of most of the requirements set forth in Table 9.4:

1. control blocks selected from in-house archives have similar, but not identical, pre-analytic phase.
2. control blocks selected from in house archives may be subjected to an identical analytic phase only if mounted on the test slide ('on-slide' as in Fig. 9.3).
3. control blocks selected from in house archives do not contain a known amount of the reference standard protein.
4. control blocks selected from in house archives are not universally available to all laboratories performing the assay; in fact, the opposite holds true, even using similar selection criteria no two control blocks within a single laboratory are the same; by extension, obviously no two labs are validated against the same control.
5. control blocks selected from in house archives are not inexhaustible; once exhausted, they must be replaced by another block selected by similar principles. Again, it is NOT the same control material. It is a new control block and unless properly validated against the exhausted control the entire assay may change.
6. control blocks selected from in house archives should be selected on a 'fit for purpose' principle, with respect to anticipated level of expression.

Attempts to extend these same types of controls into biomarker assays meet with additional difficulty because biomarker expression, almost by definition, varies from case to case, from tissue to tissue, is heterogenously expressed within a lesion, and may not be represented in normal tissue.

The 'Best Practice' guidelines in the AIMM control series (Cheung et al. 2017b; Table 10.1) attempt to remedy some of the above shortfalls, by introducing standard recommendations for the selection of control materials, which in the most complete form are represented by iCAP (immunohistochemistry Critical Assay Performance) controls (Table 10.2, Figs. 10.1, 10.2 and 10.3; Torlakovic et al. 2015).

The concept of iCAP controls embodies selection of controls for which the staining and distribution characteristics that are well known and

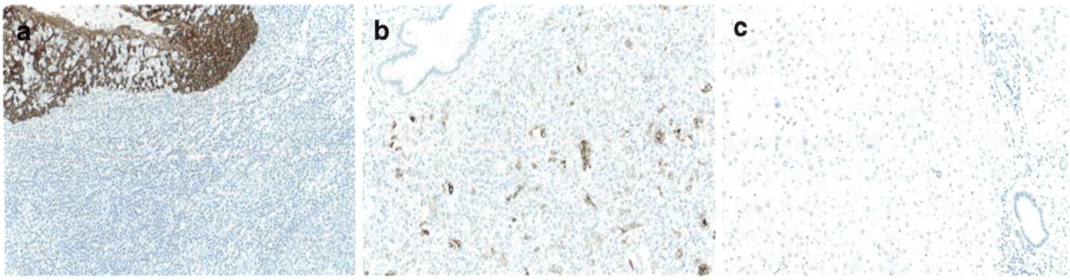

Fig. 10.1 Example: CK5 and/or CK14 (high-molecular weight cytokeratin). (**a**) Tonsil: high expressor—squamous epithelial cells show a moderate to strong cytoplasmic staining reaction. (**b**) Pancreas: low expressor (LLOD, low limit of detection); intercalated ducts must show a weak to moderate membranous staining reaction. (**c**) Liver cells: negative; no staining reaction seen. iCAPC immunohistochemistry critical assay performance controls for different expression levels (Modified from Torlakovic et al. 2015, by permission of Wolters Kluwer Health Inc.)

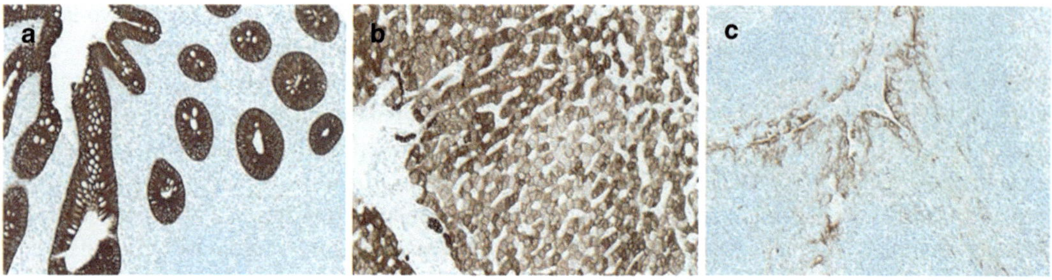

Fig. 10.2 Example: CK8 and/or CK18 (low-molecular weight cytokeratin). (**a**) Appendix: high expressor, columnar epithelial cells show a moderate to strong staining reaction. (**b**) Liver: low expressor (lower limit of detection- LLOD): majority of hepatocytes show weak to moderate cytoplasmic staining reaction. (**c**) Tonsil: scattered squamous epithelial cells show a moderate to strong cytoplasmic staining reaction: reticulum cells in germinal centers show a weak cytoplasmic reaction: low expressor (LLOD) (Modified from Torlakovic et al. 2015, by permission of Wolters Kluwer Health Inc.)

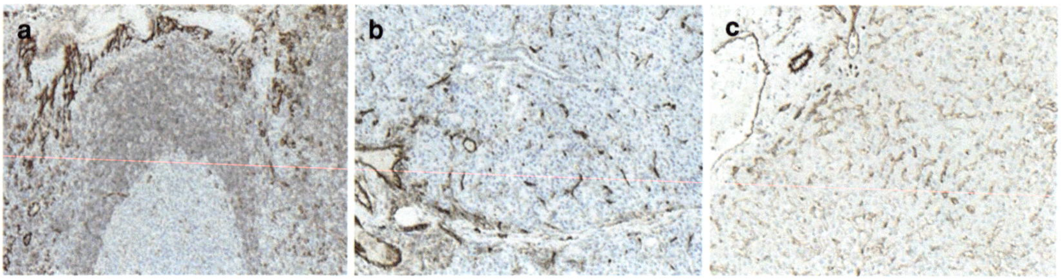

Fig. 10.3 Example: CD31. (**a**) Tonsil: mantle zone B cells show a weak to moderate membranous staining reaction (LLOD). (**b**) Pancreas: high expressor, endothelial cells show a moderate to strong membranous staining reaction. (**c**) Liver: sinusoid lining cells show a weak to moderate membranous staining reaction (LLOD) (Modified from Torlakovic et al. (2015), by permission of Wolters Kluwer Health Inc.)

documented, together with the expected expression levels of the target analyte (protein or biomarker). For biomarkers in the context of cancer treatment, the same concept is applicable, but is much more difficult to execute because of the variable expression and distribution of many biomarkers in health, as well as in disease.

The types of tissue controls that qualify for iCAP designation are highly characterized for the analyte (IHC target) in terms of staining pattern and intensity variations. Recommended iCAP controls also incorporate the idea of Low and High Expressor controls (Table 10.3; Torlakovic et al. 2015), which are chosen as appropriate for a specified IHC test. Examples of iCAP controls for IHC in general are to be found in the original AIMM Control Series (Table 10.1). The concept has been extended to the field of biomarker assays, where efforts are made to characterize control materials to the maximum extent possible, including quantification of the target analyte.

Low and high expressor controls embody the concept of 'fit for purpose' by selecting for each IHC test a control tissue known to show levels of expression of the target antigen (and thus intensity of staining) that is similar to the expression level expected (on the basis of experience and the literature) in the test tissue. The goal is to calibrate the detection sensitivity of the Total IHC test to fit the clinical purpose. Briefly the procedure is as follows: when first setting up an IHC (or IF) test, during which the optimal concentration and incubation time of the primary antibody (and the detection system) are determined by checker board titration of both primary antibody and labeling antibody (Taylor and Cote 2005).

In addition, controls are selected that show a level of expression (intensity of stain reaction) similar to that expected in the test tissue, as described above (Figs. 10.1, 10.2 and 10.3).

When an IHC test is set up using tissue that has a very high expression of the test analyte, then antibody concentrations may be reduced (that is use of high dilutions) or incubation times may be shortened to give optimal intensity of the stain reaction with minimal background; if this same test protocol is then used for clinical diagnostic testing, then cells or tissues that have lower, but still significant, expression are likely to give false negative results. The positive control paper from the International Ad Hoc Committee paper (Torlakovic et al. 2015) gives numerous examples of carefully chosen controls, to match anticipated low and high expression levels in the test specimens (Table 10.3 and Figs. 10.1, 10.2 and 10.3) and should be considered essential reading for all investigators wishing to improve IHC performance in specified applications (that is—'fit for purpose').

The concept applies even more so to biomarker expression, with controls selected to match qualitative expectations of expression (e.g. PD-L1 in normal tonsil [low level expression] versus placenta [high expression] control tissue, or more ideally by using control preparations with known expression levels such as carefully selected or bioengineered cell lines, the first example being in the approved Hercepest (see Fig. 11.1).

Details of the optimization process for tests developed within a laboratory (LDTs) are to be found in published papers (Torlakovic et al. 2015), IHC manuals (Hewitt et al. 2011) and by recourse to the major external QC organisations referenced previously. The use of carefully selected control tissues with low or high expressor as appropriate for the intended use, is recommended as described above. If using RTU tests, optimization will have been performed in provisional fashion by the vendor. If using approved or certified biomarker assays, optimization will have been performed in final form by the vendor and will be accompanied by clinical correlates. In all cases clinical use is subject to validation by the performing laboratory using in house tissues.

The concept of variable intensity of expression (resulting in varying intensity) has been carried into several of the approved biomarker tests by the use of cell lines, that have been selected, biologically engineered, consistently to express different levels, and thus serve as semi-quantitative calibrators of assay performance (see Fig. 11.1).

10.3.2 Positive Internal Tissue Controls

As noted in Table 10.3 the cell or tissue elements present within the test section, which may be expected (with high confidence) to express the marker in question, provide an extremely valuable control for both specificity and sensitivity of the assay. They have undergone identical preanalytic and analytic phase conditions. Also, they may be adjacent to the test cells (tumor cells) of interest, allowing direct comparison of quality of stain reaction and intensity, either manually or by digital imaging and analysis.

In the earliest IHC studies of routine FFPE tissue examining putative lymphoma and myeloma for intracellular kappa and lambda light chain, the presence of residual normal plasma cells served as a control both for sensitivity and specificity (Fig. 10.4) (Taylor and Burns 1974). There was also the additional advantages of kappa and lambda antibodies each serving as the equivalent

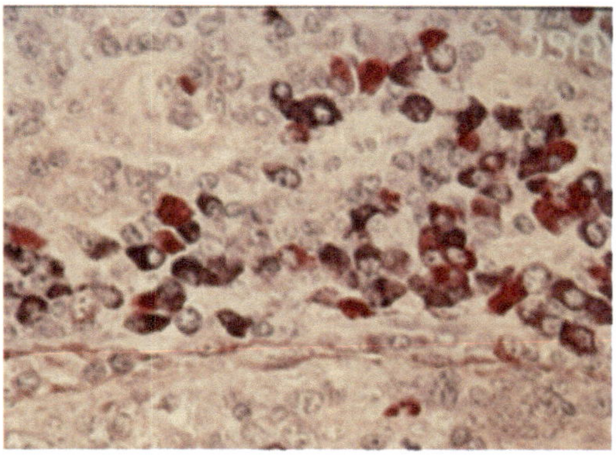

Fig. 10.4 Internal controls. Proteins (antigens/epitopes) that are ubiquitous within tissues have been utilized for 50 years as internal controls for many IHC stains, exemplified here by the staining of plasma cells for immunoglobulin The concept was described by Taylor and Burns (1974), in the first immunoperoxidase studies on routine FFPE tissue, but extending the concept to biomarkers is more difficult

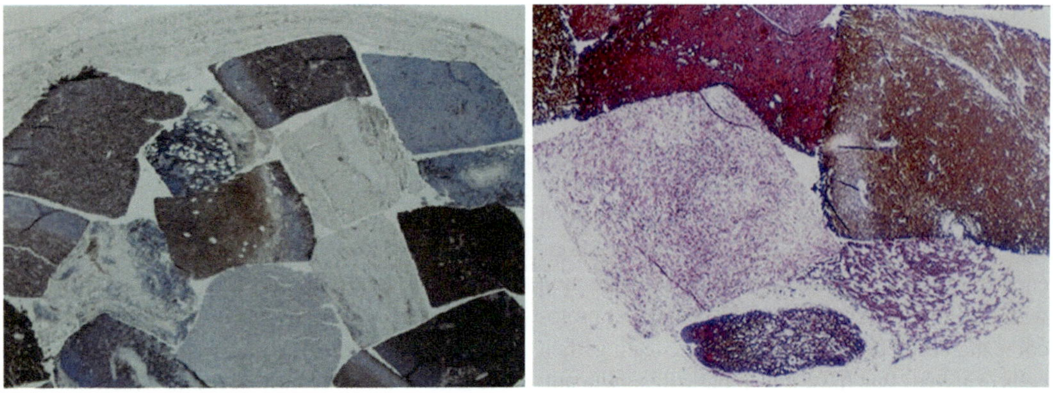

Fig. 10.5 Multi-tissue blocks in traditional sausage format. On the left, stained for CD20; on the right a duplex stain for CD20 (brown) and CD39 (red). TMAs composed of punched cores (see Figs. 7.4, 10.6, 10.7) have largely replaced this method (This figure was published in Immunomicroscopy, A Diagnostic Tool for the Surgical Pathologist. Eds. Taylor and Cote (2005); by permissions Elsevier)

of a negative reagent control, each one for the other.

Note that the use of plasma cells as an internal control for immunoglobulin (as in Fig. 10.5) also provides an example of possible false negative results that may occur if plasma cells, which contain high levels of intracellular Ig, are used to set up an IHC test for detection of surface Ig on B cells. Surface Ig is present at much lower concentrations and will not be detected (false negative), unless the test is recalibrated to a low Ig expressor (LLOD) control, exemplified by CD31 in Fig. 10.3 (this caveat holds true both for frozen sections and AR retrieved FFPE sections). This issue is discussed more fully in subsequent pages.

10.4 Tissue Micro-Arrays (TMAs): 'Sausages' and Tumor Tissue Banks

Tissue micro-arrays (TMAs) should not be confused with the use of the term 'microarrays' in molecular biology, usually with reference to gene expression microarrays or 'chips' upon which are arranged hundreds or thousands of nucleotide sequences.

Multi-tissue (sausage) blocks were introduced more than three decades ago (Battifora 1986). The original 'sausage blocks' were small tissue segments cut from fixed tissue or from FFPE blocks, bundled, held, together by small intestine (sausage skin), and re-embedded into a new paraffin block (Fig. 10.6).

This cumbersome method was replaced by the use of hollow needles to extract cores of tissue from FFPE blocks and then to 'array' these cores by re-embedding into a new receptor tissue block. The term 'tissue microarray' was introduced (Kononen et al. 1998) to describe the resulting blocks or slides that contain from as few as six to several hundred (see Figs. 7.4, 10.6, and 10.7) different tissue samples (core preparation reviewed by Skacel et al. 2002).

TMAs composed of 'cores' of normal and or tumor tissues, in duplicate or triplicate, are very useful in initial evaluation of a new primary antibody seeking a 'crash experience' of its staining characteristics on as many tissues as possible, in as short a time as possible (see verification and validation).

TMAs also are useful in research applications to test a large number of tissue samples against several different antibodies economically and efficiently, while effectively guaranteeing that each core is subject to the same analytic conditions. The utility of this approach in research of this approach was recognized two decades ago, very soon after introduction of the method, and is well illustrated by two examples. Richter et al. (2000) incorporated more than 2000 different bladder cancer specimens into just five TMAs, which were examined for cyclin E expression by FISH and by IHC. This study, which would have required over 4000 sections if performed one slide at a time, was

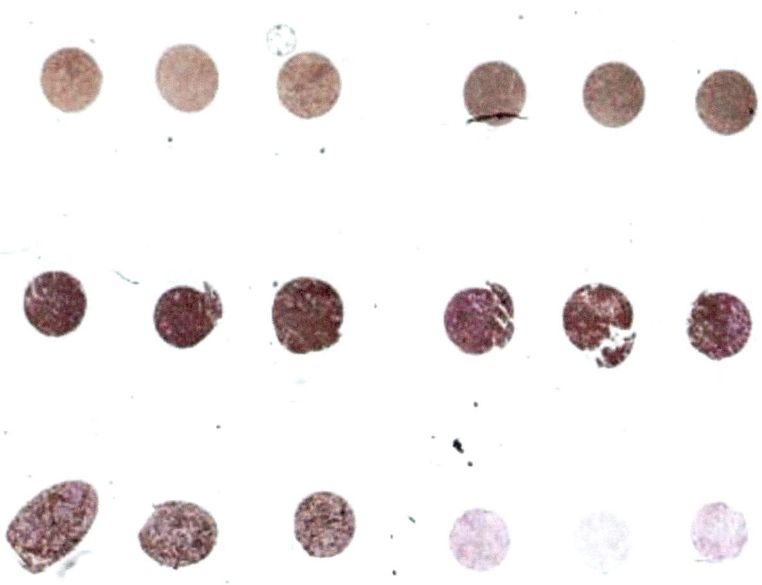

Fig. 10.6 Eighteen cores from a 210 spot TMA prepared 'in house' for research purposes, allowing study of multiple cases of disease (in this instance, Hodgkin lymphoma) by staining only a small number of slides as described in Wang and Taylor (2003)

completed in less than a week. Our own experience (Wang and Taylor 2003, Fig. 10.6) is equally dramatic. Cores from 62 cases of Hodgkin lymphoma, plus eight controls, were entered in triplicate samples into a 210 'spot' TMA using a 0.6 mm core needle. The resultant TMAs were evaluated for 15 parameters, including FISH and TUNEL, in duplicate. The whole study required less than 50 slides, as opposed to more than 6000 if cut and stained separately, for which cost alone would have been prohibitive.

Disadvantages of TMAs include the small sample size of the cores (usually between 1 mm and 3 mm) and the fact that, even when carefully prepared 'in-house', the cores from different cases do not have identical pre-analytic conditions. As already discussed, purchased TMAs may have still greater variability of fixation and other unknown pre-analytic conditions.

As described, large TMAs are very useful in initial verification and validation of a new (or replacement) primary antibody, but not necessarily as routine controls in 'day to day' laboratory practice. They, in fact, are somewhat wasteful of tissue if used to replace the orthodox single tissue positive controls listed in Tables 10.2 and 10.3. However, smaller TMAs composed of a score of representative disease cores, or as few as five or six carefully selected cores of normal tissue have been developed and promoted by NordiQC as a very effective positive tissue control that can serve for multiple primary antibody specificities (see Nielsen 2015; NordiQC. https://www.nordiqc.org/). These controls of up to two cores should for maximum effect be used as on-slide controls (Fig. 10.7).

Stores or banks of tumor (and normal) tissue specimens are, of course, a pre-requisite for construction of a TMA in house. By chance, as it were, every surgical pathology department has a tissue bank of sorts, in the form of archival FFPE blocks of specimens accessioned through the laboratory. Such blocks routinely are retained for 5 or 10 years, according to regulatory requirements, or for longer periods if there is interest in preservation of blocks for research purposes, plus available space for storage and financial resources to administer the process. These archival tissues are documented by the linked pathology reports and can be anonymized as appropriate, with patient consents obtained for certain specified purposes according to differing local and national regulations.

This archival 'bank' is by far the most common source of control materials, but as already

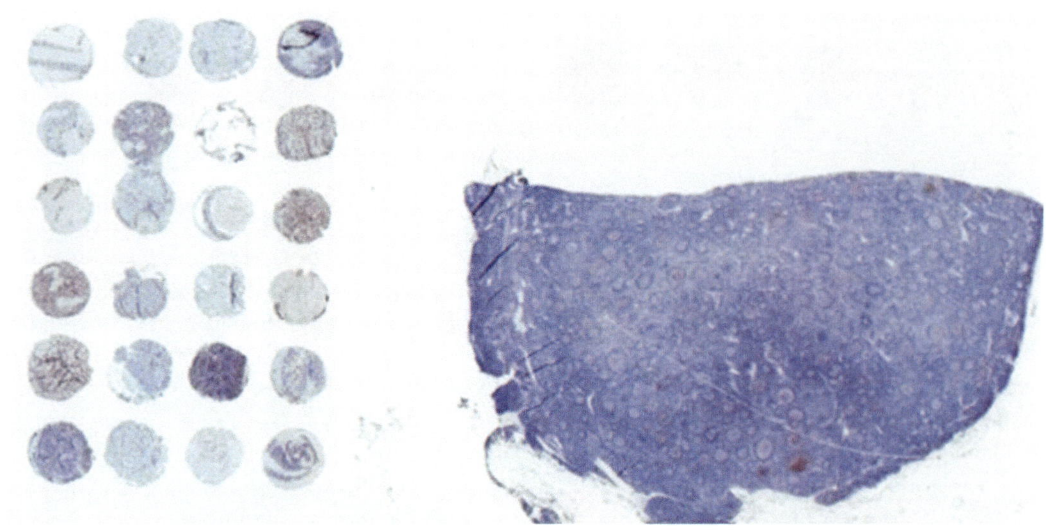

Fig. 10.7 Onslide TMA control for CD10, consisting of 24 cores of normal and pathologic tissue. The known patterns of staining in the cores serve as both specificity and sensitivity controls (Courtesy of DR. Regan Fulton, Array Science)

discussed it does not meet all of the desired characteristics of controls; pre-analytic conditions are not identical, but only similar (probably), albeit much better than procuring control materials from external sources; the bank is available only locally and is not inexhaustible; also the actual amount of target analyte in each archival block is unknown. Lastly archival tissue blocks are only fit for purpose if the purpose is limited to the testing of FFPE tissues, including extracts. For all other applications that do not utilize FFPE tissues the archival bank of FFPE blocks is of no value.

This last limitation was recognized many years ago, and led some institutions, particularly Cancer Centers, to initiate new and separate tissue banks, seeking to procure excess tissues at the time of surgery, and bank them by a variety of methods, including liquid nitrogen storage, for study of frozen tissues or extracts. Detailed collection protocols were devised with intended use in mind, with a growing consensus as to collection and storage procedures. Liquid nitrogen (snap frozen) stored tissues are fit for certain research purposes, but the material from these banks should not then be used as control material for FFPE based testing, even if subsequently FFPE processed, because of additional unknown changes in protein (antigen) preservation and diffusion during the freezing, thawing process. Frozen tissue reprocessed into FFPE blocks and H&E sections also have been used in research publications for digital morphometric and machine learning studies, which is not a recommended practice because the freezing prior to processing to FFPE sections greatly distorts the morphology (Part IV).

There are several excellent reviews of tissue banking procedures (McDonald 2010; Bevilacqua et al. 2010; NCI 2007, 2011; Sheppard et al. 2020), among which the report of NCI-NIST workshop of 2010 provides one of the most detailed 'Best Practice' assessments for establishing and managing tissue banks (Biospecimen repositories) including pre-analytic, biosafety and intended use recommendations (NCI 2011; Taylor 2011). For use in FFPE applications the pre-analytic recommendations are updated in Chaps. 5, 6, and 7. It is important to note in terms of semantics that the recommendations discussed here are distinct from those of AATB (The American Association of Tissue Banks), which relates primarily to tissues for transplantation and has mandatory, legally framed standards.

Unfortunately, many research projects that use FFPE tissues, together with pharmaceutical companies engaged in test development (of FFPE biomarker tests), and companies who serve as vendors of TMAs utilize tissues have in the past collected materials by undefined (and uncontrolled) approaches, as the basis for test R&D (research and development) and TMA construction. Results obtained using these materials should be interpreted with extreme caution, including especially those TMAs where documentation and the provenance of each core is not available. Simply to state that the tissues are 'formalin fixed' does not suffice, especially considering that many banks include previously frozen tissues, which are then formalin fixed, or tissues long held in formalin (e.g. autopsy tissues), or tissues obtained from foreign sources, in all of which the pre-analytic issues are unknown, and thus the state of preservation of biomarkers is unknown.

References

Battifora H. The multitumor (sausage) tissue block: novel method for immunohistochemical antibody testing. Lab Investig. 1986;55:244–8.

Bevilacqua G, Bosman FT, Dassesse T, Höfler H. The role of the pathologist in tissue banking: European consensus expert group report. Virchows Arch. 2010;456:449–54. https://doi.org/10.1007/s00428-010-0887-7.

Canadian Biomarker Quality Assurance—Programme canadien d'assurance de la qualité des biomarqueurs. https://www.cbqa.ca/

Cartun R, Taylor CR. Techniques of immunohistochemistry: principles, pitfalls and standardization. In: Dabbs DJ, editor. Comprehensive diagnostic immunohistochemistry. 5th ed. Amsterdam: Elsevier; 2018.

Cheung CC, D'Arrigo C, Dietel M, et al. Evolution of quality assurance of clinical immunohistochemistry in the era of precision medicine—part 1: fit-for-purpose approach to classification of clinical immunohistochemistry tests. From the international society for immunohistochemistry and molecular morphology (ISIMM) and international quality network for pathology (IQN path). Appl Immunohistochem Mol Morph. 2017a;25:4–11.

Cheung CC, D'Arrigo C, Dietel M, et al. Evolution of quality assurance for clinical immunohistochemistry in the era of precision medicine—part 4: tissue tools for quality assurance in immunohistochemistry. From the international society for immunohistochemistry and molecular morphology (ISIMM) and international quality network for pathology (IQN path). Appl Immunohistochem Mol Morph. 2017b;25:227–30.

College of American Pathologists Accreditation Checklists. 2020. https://www.google.com/url?sa=t&rct=j&q=&esrc=s&source=web&cd=&ved=2ahUKEwizm5r1x4XvAhXRIDQIHQcLBDYQFjABegQIAhAD&url=https%3A%2F%2Fdocuments.cap.org%2Fdocuments%2Fcap-accreditation-checklists.pdf&usg=AOvVaw2x4EVwmVwK98oVt8QiUyZG

Hewitt SM, Robinowitz M, Bogen SA, Gown AM, Kalra KL, Otis CN, Spaulding B, Taylor CR. Quality assurance for design control and implementation of immunohistochemistry assays: approved guidelines, vol. 31. 2nd ed. Wayne, PA: Clinical Lab Standards Institute; 2011. p. 4.

Kononen J, Bubendorf L, Kallioniemi A, Barlund M, Schraml P, Leighton S, Torhorst J, Mihatsch MJ, Sauter G, Kallioniemi OP. Tissue microarrays for high-throughput molecular profiling of tumor specimens. Nat Med. 1998;4:844–7.

McDonald SA. Principles of research tissue banking and specimen evaluation from the pathologist's perspective. Biopreserv Biobank. 2010;8:197–201.

National Cancer Institute Best Practices for Biospecimens. Resources. 2007. http://biospecimens.cancer.gov/global/pdfs/NCI_Best_Practices_060507.pdf

National Cancer Institute Best Practices for Biospecimens. Report of the NCI-NIST biospecimen quality assessment & standards development workshop (Washington DC). 2011. https://biospecimens.cancer.gov/bestpractices/2011-NCIBestPractices.pdf. Accessed 20–22 Oct 2010.

Nielsen S. External quality assessment for immunohistochemistry: experiences from NordiQC. Biotech Histochem. 2015;90:1–10. https://doi.org/10.3109/10520295.2015.1033462.

NordiQC. https://www.nordiqc.org/

Richter J, Wagner U, Kononen J, et al. High-throughput tissue microarray analysis of cyclin E gene amplification and over expression in bladder cancer. Am J Pathol. 2000;157:787–94.

Sheppard E, Madej RM, Alfaro MP, et al. Collection, transport, preparation, and storage of specimens for molecular methods. 2nd ed. Wayne, PA: Clinical Lab Standards Institute; 2020. MM13

Skacel M, Skilton B, Pettay JD, Tubbs RR. Tissue microarrays: a powerful tool for high-throughput analysis of clinical specimens. Appl Immunohistochem Mol Morph. 2002;10:1–6.

Taylor CR. Focus on biospecimens: the issue is the tissue. Observations on the "NCI-NIST fitness for purpose quality assessment and standards workshop". October 2010. Appl Immunohistochem Mol Morph. 2011;19:95–8.

Taylor CR, Burns J. The demonstration of plasma cells and other immunoglobulin-containing cells in formalin-fixed, paraffin-embedded tissues using peroxidase-labelled antibody. J Clin Pathol. 1974;27:14–20.

Taylor CR, Cote RJ, editors. Immunomicroscopy: a diagnostic tool for the surgical pathologist. 3rd ed. Saunders, PA: Elsevier; 2005. (1st edition, Taylor was 1986; 2nd edition, Taylor and Cote was 1994)

Torlakovic EE, Francis G, Garratt J, Gilks B, Hyjek E, Ibrahim M, Miller R, Nielsen S, Petcu E, Swanson P, Taylor CR, Vyberg M. Standardization of negative controls in diagnostic immunohistochemistry: recommendations from the international ad hoc committee. Appl Immunohistochem Mol Morph. 2014;22:241–52.

Torlakovic EE, Francis G, Garratt J, Gilks B, Hyjek E, Ibrahim M, Miller R, Nielsen S, Petcu E, Swanson P, Taylor CR, Vyberg M. Standardization of positive controls and introduction of immunohistochemistry critical assay performance controls (iCAPCs) in diagnostic immunohistochemistry: recommendations from the international ad hoc committee. Appl Immunohistochem Mol Morph. 2015;23:1–18.

Torlakovic EE, Cheung CC, D'Arrigo C, et al. Evolution of quality assurance of clinical immunohistochemistry in the era of precision medicine—part 2: immunohistochemistry test performance characteristics. From the international society for immunohistochemistry and molecular morphology (ISIMM) and international quality network for pathology (IQN path). Appl Immunohistochem Mol Morph. 2017a;25:79–85.

Torlakovic EE, Cheung CC, D'Arrigo C, et al. Evolution of quality assurance for clinical immunohistochemistry in the era of precision medicine—part 3: technical validation of immunohistochemistry (IHC) assays in clinical IHC Laboratories. From the International Society for Immunohistochemistry and Molecular Morphology (ISIMM) and international quality network for pathology (IQN path). Appl Immunohistochem Mol Morph. 2017b;25:151–9.

UKNEQAS. Immunocytochemistry and in situ hybridization. https://ukneqasiccish.org/

Wang J, Taylor CR. Apoptosis and cell cycle-related genes and proteins in classical Hodgkin lymphoma: application of tissue microarray technique. Appl Immunohistochem Mol Morph. 2003;11:206–13.

11 Analytical Phase: Alternative and New Control Systems

11.1 Alternative and New Control Systems

The external controls discussed in Chap. 10 are derived from normal and/or pathologic archival tissues or more ideally from excess tissues specifically selected and processed for the purpose, with a pre-analytic process matching the test tissues as closely as possible. Reference to Table 9.4 shows that such tissues have limitations, with reference to cost, need for periodic replacement of exhausted blocks and availability (confined to the lab that produces them).

The burgeoning interest in companion diagnostic tests that purport to classify patients into 'responders' and 'non responders' for a specified 'targeted' therapy, has resulted in a demand for methods that 'quantify' the corresponding target molecules in tumors from these patients. (Bogen 2019; Cheung et al. 2017; Taylor 2006, 2014, 2015, 2019; Taylor and Levenson 2006).

This demand has created great pressure for the development of new control systems that not only address the issue of universal access to identical control materials, but also meets the needs of true quantification (by weight) through access to standard calibration controls.

With respect to companion diagnostics different methods are employed depending upon the nature of the target, whether protein, nucleic acid, or mutational event producing dysregulation of cell control pathways. In those instances where the candidate therapeutic agent targets abnormal expression of a protein, then labeled antibody methods, either immunofluorescence or immunohistochemistry (IHC), in theory represent the methods of choice (Gu and Taylor 2014). Each method has intrinsic advantages and drawbacks, and each is limited by the types and quality of control materials.

For all methods a true quantitative assay requires quantifiable controls and calibration standards, much as employed in Clinical Chemistry. Bogen (2019) provides an excellent discussion of the topic as a means of increasing accuracy of IHC.

Alternative approaches that have been developed to meet some of these deficiencies are discussed in the following pages, and alluded to in Part III as one of the areas in which only the pathologist can assure quality.

11.2 Cell Lines

Early attempts to develop commercially available cell line controls are exemplified by Quicgel™ (Riera et al. 1999), which is essentially an artificial tissue control block incorporating a cell line, which may processed in parallel to test tissue to yield an FFPE block.

The use of cell lines *per se* has also been employed for a FDA approved HER2 'staining test' kit (Dako, HercepTest ™), which served as

B. Jasani et al., *Precision Cancer Medicine*, https://doi.org/10.1007/978-3-030-84087-7_11

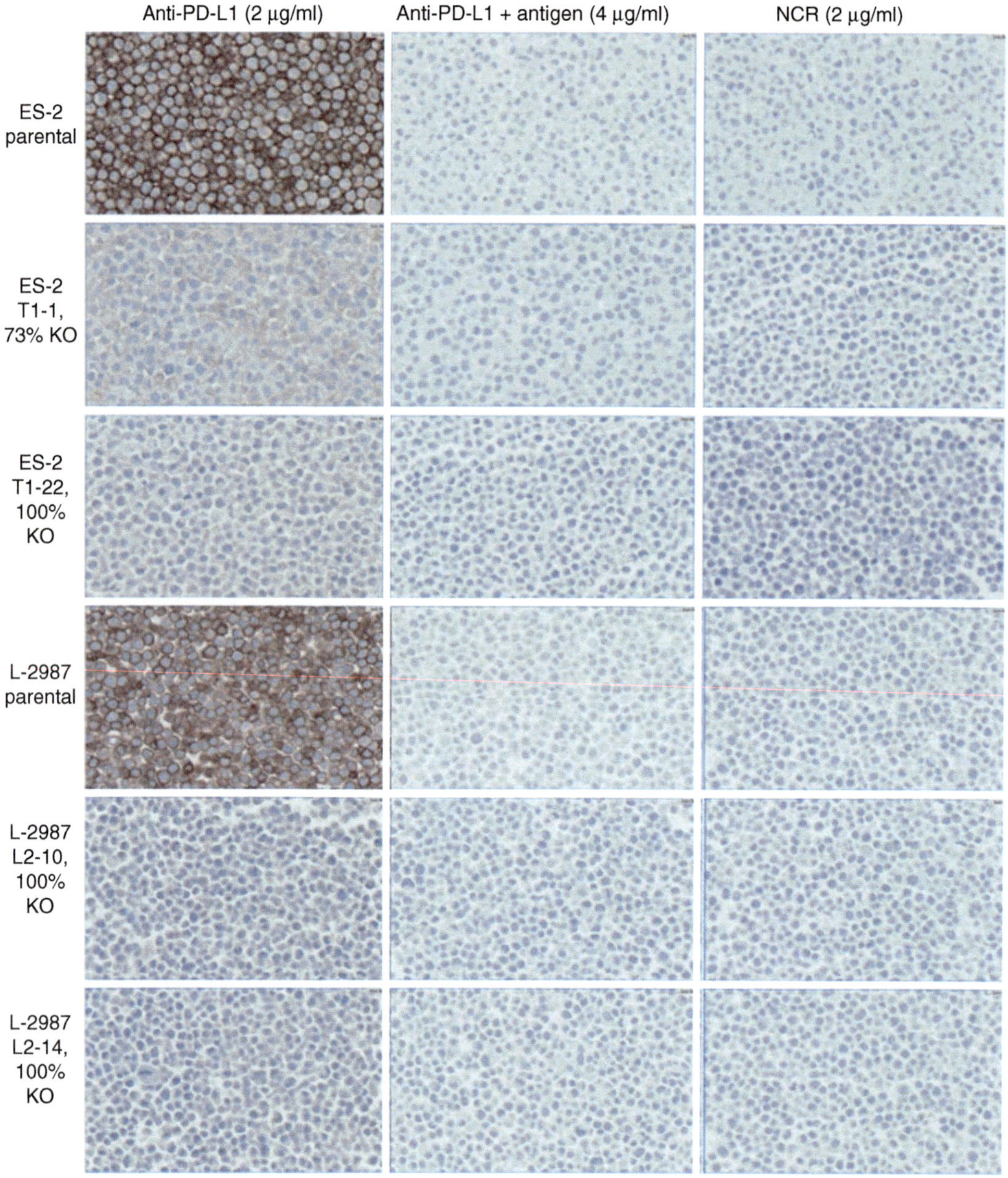

Fig. 11.1 Bioengineered cell lines for PD L1 provide more consistency of staining than normal tissue controls (discussed below) but the pattern of expression differs significantly. The left column shows staining with PD-L1 antibody; the center column, the antibody absorbed with excess antigen; the right hand column is the negative control reagent. Cell line ES-2 is depicted in the top three blocks, and L-2987 in the bottom three. KO signifies knockout cell lines, with absence of PD L1; all are FFPE processed pellets and are the equivalent of tissue positive and negative controls (Chap. 10) (From Philips et al. 2015, by permission of Wolters Kluwer Health Inc.)

the prototype for much of what was to follow. The HercepTest kit contains three cell line controls placed on the same slide: a negative, a 1+ (low or weak) and a 3+ (high or strong). Results are read by the eye of the pathologist and are semi-quantitative. It is vital to remember that these cell lines preparations control for the analytic phase of the test, but not the pre-analytic phase. In addition, interpretation has sometimes been difficult among laboratories and pathologists, in part because patterns of stain reaction in the cell line controls do not closely match those seen in FFPE sections.

The manufacturer stresses that the levels of expression of the HER2 cell lines, while known, cannot be used for direct indication of expression in FFPE tissue sections (*negative: MDA-231, 21,600 HER2 receptors per cell: 1+ weak MDA-175, 92,400 HER2 receptors per cell: and 3+ strong SK-BR-3, >1,400,000 HER2 receptors per cell). The Roche/Ventana's Pathway *Her2* test is another early example. Jensen et al. (2017) provide an example as to how a quantitative IHC method may be developed beginning with characterized cell lines; a topic that will be revisited later on this chapter.

Subsequently a number of other approved companion diagnostics have included characterized cell lines in ready to use (RTU) test kits, especially when graded interpretation (semi-quantitative) is required (see Fig. 11.1). Quality controlled cell line preparations with various degrees of documentation of expression levels are also available separately for a number of other biomarkers (e.g. Horizon; https://horizon-discovery.com/en/engineered-cell-lines: Amsbio; https://www.amsbio.com/ffpe-cancer-cell-line-controls/). All must be validated for the intended use.

As with tissue controls, cell line controls may be positive or negative. Positive cell line controls monitor technical (analytic) performance, which can include AR, blocking, reagents and protocol. In some instances, positive controls with different documented levels of expression are available, much as with 'low and high expressor' tissue controls described in Chap. 10, but in the case of cell lines the designation is based on documented manufacturing QC (as for the HercepTest™ described above). Negative cell line controls may totally lack the protein of interest and may be bioengineered as in the example of the HercepTest™ to yield no detectable staining if the assay is correctly performed; that is, some HER2 is in fact present, but it should not be visualized if the test is performed at the proper level of detection sensitivity.

Cell line controls can assess both technical sensitivity and specificity depending on the performance characteristics of the cell lines that are used. As with external tissue controls, cell line controls do not serve to control for pre-analytic variables; only internal controls do that. Also, interpretation is not exactly the same, especially for biomarkers expressed at the cell membrane, which will appear different in most cell line preparations as opposed to tissue sections. Faux tissues, discussed below, seek to restore the morphologic comparison.

11.3 Faux or Pseudo-Tissues

Faux tissues are a variant of cell line controls, in which an attempt is made to produce a form of 3D pseudo-tissue, which can be processed by FFPE and then sectioned to yield morphologic features and patterns of IHC staining that are similar to real tissues. Two different approaches have shown success.

One approach is to use tissue slice cultures (TSC) grown in a rotary culture mode so as to allow growth of several cell types (including epithelial and stromal cells) and encourage their arrangement into three dimensional 'tissue-like' forms. Maund et al. (2014) used 300 μm thick slices of cores from fresh prostatectomy specimens, both benign and malignant, and were able to maintain mixed cultures of stromal and epithelial cells for several days. This model appears more suited for functional studies of cell interactions than for production of standardized control materials. As described initially the method falls short in terms of establishing long term cultures in a reproducible manner.

A second approach is to take individual cell lines selected on the basis of known expression of analyte(s) of interest, and then co-culture with mesenchymal cells, such as fibroblasts or endothelial cells. In early studies cells were grown in rotational culture, initially to mimic low gravity conditions by as part of NASA's interest in cell growth characteristics in space (Ingram et al. 2010; Kaur et al. 2011) (see Fig. 11.2). Using this approach, three-dimensional "faux tissue" pellets were produced containing two or more cell lines (e.g., fibroblasts, breast cancer cells, and endothelial cells), which could be aggregated into pellets and processed by the usual FFPE protocols. These aggregates were termed 'histoids' and when sectioned were shown by IHC to express analytes of interest displayed in the context of morphologic features and patterns of expression that resembled human tissues.

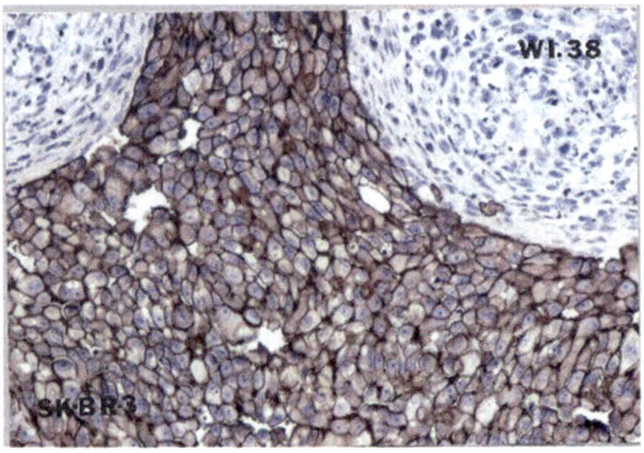

Fig. 11.2 Histoid' stained for HER2 and showing tissue like morphology: composed of SK-BR-three breast cancer line and WI.38 fibroblasts. (Ingram et al. 2010. NIH 'Retrieval of DNA, RNA and protein from archival tissue' PI. CR Taylor). (Figure from Taylor and Cote 2005) (This figure was published in Immunomicroscopy, A Diagnostic Tool for the Surgical Pathologist. Eds. Taylor and Cote (2005); by permissions Elsevier)

Histoids meet most of the requirements spelled out in Table 9.4 and show great potential to serve as reference standards for many commonly employed antibodies and staining protocols, including control of tissue fixation and processing steps. FFPE processed Histoids, like matrix models, theoretically are available in unlimited quantities and may be mounted directly the on the slide with the 'test tissue' serving as a control tissue (both positive and negative) (see Fig. 11.3). Pelleted Histoids, in theory, may also be added to the tissue cassette containing the clinical biopsy specimen, then to undergo all stages of processing and staining in a manner identical to the test tissue, although logistical challenges are in practice daunting. Cultured xenograft tumors represent still another approach with the potential to yield control materials that retain architectural features that are similar to the tissue specimen being tested.

As noted, faux tissue have the potential to meet most or the required characteristics set forth in Table 9.4, including universal availability, though affordability remains an issue. For 'faux' tissues as for cell line blocks the practical issues of scale up to a commercial level of production and distribution in a form that could incorporated in all stages of sample preparation (FFPE), are challenging.

Prototypic faux tissues in the form of FFPE sections (or blocks) are available commercially (StatLab: https://www.statlab.com/; Amsbio: https://www.amsbio.com/ffpe-cancer-cell-line-controls/) and may be used as more standardized forms of positive and negative controls, which are essentially the same from lab to lab; that is they are identical within limits of batch reproducibility and a manufacturing QC, whether evaluated light microscopic examination of IHC pattern and stain intensity, or better by digital

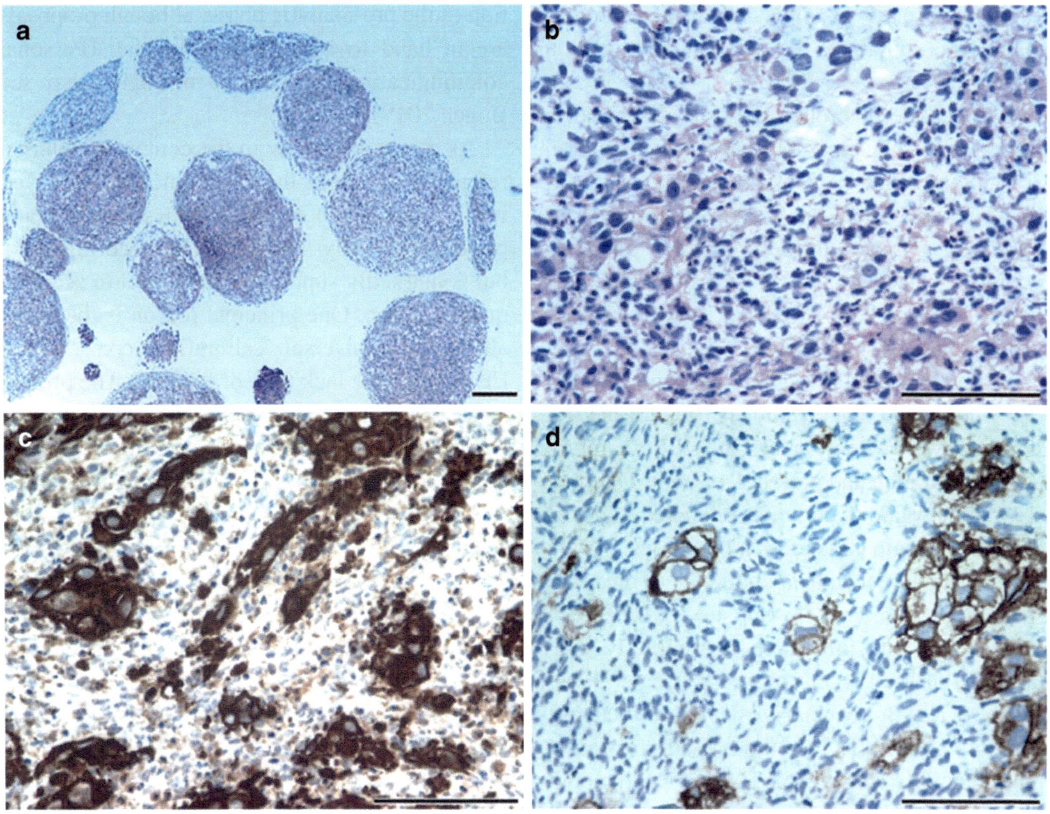

Fig. 11.3 Histoid of breast MCF7 and fibroblast stroma. Images (**a**) and (**b**) show H&E stains at low and high magnification, with good representation of morphology. An IHC stain for 'pan-keratin (**c**) highlights the 'invasive appearance of the breast cancer cells. The HER2 IHC stain (**d**) shows a staining pattern closely resembling breast cancer as depicted with the HercepTest (Fig. 4.2b). Bars 200 μm (Cell blocks prepared by Dr. A. Imam: adapted from Taylor 2015. Permission Springer Nature)

algorithm analysis (Part IV). Faux tissues currently may be distributed in the form of FFPE cut sections (or better, as blocks). As such they 'control' the Analytic Phase, but provide only limited assurance for pre-analytic failure (bad fixation) in the test section. To use faux tissues as calibration controls in order to measure the absolute amount of target analyte present per specified cell type is a challenge for the future, that will require strict control of culture and preparation conditions, quantification of analyte present and digital image analysis (rather than by the eye of the observer). These demands are not presently achievable for faux tissues.

11.4 Protein Spots

The problems of developing purified protein standards for routine use, are both similar and different to those discussed for faux tissues. The logistics of distributing any reference standard and incorporating the appropriate standard into FFPE blocks routinely (for each different stain) are daunting, but progress has been significant with respect to technical issues.

The idea is not new, but execution has proven difficult. The 'step wedge' tested by Millar and Williams (1982, reviewed Jasani et al. 1992) and matrix models (van der Ploeg and Duijndam

1986) were early examples of artificial control media incorporating the protein (antigen) in question.

The peptide or protein deposits described by Bogen and colleagues (Bogen and Sompuram 2004; Sompuram et al. 2006; Vani et al. 2008) (see Fig. 11.4) represent a more recent and very promising approach in the production of known reference standards. As an early example, this group of investigators (Vani et al. 2008) employed peptide slides as standards in an elegant study that compared the proficiency of different laboratories. They found that the almost 100% of the IHC 'failures' were due to errors in AR, or errors in antibody titration and protocol, or both. The study showed the value of common reference standards that can be compared across laboratories.

Although the technical challenge to preparing standard protein deposits that survived the FFPE process met with limited success initially, there has been marked recent progress (Bogen 2019). In his review Bogen analyzes some of the shortfalls of current IHC methods with respect to reproducibility and accuracy, in a revealing comparison with clinical laboratory practices.

One significant drawback of the protein spot method is that the nature of the peptide material control does not yet allow routine direct evaluation of the pre-analytic phase, although proposals are in hand to address that shortfall (Personal communication, Steve Bogen 2019—also see Bogen 2019).

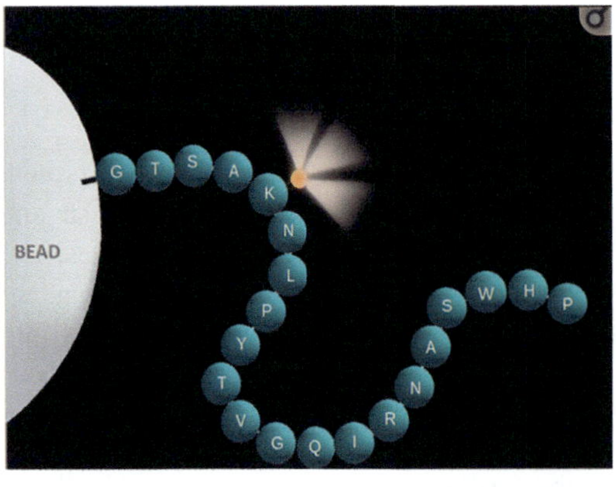

Fig. 11.4 Protein deposits or spots; here showing a peptide attached to a glass bead that can be deposited on the slide. The peptide is given a fluorescent label. The direct relationship between intensity of fluorescence and amount of peptide (and protein) allows for accurate quantification of the standard (for details see Bogen 2019, by permission of Wolters Kluwer Health Inc.)

As discussed below in the context of internal reference standards, the ELISA method employed in the clinical laboratory employs reagents and principles closely similar to IHC (see Fig. 3.3), but is markedly superior with respect to accurate quantification. One principal reason is the availability of universal calibration controls for ELISA and the lack thereof for IHC. The protein spots described above show promise in closing this performance gap, an essential step delivering an IHC quantitative assay, as described below.

11.5 Internal Controls and Internal Reference Standards

The idea of utilizing 'internal controls' for IHC is not at all novel (Figs. 10.5 and 11.5). IHC stains are performed on a tissue section that usually contains multiple cell types and tissue elements, which in turn contain numerous antigens (proteins, analytes) in addition to the antigen (protein, analyte) under investigation. The degree to which normal cells display, or fail to display, the expected pattern and intensity of reaction for many of these 'internal control' antigens is routinely employed by pathologists in assessing both sensitivity and specificity of each IHC stain.

However, effective evaluation of these internal controls does require that the pathologist has both experience and a complete knowledge of the expected staining patterns. This last factor is essential to delivery of a Precision Pathology diagnostic service, to the extent that the reliability and validity of IHC biomarker results that are not backed by such experience is questionable. The same is in fact true for all IHC testing, whatever the protein (antigen) stained. Unfortunately, many research publications lay heavy emphasis on choice of reagents (such as antibody clones) and little upon the credentials and experience of those reading the end results. Of course, the advent of fit for purpose AI driven algorithms will in future go some way to alleviating this concern (Chaps. 13 and 14; Part IV).

There is, in fact, an extensive historical experience of the use of internal controls, both positive and negative, in traditional qualitative IHC staining. As noted in the preceding pages, examination of differential plasma cell staining for kappa light chain versus lambda light chains was an intrinsic part of proof of principle in the first routine immunoperoxidase (IHC) stains of FFPE tissues (Fig. 10.5) (Taylor and Burns 1974).

Subsequently vimentin was employed by Hector Battifora with a slightly different intent, namely as an internal control to assess overall 'loss of antigenicity' in FFPE tissues (Battifora 1991). The rationale was that the intensity of staining of vimentin, which is present in almost all tissue samples and may be regarded as 'formalin sensitive,' would serve as an indicator of the extent of conservation, or loss, of proteins in general. In short, if the IHC method could not detect vimentin, it would be unlikely to detect anything else! The converse is less true.

These concepts extend into the realm of biomarker evaluation. In the process of interpretating ER/PR IHC stained sections, identification of positive nuclear staining in residual normal breast duct elements provides some assurance that the Total Test is valid (pre-analytic and analytic phases), and that the negative appearing cancer cells are biologically negative.

The manifold challenges to standardizing assessment of any biomarker, are well illustrated by Ki67, which is the subject of a superb series of papers in the February 2021 issue of AIMM, edited by Regan Fulton (Fulton 2021), and compulsory reading for anyone and everyone who even considers attempting to develop and standardize any biomarker.

Interpretation of Ki67 IHC staining requires detailed knowledge of the expected staining patterns of Ki67 in any normal cells present within the section. Even then tissue controls demonstrate only an expected range of staining. For example, proliferative rates vary in normal tonsil, which is the control most often used. In addition, UKNEQAS data reveal that different clones of KI67 antibodies produce differing results (Parry et al. 2021), a problem that is compounded by multiple protocols and staining platforms, and the absence of a uniform reference control to bring disparate tests into concordance. Cell line-based controls provide a potential solution (Roge et al. 2021a), especially if defined by image analysis methods. These challenges are, however, dwarfed by the greatest problem of all, namely the disparate methods of scoring, interpreting and reporting Ki67 results (Roge et al. 2021b; van den Berg et al. 2021), which are so far lacking in agreement and reproducibility from lab to lab as to seriously degrade the possible value of a Ki67 'score.'

The authors of this book believe that the only realistic approach to resolving this last issue is by whole slide AI guided image analysis methods as discussed in Part IV, but success of such an approach is of course predicated upon laboratories being able to perform well controlled reproducible Ki67 assays, which, as noted, is not a *fait accompli*.

With respect to other biomarkers the situation is much more complex, again in large part because of lack of predictable expression of the biomarker in any normal tissue elements that may be present within tumor section. For example, the PD- L1 test seeks to evaluate expression

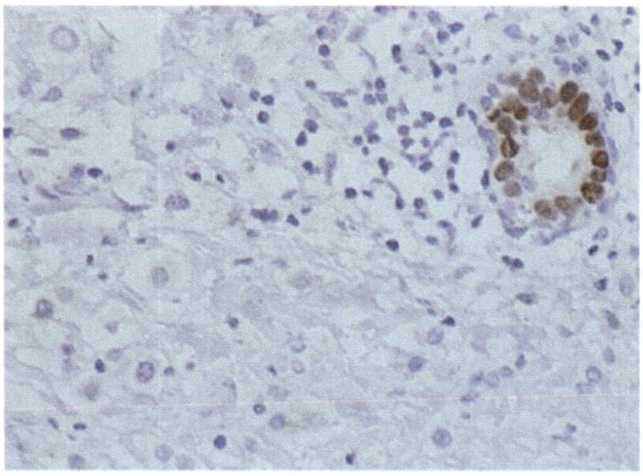

Fig. 11.5 IHC for ER (estrogen receptor). Breast cancer cell nuclei (lower left of field) show no evidence of brown staining, in contrast to a residual normal duct (upper right) that shows moderate to strong reactivity, providing evidence that the Pre-analytic and Analytic phases met anticipated performance, and that the breast cancer is negative for ER (within the test parameters). Personal collection of author CRT

by tumor cells and, in some instances, also by immune cells. Observation of positive staining in the tumor cells of interest provides only general assurance that the test 'has worked' and complete lack of staining in a section is not evidence of test failure; the cells may be biological non-expressors, meaning that the test result must be interpreted in the presence of proper control results. Also, detection of positive staining provides no assurance of the appropriate level of sensitivity or specificity, because levels of expression in tumor and immune cells vary so widely that results are by definition not predictable.

It is true that experience and knowledge of the expected patterns (and intensity) of PD- L1 expression of certain normal cell types has been exploited to serve as an external tissue positive (and negative) control, namely the observed intensity of reaction of squamous epithelium in the crypts with a weaker reaction in the germinal center histiocytes in sections of tonsil subjected to standard FFPE processing. However, utilization of these same cell types as internal tissue controls is precluded by the fact these cells are not always present in tumor sections being tested, and even when present show variations in PD- L1 expression that are not totally consistent from one control sample to another, varying widely also with different antibody clones and test systems (Fig. 11.6). With this wide degree of variation in intensity in control tissues, interpretation of expression in pathologic specimens is difficult, and comparison across different laboratories near impossible.

The study led by one of the authors (BJ) (Koppel et al. 2018), showing that expert pathologists can optimize different IHC methods to achieve some level of concordance, in spite of the

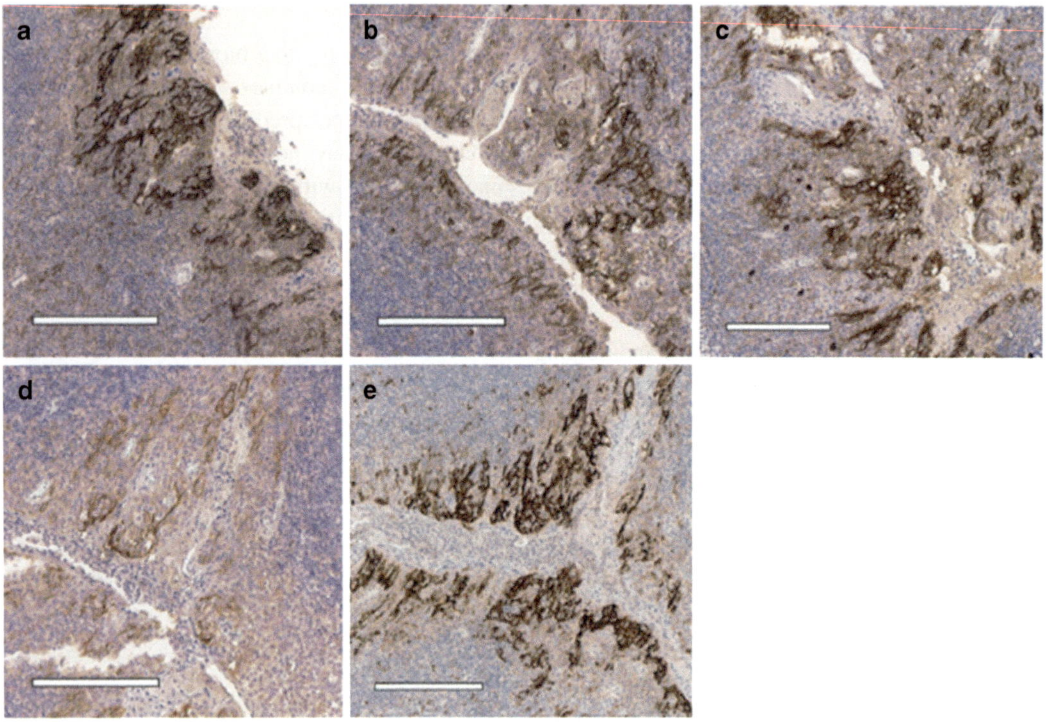

Fig. 11.6 Tonsil squamous epithelium showing variation in staining of tonsil squamous epithelium for PD-L1 with clone 28-8 and different detection systems: (**a**) Dako PD L1 (clone 28-8) Pharma Dx kit was taken as the standard. The Abcam 28-8 antibody was then employed on four different platform/detection systems—(**b**). With Dako autostainer link 48; (**c**) with Dako Omnis stainer; (**d**) with Leica Bond III; (**e**). with Ventana BenchMark Ultra (From Koppel et al. 2018; by permission of Springer Nature)

difficulties in establishing comparable controls, likely attests more to the ingenuity and perseverance of the pathologists than to the uniformity of the controls or the overall quality and reproducibility of these IHC methods for PD L1 (Fig. 11.6). Notably the optimization procedures used by Koppel and colleagues to achieve this degree of concordance among the methods were extensive and complex beyond the capabilities or economic resources of most service laboratories; the original paper should be consulted for details (Koppel et al. 2018).

11.6 Quantifiable Internal Reference Standards (QIRS)

As currently constituted the usual positive controls, cell lines, and faux tissues, are all in reality 'qualitative' controls (Chap. 10). When scored by the eye of the pathologist they at best provide a semi-quantitative result in terms of intensity of stain. Positive controls are selected to contain sufficient analyte to produce intense staining (the common situation, high expressors), or for producing low intensity staining (low expressors), for reasons expounded in the discussion of positive controls (Figs. 10.1, 10.2 and 10.3). In either case exactly how much of the analyte (antigen, protein) is present in the 'control' is entirely unknown. This approach fails in significant ways to meet the required characteristics set forth as Table 9.4, because there are no accurate data as to the measured amount of the test analyte present in the control, which is a critical requirement for the purposes of quantification.

Protein spots are at present the only control materials that are able to provide absolute data on amount of analyte present; however, as noted above, these are external controls and provide no assurance with respect to the pre-analytic phase, falling short of another important requirement, integration into all phases of the assay (Table 9.4).

There is, however, one control method that has the potential to meet all required characteristics (table), namely a system based upon use of internal controls (Taylor 2006; Taylor and Levenson 2006; Taylor and Becker 2011; Neumeister et al. 2014) (see Fig. 11.7). For an internal reference standard to be effective it should be demonstrated in the same FFPE section, alongside the antigen under study (test analyte). By definition an internal control then is subject to identical pre-analytic, analytic and post-analytic phases, and is available to all laboratories, inexhaustible and inexpensive, because it is to be found in the section being tested. Internal controls can also be utilized in a fit for purpose mode, designed for each target antigen (analyte). The one characteristic that currently is lacking is that data do not exist with respect to the absolute amount of the reference standard protein that is present in the selected internal control cell (tissue). Ideally such quantitative data should be available at key points in the Total Test process; from the moment of taking the tissue from the body, at the beginning of the pre-analytic phase, and at the point when interpretation begins (after the analytic phase) (see Fig. 7.1).

As already noted, IHC stains are performed upon tissue sections that are rich in antigens (proteins, analytes). The question then arises as to whether any one, or more, of these numerous 'background' proteins might be 'universally present' (or nearly so) in diverse cells or tissues, and if so, whether the amount present can be reliably measured, and its survival characterized before and after fixation and processing (post-FFPE). Put simply, is it possible to exploit the presence of widely distributed cellular proteins to develop a system or panel of 'quantifiable internal reference standards'?

In order to evaluate simultaneously both the test analyte and the control the new IHC 'assay' would need to be performed as a standardized tightly controlled 'double IHC stain reaction', including a 'stain' for the unknown 'test' analyte, and a second 'stain' for an internal reference analyte. For accurate quantification relative intensities would be determined by quantitative image analysis, for example by comparative quantitative spectral imaging (Taylor and Levenson 2006) (see Fig. 11.8), not the naked microscopic eye.

Recent advances in IF (immunofluorescence) methods, coupled with digital reading, may render the multiplex IF method more effective for

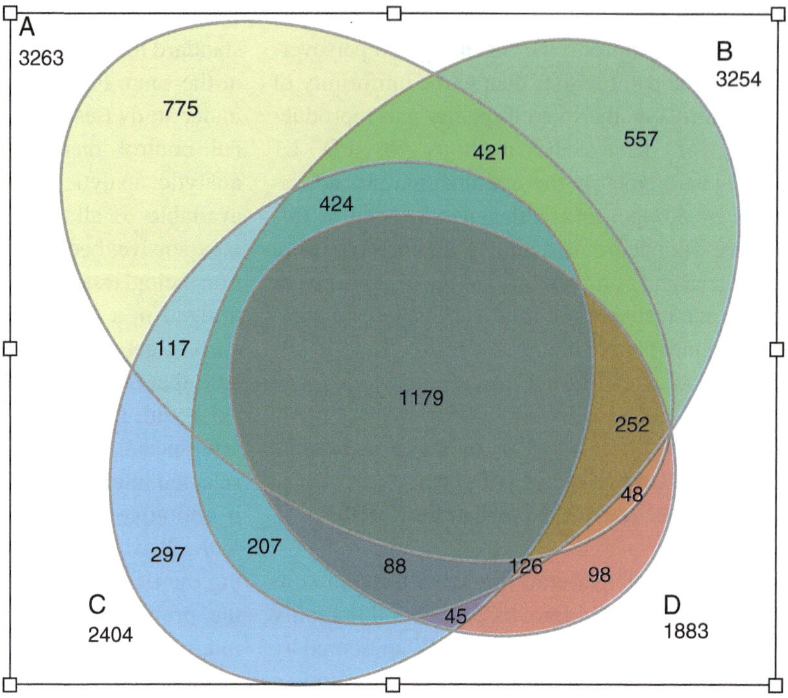

Fig. 11.7 Four extracts of the same renal carcinoma showing the large number of proteins identifiable in FFPE tissue by Mass Spectrometry. Samples A and B were extracted from FFPE tissue by a heat induced AR method using Tris-HCl buffer containing 2% SDS (pH 9 for A; pH 7 for B). Sample C was extracted from fresh tissue. Sample D was extracted from FFPE tissue by a protocol without heating treatment as originally described in Shi et al. (2006); figure from Taylor (2019), by permission of Springer Nature

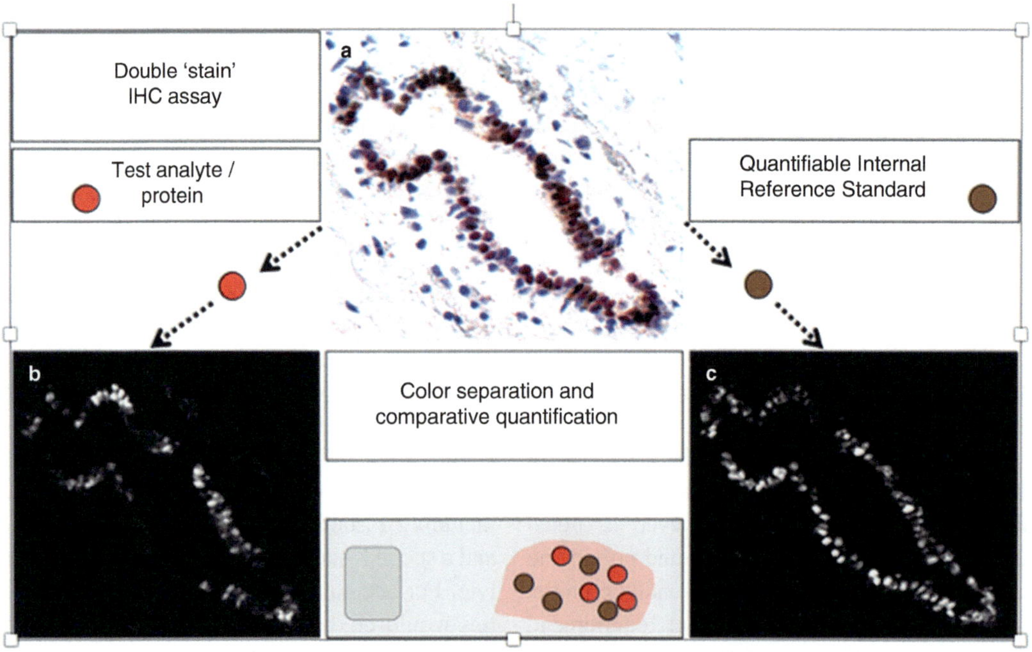

Fig. 11.8 By performing a rigorously controlled double IHC assay with a brown chromogen (diaminobenzidine) for the quantifiable internal reference standard (QIRS) and a red chromogen (Fast red) for the test analyte/protein, the intensity patterns of the two proteins can be separated and compared one against the other in a quantifiable manner as proposed by Levenson in 2006 (Taylor and Levenson 2006; figure from Taylor 2015, by permission Springer Nature)

this purpose, not least because the intensity of the IF signal (including in calibration controls) can more readily be made directly proportionate to the true amount of target analyte present in the test section (Chaps. 13 and 14, Part IV).

Just as with the usual qualitative internal controls, a detailed knowledge of expected patterns of staining is a prerequisite, and it would need to extend beyond expected relative levels of intensity to direct quantification of the proteins present in the internal controls (i.e. calibration). A system of quantitative internal reference standards (QIRS) would also be able to control for methodologic variations across the Total Test, including pre-analytic, analytic and post-analytic phases, such that intensities of IHC stain reaction (or fluorescence) detected at completion of the test would reflect the biologic condition of the cells, not methodologic variation. Proposed approaches envisage the setting up of a reference library of internal protein standards based upon a few ubiquitous proteins that are present in relatively consistent amounts in known cell types, a system analogous to the use of 'house-keeper' RNA or protein controls in molecular assays. Proposed approaches have been discussed elsewhere, to which the interested reader is referred (Taylor 2015, 2019). Multiplex IHC methods that incorporate digital display and image analysis lend themselves to this approach (Chaps. 13 and 14).

The direction that might be taken is illustrated by a collaboration initiated by Richard Cote from the laboratory of one of the author (CRT) at USC, with the goal of identifying quantifiable internal standards for FFPE tissues, both proteins and RNA (Pagliarulo et al. 2004; Capodieci et al. 2005). These investigators described a prototypic method, which they called RNA peT-FISH (paraffin embedded Tissue-FISH), for demonstrating RNA gene expression profiles in individual cells in FFPE sections. The method yielded predictive quantitative gene expression signatures in a variety of FFPE tissues. The approach employed ubiquitous house-keeping gene RNAs as internal reference standards, that in theory could be developed to provide the basis of a validated quantitative ISH method. In another example, standardized RT-PCR (StaRT PCR) method can be rendered quantitative by the use of internal actin RNA (widely distributed in different cells) as the reference control. This approach was successfully employed to quantify transcripts in bladder cancer cell lines and tumor tissues, and demonstrated its superior reproducibility and consistency in relation to real time PCR (Pagliarulo et al. 2004).

By analogy, is it possible to identify equivalent 'house-keeping' or structural proteins that are present in relatively constant amounts in specific cell types that enjoy a wide tissue distribution? More than a decade ago, it was shown there is a sufficient variety of proteins present in FFPE tissues to provide a basis for selection of a limited panel to serve as QIRS (Fig. 11.7; Shi et al. 2006). Given that such proteins could be identified in all (almost all) tissue sections, there is the potential to develop internal control system.

The initial goal for a quantitative biomarker assay should be to achieve results that are superior to current semi-quantitative IHC measurements, while at the same time controlling for vagaries in sample preparation, and the lack any objective (quantifiable) reference standard whatsoever. Once a 'quantifiable internal reference standard' is established in cell types adjacent to the tumor cell(s) containing the 'test' analyte within an FFPE section, then other confounding issues, such as variation in section thickness or the exact plane of transection of individual cells, can be addressed, in the manner of 'background noise', by computer assisted image analysis systems.

11.7 Quantitative In Situ Proteomics (QISP)

Here the advice of Sherlock Holmes comes to mind,

> —whenever one has excluded the impossible, whatever remains, however improbable, must be the truth. [Conan Doyle 1892].

In order to begin to appreciate this 'truth' we must first go "back to the future," and take a look into the past. Some 15 years ago one of the authors (Taylor 2006), in considering the "enormity of the task' of ever achieving anything approaching uniform pre-analytic conditions, or standard controls in even his own institution, wrote as follows:

"If sample preparation is unlikely to reach a meaningful level of standardization in the near future (i.e. is presently impossible), and if universal tissue reference standards, meeting the criteria expounded in Table 9.4, are remote in prospect (i.e. are almost impossible), what other alternatives are there? Perhaps only those that are "improbable," or radically different" (De Bono 1970).

"Edward De Bono may have reached a similar conclusion (to that of Holmes), again by logic, that when conventional methods have foundered, a radically different approach is necessary. Hence the hypothesis of *"quantifiable internal reference standards"* is offered."

Today, the future has arrived, and the truth is staring us in the face, namely that:

1. IHC methods, being rapid and inexpensive, increasingly will be applied as companion diagnostics.
2. In spite of the fact that the IHC method, as routinely performed, is inadequate to the task.
3. However, a quantitative IHC method is possible, given rigorous protocols, plus an improved system of controls that includes the pre-analytic and universal calibration controls.
4. The requirement for precise quantification will render obsolete current manual methods of semi-quantitative (+ to +++) scoring.
5. True quantification of biomarkers will require that the eye of the pathologist is supported by AI derived digital image analysis.

This book is a direct response to this truth and to the fact that changes in anatomic pathology already are so far advanced as to be unstoppable. The pharmaceutical companies will continue the race to develop targeted therapies as part of Precision Medicine. They and their partners who are evaluating IHC based companion diagnostics to meet the scrutiny of regulatory authorities in the US and elsewhere (Mire-Sluis et al. 2014a, b) are providing the foundations of Precision Pathology.

The current status and progress in the pre-analytic and analytic phases have been discussed in Chaps. 5, 6, 7, 8, 9, 10, and 11. The ongoing development of improved sensitive IHC assay methods, coupled with the use of universal quantitative reference standards and calibrated image whole slide analysis will ultimately produce IHC methods that are precise and accurate. The following Chaps. (12 and 13) relating to the post-analytic phase include discussion of the ability to combine precise morphologic resolution on a cellular and sub-cellular level, with accurate measurement of minute amounts of protein in defined microanatomic locations. Together these capabilities create the new field of Quantitative In Situ Proteomics (QISP), which will be applied to generate a range of quantitative biomarker assays directly on the tissue sections by the next generation of surgical pathologists.

"If in the fullness of time it transpires that pathologists come to regard IHC (and ISH) methods not simply as stains, but as cell-based quantitative assays, then we will have achieved more than transforming the concept of the stain, we will have accomplished the transmutation of the pathologists themselves." (Taylor 2006).

References

Battifora H. Assessment of antigen damage in immunohistochemistry. The vimentin internal control. Am J Clin Pathol. 1991;96:669–71.

Bogen SA. A root cause analysis into the high error rate in clinical immunohistochemistry. Appl Immunohistochem Mol Morph. 2019;27:329–38.

Bogen SA, Sompuram SR. Recent trends and advances in immunodiagnostics of solid tumors [review]. BioDrugs. 2004;18:387–98.

Capodieci P, Donovan M, Buchinsky H, et al. Gene expression profiling in single cells within tissue. Nat Methods. 2005;2:663–5.

Cheung CC, D'Arrigo C, Dietel M, et al. Evolution of quality assurance for clinical immunohistochemistry in the era of precision medicine—part 4: tissue tools for quality assurance in immunohistochemistry. From the international society for immunohistochemistry and molecular morphology (ISIMM) and international quality network for pathology (IQN path). Appl Immunohistochem Mol Morph. 2017;25:227–30.

Conan Doyle A. The adventures of Sherlock Holmes. Adventure XI. The adventure of the Beryl coronet. Strand Mag. 1892;3:511–25.

De Bono E. Lateral thinking. London: Pelican Books; 1970.

Fulton R. Getting a grip on Ki67. Appl Immunohistochem Mol Morph. 2021;29:83–5.

Gu J, Taylor CR. Practicing pathology in the era of big data and personalized medicine. Appl Immunohistochem Mol Morph. 2014;22:1–9.

Ingram M, Tachy GB, Ward BR, et al. Tissue engineered tumor models. Biotech Histochem. 2010;85:213–9.

Jasani B, Thomas ND, Navabi H, Millar DM, Newman GR, Gee J, Williams ED. Dinitrophenyl (DNP) hapten sandwich staining (DHSS) procedure: a 10-year review of its principal reagents and applications. J Immunol Methods. 1992;150(1–2):193–8.

Jensen K, Krusenstjerna-Hafstrøm R, Lohse J, Petersen KP, Derand H. A novel quantitative immunohistochemistry method for precise protein measurements directly in formalin-fixed, paraffin-embedded specimens: analytical performance measuring HER2. Mod Pathol. 2017;30:180–93. https://doi.org/10.1038/modpathol.2016.176.

Kaur P, Ward B, Saha B, Young L, Groshen S, Techy G, Lu Y, Atkinson R, Taylor CR, Ingram M, Imam A. Human breast cancer histioid: an in vitro 3D coculture model that mimics breast tumor tissue. J Histochem Cytochem. 2011;59:1087–100.

Koppel C, Schwellenbach H, Zielinski D, Eckstein S, Martin-Ortega M, D'Arrigo C, Schildhaus H-U, Ruschoff J, Jasani B. Optimization and validation of PD-L1 immunohistochemistry staining protocols using the antibody clone 28-8 on different staining platforms. Mod Pathol. 2018;31:1630–44.

Maund S, Nolley R, Peehl D. Optimization and comprehensive characterization of a faithful tissue culture model of the benign and malignant human prostate. Lab Investig. 2014;94:208–21. https://doi.org/10.1038/labinvest.2013.141.

Millar DA, Williams ED. A step-wedge standard for the quantification of immunoperoxidase techniques. Histochem J. 1982;14:609–20. https://doi.org/10.1007/BF01011893.

Mire-Sluis A, Ritter N, Cherney B, Schmalzing D, Blumel M. Reference standards for therapeutic proteins: current regulatory and scientific best practices and remaining needs. Part 1. BioProcess Int. 2014a;12(3):26–36. https://bioprocessintl.com/upstream-processing/assays/reference-standards-for-therapeutic-proteins-350518/

Mire-Sluis A, Ritter N, Cherney B, Schmalzing D, Blumel M. Reference standards for therapeutic proteins: current regulatory and scientific best practices and remaining needs. Part 2. BioProcess Int. 2014b;12(5):12–38. https://bioprocessintl.com/2014/reference-standards-for-therapeutic-proteins-351584/

Neumeister VM, Parisi F, England AM, et al. Models and techniques. A tissue quality index; an intrinsic control for measurement of effects of pre-analytic variables on FFPE tissue. Lab Investig. 2014;94:467–74.

Pagliarulo V, George B, Beil SJ, Groshen S, Laird PW, Cai J, Willey J, Cote RC, Datar RH. Sensitivity and reproducibility of standardized competitive RT-PCR for transcript quantification and its comparison with real time RT-PCR. Mol Cancer. 2004;3:5. https://doi.org/10.1186/1476-4598-3-5.

Parry S, Dowsett M, Dodson A. UKNEQAS ICC & ISH Ki67 data reveals differences in performance of primary antibody clones. Appl Immunohistochem Mol Morph. 2021;29:86–94.

Phillips T, Simmons P, Inzunza HD, Cogswell J, Novotny J, Taylor CR, Zhang X. Development of an automated PD-L1 immunohistochemistry (IHC) assay for non small cell lung cancer. Appl Immunohistochem Mol Morph. 2015;23:541–9. https://doi.org/10.1097/PAI.0000000000000256.

Riera J, Simpson JF, Tamayo R, Battifora H. Use of cultured cells as a control for quantitative immunocytochemical analysis of estrogen receptor in breast cancer. The Quicgel method. Am J Clin Pathol. 1999;111:329–35.

Roge R, Nielsen S, Riber-Hanssen R, Vyberg M. Image analysis assessed cell lines as potential performance controls of Ki67 immunostained slides. Appl Immunohistochem Mol Morph. 2021a;29:95–8.

Roge R, Nielsen S, Riber-Hanssen R, Vyberg M. Ki67 proliferation index in breast cancer as a function of assessment method: a NordiQC experience. Appl Immunohistochem Mol Morph. 2021b;29:99–104.

Shi S-R, Liu C, Balgley BM, Lee C, Taylor CR. Protein extraction from formalin-fixed, paraffin embedded tissue sections: quality evaluation by mass spectrometry. J Histochem Cytochem. 2006;54:739–43.

Sompuram SR, Vani K, Hafer LJ, Bogen SA. Antibodies immunoreactive with formalin-fixed tissue antigens recognize linear protein epitopes. Am J Clin Pathol. 2006;125:82–90.

Taylor CR. Quantifiable internal reference standards for immunohistochemistry: the measurement of quantity by weight. Appl Immunohistochem Mol Morph. 2006;14:253–9.

Taylor CR, Cote RJ, editors. Immunomicroscopy: a diagnostic tool for the surgical pathologist. 3rd ed. Philadelphia: Elsevier Saunders; 2005. (1st edition, Taylor was 1986; 2nd edition, Taylor and Cote was 1994).

Taylor CR. Predictive biomarkers and companion diagnostics. The future of immunohistochemistry—'in situ proteomics', or just a 'stain'? Appl Immunohistochem Mol Morph. 2014;22:555–61.

Taylor CR. Quantitative in situ proteomics; a proposed pathway for quantification of immunohistochemistry at the light-microscopic level. Cell Tissue Res. 2015;360:109–20.

Taylor CR. Introduction to predictive biomarkers: definitions and characteristics. In: Badve S, Kumar G, editors. Predictive biomarkers in oncology: applications in precision medicine. Berlin: Springer Sciences; 2019.

Taylor CR, Becker KF. Liquid morphology: immunochemical analysis of proteins extracted from formalin fixed paraffin embedded tissues: combining proteomics with immunohistochemistry. Appl Immunohistochem Mol Morph. 2011;19:1–9.

Taylor CR, Burns J. The demonstration of plasma cells and other immunoglobulin- containing cells in formalin-fixed, paraffin-embedded tissues using peroxidase-labelled antibody. J Clin Pathol. 1974;27:14–20.

Taylor CR, Levenson RM. Quantification of immunohistochemistry—issues concerning methods, utility and semiquantitative assessment. Histopathology. 2006;49:411–24.

Van den Berg EJ, Duarte R, Dickens C, et al. Ki67 immunohistochemistry quantification i breast carcinoma: a comparison of visual estimation, counting and immunoratio. Appl Immunohistochem Mol Morph. 2021;29:105–11.

Van der Ploeg M, Duijndam WAL. Matrix models: essential tools for microscopic cytochemical research. Histochemistry. 1986;84:283–300.

Vani K, Sompuram SR, Fitzgibbons P, Bogen SA. National HER2 proficiency test results using standardized quantitative controls: characterization of laboratory failures. Arch Pathol Lab Med. 2008;132:211–6.

12 Post-Analytic Phase: Interpretation, Scoring and Reporting of Biopsy Results

12.1 Assessment of Controls

> An expert is a person who tells you a simple thing in a confused way, in such a fashion as to make you think the confusion is your own fault.
> W. B. Castle, 1955 (Source: Strauss MB, Familiar Medical Quotations. Little Brown, Boston, 1968)

Interpretation is more easily said than done. The task itself is complex and decisions may be difficult (Part III). Furthermore, the intent of the expert pathologist, set forth in writing, is not always decipherable by clinicians and patients. Also, there is dawning recognition that the opinions of different experts are not necessarily in harmony, whether in regard to the interpretation of the basic H&E stained material, or the interpretation and significance of IHC biomarker results.

Initial evaluation of the results of negative and positive and controls is normally performed by technologists/biomedical scientists within the IHC laboratory before the slides (or digital scans) are released to the pathologists. If the performance of the controls does not meet specifications, the test should be repeated after investigation, and correction, of possible cause.

Further evaluation of the controls by the pathologist is a critical part of clinical interpretation of the IHC results. Many QC and QA agencies require documentation of review and approval of such controls on a daily basis. Clearly the level of experience of both technologist and pathologist is critical to proper interpretation.

12.2 Sensitivity and Specificity

12.2.1 Positive and Negative Results in Relation to Controls

There is some uniqueness in the traditional manner of use of the terms 'sensitivity' and 'specificity' with respect to anatomic pathology and the IHC method (see Table 10.1; and Torlakovic et al. 2015).

12.2.2 Sensitivity

In the context of IHC the term sensitivity usually refers to 'technical sensitivity' meaning the extent to which the primary antibody can be diluted and still achieve target recognition, when using a specified detection system. It is in effect a surrogate for the technical 'sensitivity' of the Total Test. In some circumstances (research papers, vendor's information or package inserts) the term sensitivity may refer to the detection system alone, ranging from low to high sensitivity (e.g. direct conjugate method vs ABC method vs polymer-based labels vs tyramide amplification etc. see Chap. 9). The optimal dilution of a specified primary antibody might vary from 1:20 for a direct conjugate method (low sensitivity detection method) to 1:1000 or more in polymer based or tyramine amplification methods (high sensitivity detection). The implication of technical sensitivity is generally understood within this

B. Jasani et al., *Precision Cancer Medicine*, https://doi.org/10.1007/978-3-030-84087-7_12

context, but it differs from the use of the term sensitivity in clinical laboratory tests, which usually addresses diagnostic or clinical sensitivity in a patient population.

12.2.3 Specificity

Similarly in the clinical laboratory use of the term specificity usually implies 'diagnostic specificity,' or the ability of a test to detect true positives in a population, in the absence of false positives. By Predictive Value Theory specificity is defined as the percentage value TN/(TN + FP) × 100%, where TN, total true negatives, is the number of patients who do not have the disease and FP, false positives, is the number of patients identified by the test as positive, but who are not diseased.

In IHC 'specificity' is usually used in a more restricted manner, again limited to 'technical specificity,' meaning the ability of an antibody (and detection system) to bind exclusively to its particular antigen in the absence of staining of other molecules.

The (technical) sensitivity and specificity of the total IHC test are assessed by use of positive and negative reagent and tissue controls, as described previously (Chaps. 9 and 10).

The true diagnostic sensitivity and specificity of IHC stains are not usually evaluated by the performing laboratory by the formal testing of clinical case populations. Therefore, the pathologist making an interpretation of the diagnostic import of an IHC stain uses her (his) knowledge of case populations from experience and from the literature; that is their understanding of the percentages of cases showing positive or negative reaction for the stain (marker) in question, as discussed further in Part III. For example, in the case of anaplastic tumors of unknown origin, the relative percentages of cases reported in literature to be positive (or negative) for Pan-keratin, CD45, vimentin and S100 etc. may be used by the pathologist in reaching a diagnostic conclusion (for an overview and details regarding major tumor types see Simental-Pizarro et al. 2016; Dabbs 2018).

Diagnostic sensitivity and specificity in IHC are thus inferential, derived from published data on relative frequency of positive/negative marker results in tests presumed to have been properly performed and validated.

This consideration of sensitivity and specificity is a key example of how biomarker assays are posing new and more exacting demands for IHC. The linked approval of targeted drug and companion biomarker test in clinical trials generates sensitivity and specificity data at both the technical (detection) and clinical (diagnostic) levels. Validation of an approved biomarker kit (FDA or CE mark) by the performing laboratory provides confirmation of technical sensitivity and specificity with reference to proper controls (as initially established by the manufacturer), while the clinical diagnostic specificity and specificity are drawn from the trial data.

For comparable biomarker LDTs (home brew tests) the demands on the performing laboratory are higher, because the laboratory is unlikely to have clinical trial data directly linked to the internally developed test. The LDT developer thus has two choices. Either the LDT must be validated directly against a suitable case population, that is sufficient in terms of case mix and numbers so as to be acceptable to regulatory agencies (difficult). Or alternatively, the LDT must be cross validated in a sufficient number of patients against or an established and independently validated test, which generally means a test which itself is already approved (by FDA, CE or the appropriate equivalent), and is performed in an approved certified laboratory (as defined in different countries), but definitely not a research lab.

12.3 Verification and Validation IHC Biomarker Assays

Verification and validation are discussed in some detail with reference to IHC, but the same principles apply to IF and ISH methods applied to tissue sections, and in fact to all biomarker assays, including extraction based proteomic and genomic sequencing methods. Each reagent must be verified for use in the selected test system and all components of the Total Test, all equipment and reagents must be validated for performance in the intended use. Verification and validation are essential parts of the pre-analytic and analytic phases, but are again discussed briefly here, because they can only be completed when the Total Test is completed. Table 12.1 includes a summary of validation requirement. A more detailed discussion related to different specified biomarker tests in clinical use will be included in Part III.

12.3.1 Verification

Verification is an initial step in IHC test development and implementation. It involves the collection of evidence that each component of an IHC test, and the finally the completed assay (Total Test), meets performance expectations. The great majority of laboratories obtain reagents commercially, in which case the vendor package insert will (should) contain details of verification. For component reagents, such as the primary antibody, verification may involve testing for technical sensitivity and specificity of the antibody against the target antigen by Western Blot, and in arrays of frozen tissues. If the primary antibody is to be used for FFPE tissues (as is the case for most biomarker testing) then verification of performance in FFPE specimens must be included. Each component reagent must be verified prior to incorporation in the test protocol. Lastly the Total Test is verified by performance on known positive and negative tissue.

Table 12.1 Representative examples of instances when a laboratory should conduct a formal validation process

Whenever a new IHC test (stain or biomarker assay) is developed and brought online, whether LDT, RTU or approved assay.
Whenever any part of an existing IHC test is changed, whether primary antibody, batch, clone or source, or detection system, or protocol (including AR method or incubation time).
Whenever a new control (tissue block) is introduced performance must be validated with reference to the previous control block.
Whenever a new staining platform is introduced; or any other instrument that is part of the protocol (e.g. a tissue processor).
Whenever a manual protocol is replaced by an automated protocol (or vice versa)
Whenever new software is brought online for any instrument that is part of the protocol.
Whenever there is any change is pre-analytic steps, especially in fixation time (or fixative type or in additional processes such as decalcification etc.).
• Formal validation is necessary prior to bringing any lab test into service. The type and extent of validation varies, being greatest for introduction of a new test, but less extensive for more minor changes in reagents or protocol. The validation method and results should be recorded.

12.3.2 Validation

Validation is the second step in the process of establishing that the performance characteristics of each component as well as the finished verified assay (Total Test) meet the requirements of the intended use in clinical specimens. Typically, the verified test is run in a blinded manner against a set of clinical specimens of known status with respect to the biomarker being tested, as determined by an independent laboratory or an independent method. The number of specimens required for validation varies, generally being fewer for an FDA approved test (e.g. 30) and an RTU (30–50), where verification of component parts, plus extensive test validation, will have been performed by the vendor, than for a test that is developed wholly within the laboratory (LDT). For an LDT the onus for validating each reagent, plus the Total Test performance with respect to intended use is on the laboratory that develops the test (and generally 50 or more specimens).

The number of specimens used for validation should be representative of the anticipated clinical practice, and will vary with the level of 'claim' made for the test. The College of American Pathologists (Fitzgibbons et al. 2014) has published extensive validation guidelines, with recommendations of a minimum of ten positive and ten negative cases for some lower level IHC tests; for biomarker stand-alone tests these number obviously are higher.

12.4 Practical Issues in Validation

A formal validation process is essential for each laboratory to ensure that each reagent separately and the final completed test gives consistent and diagnostically useful results on tissues (FFPE) that present to the laboratory.

Performance validation of each component includes automated tissue processors and autostainers, as well as all reagents. The approaches to validating instruments vary. It is recommended to follow the manufacturer's guidelines: the goal is to demonstrate and document that the instrument is working as expected, repeatedly and reliably in the user's laboratory. Detailed requirements vary according to laboratory accreditation practices in different countries and regions; in which case local guidelines are available and should be followed.

Clearly published information regarding reagents and protocol is of value in guiding test development, whether basic IHC stain or biomarker assay. Information gleaned from research papers should be carefully scrutinized as to whether the published method itself has been validated adequately, for often it is not, at least to the rigorous level required for clinical service. As already noted, product inserts, as well as guidelines and assay manuals, also are useful in providing a start point as to how to eliminate some of the variables. Another useful available option is to access published information provided by high quality external peer review organizations, such as NordiQC, UKNEQAS, CAP and other similar QC bodies, which often include real life performance data and recommendations for best practice. These information sources help reduce the unknown variables, and have the potential to reducing effort, set up time and costs; but they do not obviate the need for final in-house validation of the completed assay.

Similarly, for individual reagents and for kits (RTUs) it is again recommended to follow the manufacturer's guidelines: the goal here is to demonstrate and document that the reagent (kit) performs reliably in the user's laboratory. At this stage validation should include establishing limits within which optimum performance may be expected, including cold ischemia time, fixation type and times (minimum and maximum), AR method, primary antibody and detection system (dilutions and incubation times).

As noted, validation of the primary antibody is a critical step in setting up a traditional IHC stain, and equally or more so in establishing an IHC biomarker assay. The technical performance of the primary antibody (usually monoclonal, but in some instances a polyclonal antiserum) will have been demonstrated by the producer of the antibody. It may involve in vitro testing of purity, sensitivity and specificity testing (e.g. Western blots) and often vendor testing of tissue sensitivity and specificity on FFPE tissues, including TMAs. This information will be provided in the package insert and serves as a guideline only. It does not obviate the need for in-house validation on FFPE tissues.

If a primary antibody is obtained from a research laboratory then the extent of testing by the researcher supplying the antibody maybe very limited in the context of FFPE specimens, and extreme caution should be exercised in considering such a reagent for clinical use. Even when transferred to and produced by a qualified manufacturer the FDA classifies such reagents as RUOs, Research Use Only, stating that such reagents are not to be used in the rendering of clinical decisions. Of course, a reagent that is first shown to be of interest in a research environment (publication) may eventually enter clinical use, but only after fulfillment of rigorous GMP manufacturing requirements by the producer (manufacturer) and validation of both technical and clinical performance.

12.5 Validation of Pre-Analytical and Analytical Phases: LDTs, RTUs and Approved Biomarker Tests

Final validation of the Total Test results must of course include interpretation and scoring methods that will discussed briefly below and visited in more detail in Part III with respect to current diagnostic practice, and in Part IV with reference to computer assisted algorithms. The present discussion deals primarily with validation of pre-analytic and analytic components.

Unfortunately, IHC has a long legacy of use as a simple stain, with qualitative assessment of staining results, using control tissues that vary from lab to lab and are themselves established in a qualitative manner as described in Chap. 9. This traditional approach may suffice for use of IHC as a qualitative stain—"Is there brown staining?" However, it must be recognized that they do not serve for biomarker assays, where the question is different—"How much brown staining is there?"

The lack of widespread rigorous validation in the past has been responsible for IHC acquiring a reputation, in the minds of some, of being unreliable or unrepeatable, non-specific or low in sensitivity. Scrutiny of such claims, where published and not simply verbal, reveals that in many instances the judgement of 'poor performance' is based upon IHC tests that were not properly performed, and not well validated, or even validated at all with respect to pre-analytic factors (other than being 'formalin fixed') and lacked proper or even adequate controls. The fault is not in the principle of the IHC test per se, but rather that the user has not performed adequate validation and control of the test (Table 12.1).

In the context of this book all prognostic and predictive biomarkers are Class II or Class III targets as described in Section I (see also Torlakovic et al. 2015). Validation of the final completed Total Test (assay), incorporating validation of the primary antibody and all instruments and reagents, requires a minimum of 25–100 cases according to ASCO/CAP recommendations, the exact number required depending upon the intended use. The validation case population should be representative of the (anticipated) experience of the laboratory and must include a sufficient number of cases with scores close to the test threshold, that is cases in the low positive and negative range for expression of the biomarker in question (for real time examples—see Phillips et al. 2015, 2018). This is an ever changing field, and in each instance up to date regulatory guidelines that are specific for each region or country should be sought and followed.

Validation is time consuming and expensive, in terms of technician and pathologist effort, reagents and materials. It may also be technically difficult, especially with internally developed IHC tests (LDTs) for which the ability accurately to perform a series of titration dilutions is essential. Once the validated test has been placed in service, ongoing performance must be monitored internally by reference to established controls and also by participation in external QC programs, such as UKNEQAS, NordiQC and CAP (discussed below) (see Fig. 12.1). Once the test has been placed in service, ongoing external QC monitoring also has its costs.

As already described (Chap. 9), as an alternative to the challenge of setting up the entire stain or test 'in-house' (as an LDT), users may choose a system (kit) that includes all of the principal reagents and a standardized and validated protocol developed by the vendor, the so called RTU (Ready To Use) approach. Commercially available RTU kits are usually coupled to recommended staining platforms and, when utilized exactly as described in the package user information, are 'guaranteed' (within limits) to provide diagnostically useful results. RTU kits, directed against the more common IHC targets of interest (stains) are widely available from many manufacturers. When an RTU kit fails to perform to the anticipated standard the problem most often relates to the pre-analytic phase, particularly fixation, or to non-adherence to protocol, especially if the test is performed manually, where strict adherence to incubation times for every slide is impossible. Platform failure is less common and is identified by proper control systems, including on slide controls (Chap. 10). FGor more extensive discussion see Torlakovic et al. (2015), Vyberg and Nielsen (2016) and Cartun and Taylor (2018).

Approved biomarker tests (striving to purpose as assays) assays) take the RTU concept to a higher level by the incorporation of clinical outcome performance data derived from combined clinical trials that are a necessary part of seeking certification of approval from regulatory bodies (e.g. FDA, CE Mark).

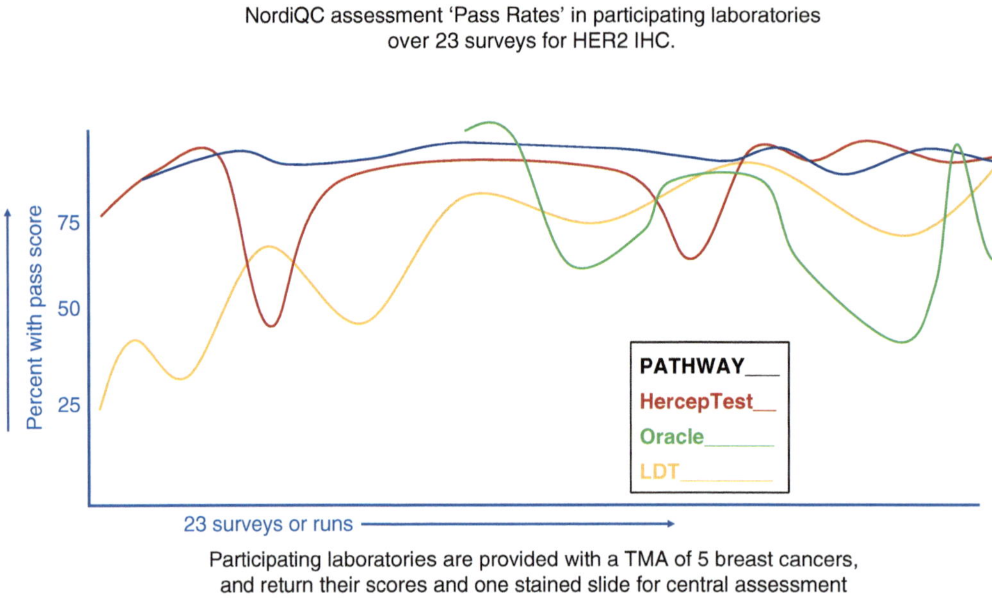

Fig. 12.1 Revealing summary data from NordiQC surveys showing relative performance of three approved HER2 tests over time, and corresponding performance of labs using LDTs against HER2. Note that over time the performance of LDTs improves as QC feedback occurs within the program, almost reaching the levels of approved tests, which show some fluctuation, apparently reflecting extent of adherence to strict protocol. Data drawn from NordiQC Assessments https://www.nordiqc.org/epitope.php

It is important to recognize that use of an approved test of itself does not guarantee superior, or even satisfactory performance. Nor, conversely, is an LDT always inferior. In each instance the final quality outcome is determined by degree of adherence to protocol, proper controls and QC (Fig. 12.1).

Today there are many examples of approved biomarker tests from a broad range of manufacturers, directed against a wide range of biomarkers. Well established examples include ER/PR, HER2, PD- L1 as will be discussed individually in Part III. Once more, it must be emphasized that while approved test have been extensively validated by the vendor for technical performance and tested for clinical performance in conjoint trials, the individual laboratory user still must conduct a sufficient internal validation to ensure quality outcome, (Fig. 12.1) as described above.

12.6 Quality Management Systems (QMS): Quality Assurance (QA), Quality Control (QC)

ISO 9000 defines QA as "part of quality management focused on providing confidence that quality requirements will be fulfilled", and QC as "part of quality management focused on fulfilling quality requirements." (https://www.iso.org/iso-9001-quality-management.html). QA is concerned with the development and selection of documented processes, protocols and standards in order to achieve a quality result. QA includes QC, which is the system of checks and tests of each component and step, and the Total Test, to show that the desired level of quality has actually been achieved (Table 12.2).

Table 12.2 Parts of the total test procedure covered by quality management systems

Elements of testing process	Quality assurance issues	Responsibility
1. Test selection: the clinical question	Indications for IHC. Selection of stain(s).	Surgical pathologist; sometimes clinician
2. Specimen acquisition and management	Specimen collection, fixation, processing, sectioning.	Pathologist/technologist
3. Technology/methodology	Reagents, protocols.	Pathologist/technologist
4. Analytical issues	Sensitivity and specificity. Automation. Qualifications of staff. Intra-and interlaboratory proficiency testing.	Pathologist/technologist
5. Results: validation/reporting	Criteria for positivity/negativity in relation to controls. Content and organization of report. Turnaround time.	Pathologist/technologist
6. Interpretation, significance	Experience/qualifications of pathologist. Proficiency testing of interpretational aspects. Diagnostic, prognostic significance. Appropriateness/correlation with other data.	Surgical pathologist and/or clinician

12.6.1 External Quality Assessment and Proficiency Testing

Laboratory QA/QC extends to include External Quality Assessment (EQA) or Proficiency Testing (PT), which is a formalized inter-laboratory testing (and comparison) program. Certified laboratories for high complexity tests (in the US) are required to participate in external PT testing, which is defined by CLIA (Clinical Laboratory Improvement Amendments act from the US Centers for Medicare and Medicaid Services, 1988) as follows: "the testing of unknown samples sent to a laboratory by an HHS-approved PT program." (https://www.cms.gov/Regulations-and-Guidance/Legislation/CLIA/downloads/CLIAbrochure8.pdf).

PT is not a requirement for non-waived (low complexity) tests in the US but is recommended strongly. Similar requirements exist or are under development in other countries.

As already described (Chap. 2) over the past decades the IHC method has been performed routinely in anatomic laboratories worldwide as a 'special stain' and more recently has been pressed into service for biomarker testing. Conversion of IHC from a qualitative stain to a quantitative assay increased the need for effective QA and QC programs. In the eyes of the regulatory agencies (CLIA, FDA, CE Mark, CBQA etc., see Chaps. 2 and 9) the IHC method extended beyond the realm of waived tests (low complexity stains) into high complexity non-waived Class II and Class III testing (biomarker tests) (FDA 1998, 2021); a classification originating in joint deliberations with the Biological Stain Commission in the US during the 1990s (Taylor 1992, 1998). Comparable progression of regulatory oversight occurred also in other countries. Progress is ongoing, and current status should be sought by recourse to the appropriate agencies for each country.

QA, QC and PT programs have evolved *pari passu* to address these increasing performance demands. In addition to quality assurance of the actual analytic process, assessment of the interpretational and diagnostic skill of surgical pathologists is incorporated in some PT programs and has become a legitimate topic in the pathology literature (excellent review-Foucar and Foucar 2000; Renshaw and Gould 2007; Torlakovic et al. 2015). Participation in one or more of the national QC programs, is essential for all labs performing biomarker assays. It is not only essential for certification purposes, but because it is well documented that active participation in external QC programs does lead to higher levels of quality performance.

Table 8.1 (Chap. 8) is drawn from an example of a UKNEQAS survey, and shows the extreme range of reagent and technical variation among participating laboratories. Follow up studies have shown that moving towards a common 'best practice' protocol yields improved results across all participants. As an early example, one useful outcome was the identification of inadequate antigen retrieval as a principal contributor to poor reliability (Rhodes et al. 2000, 2002; O'Leary 2001; Leong 2004; Leong and Leong 2011). Almost two decades later NordiQC affirmed the critical importance of AR and identified other common error sources (Vyberg Nielsen 2016; NordiQC. https://www.nordiqc.org/). (Table 12.3). Figures 12.1, 12.2 and 12.3 also are revealing with respect to intra-laboratory variation, across space ad time.

NordiQC surveys have shown similar dramatic improvement in biomarker testing for ER, PR and HER2 again, by identifying the better performing reagents and protocols, and making that information available to all participants. (https://www.nordiqc.org/epitope.php). This interactive process allows laboratories to review their performance against others and then adjust internal practices that improve performance. The stimulus to at least match one's peers is powerful!

The CAP 'AP Survey Program' in addition to the comprehensive overall laboratory accreditation requirements (CAP 2020—updates regularly), includes several surveys that are relevant to IHC and ISH (for a subscription cost; CAP, Northfield, Illinois, USA). These include Predictive and Prognostic Markers, Her 2 IHC,

Table 12.3 NordiQC, 12 year IHC survey experience: (2003–2015). Summary of factors leading to inferior results of participating labs

Antigen retrieval, inappropriate or not optimal	27%
Wrong antibody dilution (not optimized)	20%
Choice of a poorly performing detection method	19%
Choice of a poorly performing primary antibody (or RTU)	17%
Other: including endogenous biotin, drying of slides, protocol error	17%

Data drawn from NordiQC data; Nielsen (2015), Vyberg and Nielsen (2016)

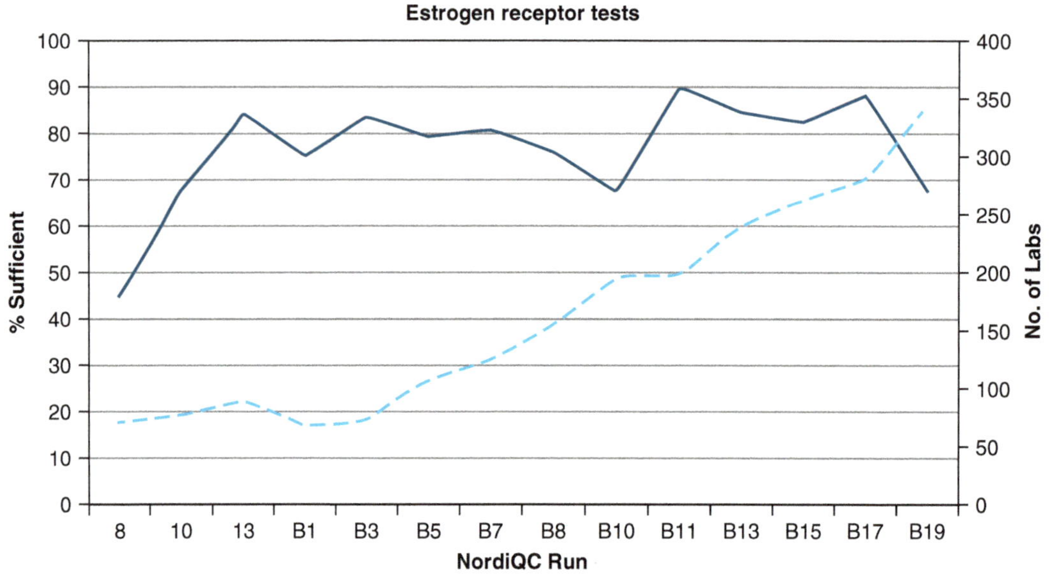

Fig. 12.2 NordiQC data showing improvement in 'sufficient' performance levels for ER among increasing numbers of participating laboratories over time (blue hatched line). Data from Vyberg, Nielsen 2016). Used under Creative Commons CC BY License, Springer Nature. Copyright is with the authors

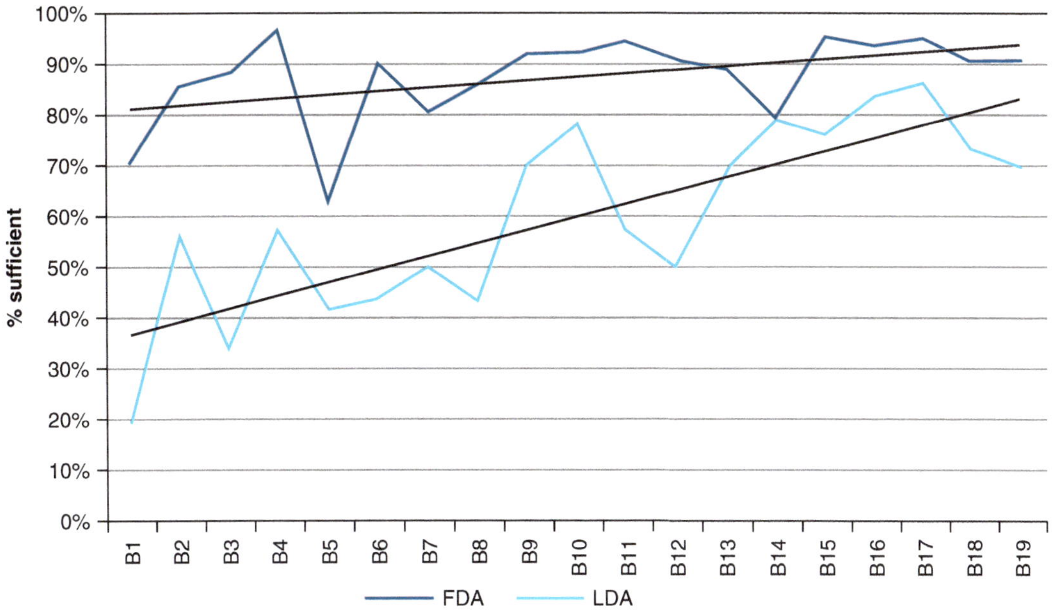

Fig. 12.3 NordiQC data showing improvement in 'sufficient' performance levels for in-house developed HER2 tests (LDTs, termed laboratory developed assays LDAs by NordiQC). Data from Vyberg, Nielsen 2016). Used under Creative Commons CC BY License, Springer Nature. Copyright is with the authors

CD117, ER, CD20 microarrays, and FISH surveys for HER2, EBV, HPV, or CMV. In each instance, cut FFPE sections are provided to participating labs with instructions as to which assays to perform. The scored results are submitted centrally, along with a basic differential diagnosis (selected from a limited multiple choice). Performance data are returned to the participants.

NordiQC (https://www.nordiqc.org/) and UKNEQAS (www.ukneqas.org.uk.) go a step further in sending the participants two unstained FFPE sections with the request as to which stain should be performed: one stained section, together with protocol details, is returned for central review by an expert panel, a procedure which allows for detailed assessment of stain quality and interpretation. Results are returned to each participant, with suggestions where improvements may be made. Data of successive surveys are made available on the respective websites (see Figs. 12.1, 12.2 and 12.3).

Finally, it is worthwhile repeating the benefit to the laboratory community and the patients) of participating in external QC programs. As recounted in Chap. 9, the proliferation of approved biomarker tests (HER2, PD LI), each with stringent specified requirements for reagents and automated platforms, effectively forced many laboratories into attempting to develop their own equivalent in-house tests.

There was, and is, genuine concern, given the enormous effort expended in research and subsequent clinical validation of approved assays, that in-house or 'home brew' Lab Developed Tests (Chap. 9) would fall far short in performance quality; and indeed, in many cases they did, at least initially. Once again, NordiQC data shows that given active, and responsive, participation in external QC programs the quality of LDTs does improve over time (seen in successive surveys) and can come close to matching that of approved tests (Fig. 12.3).

References

Cartun R, Taylor CR. Techniques of immunohistochemistry: principles, pitfalls and standardization. In: Dabbs DJ, editor. Comprehensive diagnostic immunohistochemistry. 5th ed. Amsterdam: Elsevier; 2018.

Castle WB. Harv Med Alumni Bull. 1955;29:18.
College of American Pathologists Accreditation Checklists. 2020. https://www.google.com/url?sa=t&rct=j&q=&esrc=s&source=web&cd=&ved=2ahUKEwizm5r1x4XvAhXRIDQIHQcLBDYQFjABegQIAhAD&url=https%3A%2F%2Fdocuments.cap.org%2Fdocuments%2Fcap-accreditation-checklists.pdf&usg=AOvVaw2x4EVwmVwK98oVt8QiUyZG
Dabbs DJ, editor. Comprehensive diagnostic immunohistochemistry. 5th ed. Amsterdam: Elsevier; 2018.
FDA. Guidance for submission of immunohistochemistry applications to the food and drug administration—Final guidance for industry. original issuance 1998. 1998, 2021. https://www.fda.gov/medical-devices/guidance-documents-medical-devices-and-radiation-emitting-products/guidance-submission-immunohistochemistry-applications-food-and-drug-administration-final-guidance. accessed Feb 2021.
Fitzgibbons PL, Bradley LA, Fatheree LA, et al. Principles of analytic validation of immunohistochemical assays. Arch Pathol. 2014;138:1432–43.
Foucar E, Foucar MK. Error in anatomic pathology. In: Foucar MK, editor. Bone marrow pathology. 2nd ed. Chicago: ASCP Press; 2000.
Leong AS. Quantitation in immunohistology: fact or fiction? A discussion of variables that influence results. Appl Immunohistochem Mol Morph. 2004;12:1–7.
Leong AS, Leong TY. Standardization in immunohistochemistry. Methods Mol Biol. 2011;724:37–68.
Nielsen S. External quality assessment for immunohistochemistry: experiences from NordiQC. Biotech Histochem. 2015;90:1–10. https://doi.org/10.3109/10520295.2015.1033462.
O'Leary TJ. Standardization in immunohistochemistry. Appl Immunohistochem Mol Morph. 2001;9:3–8.
Phillips T, Millett MM, Zhang X, Jansson M, Cleveland R, Simmons P, Cherryholmes G, Carnahan J, William J, Spaulding B, Satnick IR, Inzuna HD, Taylor CR, Cogswell J, Novotny J, Oroudjev E, Winther H. Development of a diagnostic programmed cell death 1-ligand 1 immunohistochemistry assay for Nivolumab therapy in melanoma. Appl Immunohistochem Mol Morph. 2018;26:6–12.
Phillips T, Simmons P, Inzunza HD, Cogswell J, Novotny J, Taylor CR, Zhang X. Development of an automated PD-L1 immunohistochemistry (IHC) assay for non small cell lung cancer. Appl Immunohistochem Mol Morph. 2015;23:541–9. https://doi.org/10.1097/PAI.0000000000000256.
Renshaw AA, Gould EW. Measuring errors in surgical pathology in real-life practice. Defining what does and does not matter. Am J Clin Pathol. 2007;127:144–52.
Rhodes A, Jasani B, Anderson E, Dodson AR, Balaton AJ. Evaluation of Her2/neu immunohistochemical assays sensitivity and scoring on formalin-fixed and paraffin-processed cell lines and breast tumors: a comparative study involving results from laboratories in 21 countries. Am J Clin Pathol. 2002;118:408–17.
Rhodes A, Jasani B, Balaton AJ, Miller KD. Immunohistochemical demonstration of estrogen and progesterone receptors: correlation of standards achieved on in house tumours with that achieved on external quality assessment material in over 150 laboratories from 26 countries. J Clin Pathol. 2000;53:292–301.
Simental-Pizarro RG, Klipfel N, Taylor CR. Tumors of unknown origin. In: Cheng L, editor. Essentials of anatomic pathology. 4th ed. New York: Humana Press/Springer; 2016.
Taylor CR. Quality assurance and standardization in immunohistochemistry. A proposal for the annual meeting of the biological stain commission, June, 1991. Biotech Histochem. 1992;67:110–7.
Taylor CR. Report from the biological stain commission: FDA issues final rule for classification/reclassification of immunochemistry (IHC) reagents and kits. Biotech Histochem. 1998;73:175–7.
Torlakovic EE, Nielsen S, Vyberg M, Taylor CR. Getting controls under control—the time is now for immunohistochemistry. J Clin Path. 2015;68:1–4. https://doi.org/10.1136/jclinpath-2014-202705.
Vyberg M, Nielsen S. Proficiency testing in immunohistochemistry—experiences from nordic immunohistochemical quality control (NordiQC). Virchows Arch. 2016;468(1):19–29. https://doi.org/10.1007/s00428-015-1829-1.

Description and Interpretation of Results; The Pathology Report

13

13.1 Content and Organization of Report

The Final Report is where the expert pathologist has unique and critical influence upon the entire biomarker dependent therapeutic process, integrating all components as described in Part III.

Having completed the validated IHC Total Test and evaluated the controls, all that remains is to interpret the result and present the conclusions in writing in a form that is understandable to our colleagues in pathology and in the clinical disciplines. Examination of this seemingly straight forward task revealed a number of complexities, and a woeful inconsistency in content and style (Taylor 2014).

13.1.1 Descriptive

Three decades ago, the Biologic Stain Commission sought a 'more standardized' format for the IHC report, with the result that the Association of Directors of Anatomic and Surgical Pathologists sponsored the development of simple guidelines (Table 13.1), which are still valid today, with some modification for the biomarker era.

Table 13.1 Guideline for incorporation of IHC data into surgical pathology reports[a]

The report should include all patient demographics and tissue identifiers as for any surgical pathology report *(plus all codes for billing as required in any particular country).*
1. All IHC results should be reported, whether positive, or negative, regardless of perceived significance.
2. A 'differential diagnosis', justifying 'stain selection' should be included.
3. The report should also include: (a) Nature of the specimen tested (frozen, paraffin section, cytoprep. etc.) (b) Antibodies employed; including where appropriate the clone identifier. (c) The result of staining for each antibody, including cellular localization where pertinent[b]
4. An interpretation of the findings in the context of the diagnosis and with reference to associated surgical pathology report, if such is not incorporated into the same report.
5. Exact protocols, retrieval methods etc. need not be part of the report, but should be available in laboratory manuals and records.
6. Synoptic reporting of pathology findings in cancer cases, include designated lines of entry for the descriptive and data elements listed above.

[a]Updated table, data drawn from various sources including Taylor and Cote (2005), Hewitt et al. (2011), Fitzgibbons et al. (2014) and CAP Cancer Protocols. www.cap.org/cancerprotocols

[b]Where 'thumbnails images' are included, these may fulfill this requirement

See also Table 3.1

Patient demographics and identifiers are essential, and to these must be added the necessary clinical codes and identifiers to assure reimbursement by whatever system is appropriate for the laboratory; in the US it is Medicare and other third party payers. NCCLS (National Committee for Clinical Laboratory Standards: CLSI Guidelines, Hewitt et al. (2011)) includes an updated version of these recommendations in its

B. Jasani et al., *Precision Cancer Medicine*, https://doi.org/10.1007/978-3-030-84087-7_13

IHC guidelines. The necessity for a clear report was strikingly emphasized by Powsner et al. (2000) in 'Clinicians are from Mars and pathologists are from Venus.' In a series of questionnaires that explored the degree to which clinicians understood the reports provided by their pathologists, the authors found that surgeons 'misunderstood' 30% of the time. Alternatively pathologists wrote incomprehensible reports 30% of the time. From a QA perspective the result is astonishing and dangerous. It is tempting to lay blame upon the clinical Martians, but clearly it is the pathologist who can have greatest impact by increasing the clarity (precision) of reporting.

In the experience of one of the authors (CRT) some the most spectacular examples of obfuscation by pathologists come from the field of lymphoma reporting and classification: the first cited by an eminent insightful pathologist –

> *"Nowhere in pathology has a chaos of names so clouded clear concepts as in the subject of lymphoid tumours."* (Rupert A Willis 1948), and the second, voiced by an eminent frustrated clinician again with reference to the fertile field of lymphoma nosology -
> *"Pathologists at times seem unable to understand each other."* (Alan C Aisenberg 1977).

For patients on whom biomarker testing is performed it is important that the biomarker results are made available in an easily understood form to pathologists and clinicians alike, in the context of the regular pathology report. Biomarker results often become available after the original pathology report has been issued, and then may be distributed separately. However, they should be linked, a process made more simple and more reliable with the advent of the electronic medical record and digitization of pathology, a topic that is reviewed extensively in Part IV and introduced briefly below.

13.1.2 Integrated and Standardized Reporting

Surgical pathology already is moving in the direction of more standardized reporting using templates for descriptive material and data entry, such as the Synoptic Report protocols for the different cancer types from CAP (College of American Pathologists. Resources & Publications: Cancer Protocols) www.cap.org/cancerprotocols. The dawning of digital pathology facilitates adoption of these standardized protocols, which include provision for entry of biomarker results. The process is accompanied by the growing incorporation of image analysis software for generating standardized scores and beyond, to the interpretation of IHC staining patterns. Digital analysis and report generation also fosters inclusion of 'thumbnail' imagery that illustrates the pattern of staining observed for each antibody applied and for the biomarker result as shown in an early prototypic report from our laboratory (Fig. 13.1).

Because such reports are today generated electronically, they are readily transmissible to involved clinicians and other pathologists, and form part of the electronic medical record. With appropriate hardware and software, digitized whole slide images (WSIs) of the entire tissue section, together with results of scoring algorithms can also be linked and filed with the report, also becoming part of a medical record that is immediately accessible where ever the patient goes in the future.

13.2 Scoring; Including Validation of Scoring Method

In the instance of biomarker testing by IHC, ISH and IF the descriptive findings are frequently augmented by a 'score' that gives the illusion of quantification. Today that score generally is semi-quantitative and, in reality, is one of the weakest links in achieving an accurate and reliable IHC (IF) assay.

With respect to cancer biomarkers detected in tissue sections by IHC or IF, the term quantification (or semi-quantification) does not extend to calibrated measurement, but instead simply means the counting of positive cells (i.e. cells expressing the signal above an arbitrary threshold) versus negative cells (those lacking expression or expressing below a threshold). With respect to biomarkers of tumor cells, usually the score is expressed as a percentage: numerator/denominator, where the numerator is the number

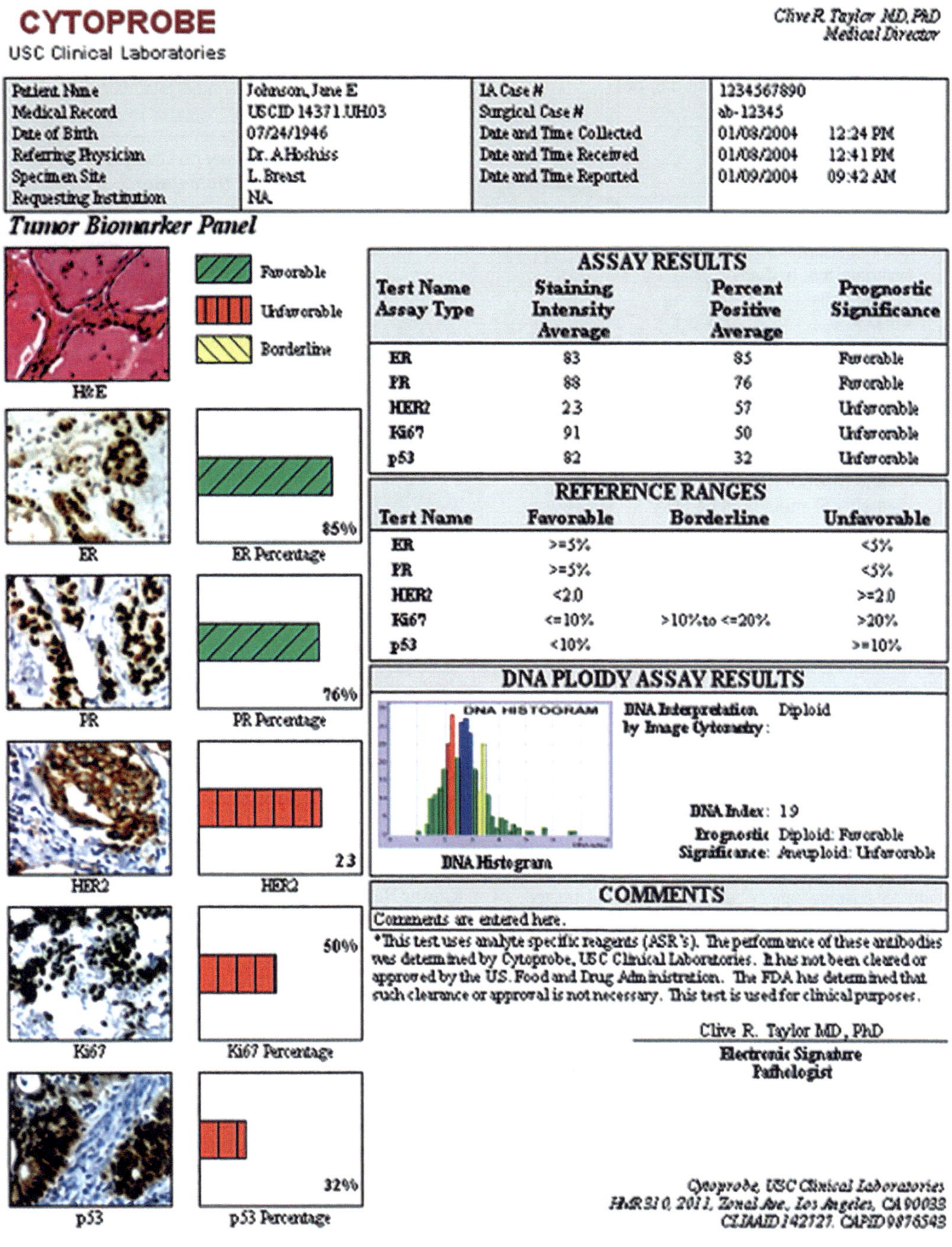

CYTOPROBE
USC Clinical Laboratories

Clive R. Taylor MD, PhD
Medical Director

Patient Name	Johnson, Jane E	IA Case #	1234567890
Medical Record	USCID 14371.UH03	Surgical Case #	ab-12345
Date of Birth	07/24/1946	Date and Time Collected	01/08/2004 12:24 PM
Referring Physician	Dr. A Hoshiss	Date and Time Received	01/08/2004 12:41 PM
Specimen Site	L. Breast	Date and Time Reported	01/09/2004 09:42 AM
Requesting Institution	NA		

Tumor Biomarker Panel

Favorable
Unfavorable
Borderline

H&E
85% ER ER Percentage
76% PR PR Percentage
23 HER2 HER2
50% Ki67 Ki67 Percentage
32% p53 p53 Percentage

ASSAY RESULTS

Test Name Assay Type	Staining Intensity Average	Percent Positive Average	Prognostic Significance
ER	83	85	Favorable
PR	88	76	Favorable
HER2	23	57	Unfavorable
Ki67	91	50	Unfavorable
p53	82	32	Unfavorable

REFERENCE RANGES

Test Name	Favorable	Borderline	Unfavorable
ER	>=5%		<5%
PR	>=5%		<5%
HER2	<2.0		>=2.0
Ki67	<=10%	>10% to <=20%	>20%
p53	<10%		>=10%

DNA PLOIDY ASSAY RESULTS

DNA HISTOGRAM
DNA Histogram

DNA Interpretation by Image Cytometry: Diploid

DNA Index: 1.9
Prognostic Significance: Diploid: Favorable
Aneuploid: Unfavorable

COMMENTS

Comments are entered here.

*This test uses analyte specific reagents (ASR's). The performance of these antibodies was determined by Cytoprobe, USC Clinical Laboratories. It has not been cleared or approved by the US. Food and Drug Administration. The FDA has determined that such clearance or approval is not necessary. This test is used for clinical purposes.

Clive R. Taylor MD, PhD
Electronic Signature
Pathologist

Cytoprobe, USC Clinical Laboratories
HMR 310, 2011, Zonal Ave., Los Angeles, CA 90033
CLIA ID 142127. CAP ID 9876543

Fig. 13.1 Prototypic example of biomarker report that includes results, interpretation and micro-images for the electronic record. Today with impending full digitization more complete and comprehensive reports are routinely available (From Taylor and Cote 2005). (This figure was published in Immunomicroscopy, A Diagnostic Tool for the Surgical Pathologist. Eds. Taylor and Cote (2005); by permissions Elsevier)

of positive tumor cells (by the scoring definition) and the denominator, the total number of tumor cells, both positive and negative cells (Fig. 13.2).

An effective scoring method should be simple to describe, easily taught, and easily learned, such that scoring is reproducible for the

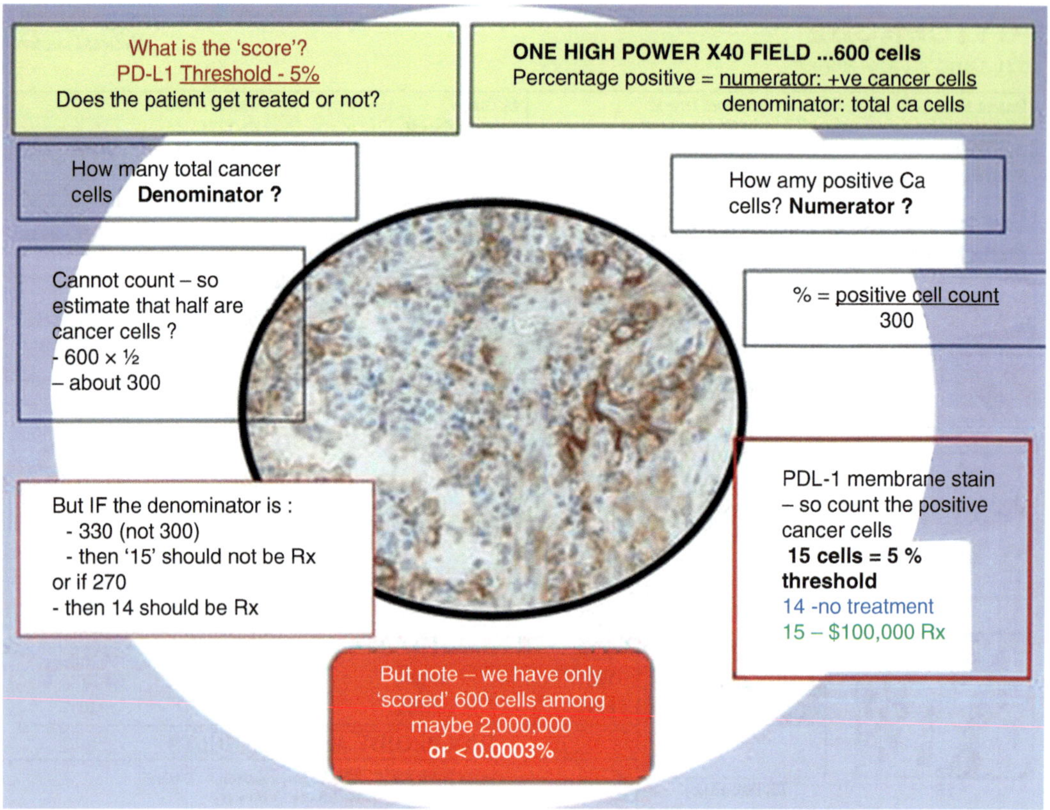

Fig. 13.2 Stylistic representation of scoring lung cancer for PD-LI. Given a 5% threshold for treatment and an 'educated guess' that there are 300 total cancer cells (the denominator) in this one high power field, then a count of 15 positive cancer cells (the numerator) gives a positive result: 15 positive cancer cells, the patient is treated; 14 not. But even then, this assumes all positive cancer cells have been clearly distinguished from positive macrophages, and that the denominator is 300, not more or less. The tasks to be completed by the scoring pathologist are outlined in the text and are impossible to complete with precision. (From Taylor 2020, by permission of Wolters Kluwer Health Inc.)

individual scorer over time, as well as among different individuals, and it should have clinical significance. Experience shows that meeting these requirements is very difficult. Almost none of the existing scoring systems meet these basic requirements.

The individual (pathologist) who is scoring the stained slide must integrate several different parameters (Fig. 13.2) to determine a positive (or negative)) result: tasks which ideally are set forth in detail in the scoring protocol, but which even then remain subjective in nature.

Tasks include the following:

1. Identification of the tumor cells separately from other cell types, including non-tumor cells of the same tissue type and, in some instances (e.g. PD L-1) immune cells.
2. Identification of tumor cells meeting the conditions for a positive cell (may be a combination of level of intensity and pattern of staining; membrane, complete or partial).
3. 'Counting' positive tumor cells, to obtain the numerator.
4. Counting the total number of tumor cells, both positive and negative, to obtain the denominator.
5. Ideally tasks 3 and 4 should be applied to the whole tissue section, but because the entire section may contain upwards of 100,000 tumor cells a complete count by eye is not possible, leading to one or more default behaviors:

(a) counting the positive tumor cells in a limited number of selected fields of view (FOVs; or Regions of Interest; ROIs), often ten, which leads to selection bias because no two scorers select the same fields. Even then, when using a ×20 objective more than 1000 tumor cells may be present in each FOV; these cannot be counted by eye and an estimate is made (Fig. 13.2).
(b) just as an accurate count of all positive tumor cells is nearly impossible, so counting the total of both positive and negative cells is even more nearly impossible, unless in a small biopsy that contains only a few 100 tumor cells.
(c) averaging the FOVs and extrapolating the count to the whole slide.
(d) in instances where it is difficult to distinguish tumor cells from other cell types that also may express the biomarker in question (e.g. normal tissue cells, macrophages and lymphocytes) then the problems are compounded, and the score really becomes an estimate, although not always recognized by everyone as such.

13.3 Scoring Systems

These overall difficulties and the resultant poor clinical performance of the test are well illustrated by scoring for ER, which in practice should be among the most straightforward biomarkers for scoring. The long term experience of the authors and the leading QC organizations is that 10% or more of ER tests give false results; either false positive or false negative. This finding led to the adoption certain practical 'solutions' in order to make effective clinical use of IHC (IF) biomarkers in tissue sections, among which are the following:

13.4 Percentage Based Scores

Raw percentage scores generally are not used directly for clinical decisions.

13.4.1 Conversion to Positive and Negative Results

A common approach is to convert the percentage score to a 'positive' or 'negative' clinical result based upon a 'threshold' value that is predictive of therapy. For ER and PR this threshold was derived from accumulated clinical experience, finally settling at 1% as a positive result. More recently the working thresholds for biomarker tests are determined in conjoint clinical trial; for example 5% or 10% or 50% (see PD-L1—Phillips et al. 2015, 2018). Different trials of different therapeutic antibodies (clones) for different (or the same nominal) biomarkers have yielded differing scoring systems, with differing thresholds for positive and negative results and for clinical significance, greatly complicating the training and learning process for pathologists, who may be expected to interpret one or more of these assays, that paradoxically, are for the same (analyte) may require different scoring approaches.

The net result of reduction of raw percentage numbers to a positive or negative result is that reproducibility of scoring is enhanced, superficially and artificially. For example, with respect to a given threshold (of say 10%), the raw percentage scores (by different observers) of 20%, 35% or 55% all exceed the threshold, therefore giving agreement for a positive clinical result; likewise raw scores of 6%, 2% or 0% all fall below the 10% threshold and all are interpreted to give a clinical negative result; that is they are 'in agreement' in spite of being wildly different.

However, if only scores close to the threshold (in this example, 10%) are compared then agreement and reproducibility suffers; no observer can reproducibly separate 8% from 11%, or 9% from 13%, in a section that contains anything upwards of a 1000 tumor cells. Reported studies of reproducibility of scoring are thus hugely influenced by the proportion of cases in the study that fall close to the threshold (whatever it is). The FDA is well aware of this issue and requires that clinical studies include threshold cases in proportion to their occurrence in the case population.

13.4.2 Percentage Combined with Intensity and/or Pattern

A second approach is to convert the raw percentage into a simplified numerical score, at the same time building in an assessment of the intensity of staining and/or pattern. Numerous research approaches to interpretation and scoring have been well reviewed in the context of bone pathology by Fedchenko and Reifenrath (2014), who also covered pre-analytic and analytic issues. The two most widely used methods are the Allred score and the H-score.

Craig Allred recognized the inconsistency of scoring for ER and PR and proposed a method (Allred et al. 1998; review Ilić et al. 2019) that took account of three levels of intensity (1 weak, 2 moderate, and 3 strong, plus) for negative), and the percentage values for each. These were arranged into buckets numbered 1–5 or 'proportion' scores (0; 1 = <1%; 2 = 1–10; 3 = 11–33; 4 = 34–66 and 5 = 67–100). The intensity number (1–3) and the proportion number (1–5) then are added, giving a range from 0 to 8. In ER scores of 0 and 2 are 'negative' in clinical import (there is no score of 1), and 3–8 are positive.

The H score is similar in principle, again requiring scoring of cells by intensity (0, 1, 2 and 3), as well as by percentage for each intensity level, and then multiplying percentage by intensity score. Possible scores range from 1 (intensity 1 × 1%) to 300 (intensity 3 × 100%); in this system a score of <1 is negative for ER in breast cancer. The method has the advantage of flexibility in application to several tasks. For example, Hirsch et al. (2003) obtained good results using H score in a study of EGFR (epidermal growth factor receptor) correlating gene copy number with protein expression.

Both these methods result in increased concordance of scores; in part through grouping of raw percentage values; in part by the greater level of scrutiny required of the observer to attempt to score different intensities; and in large part by assigning a single clinical positive or negative result in relation to a defined groups of scores.

Both methods also have been adopted in research applications for different biomarkers (usually of nuclear location), often resulting in different thresholds that define positive and negative results (e.g. FOX C1 biomarker; threshold 4) (Jensen et al. 2015). The H-score is held by many to be more useful in segregating cases that are close to the threshold and it has a greater dynamic range.

CAP and other QC organizations have weighed in with recommendations for use in breast cancer (Hammond et al. 2010; Daltoé et al. 2013; Fitzgibbons et al. 2014).

13.4.3 Concordance Training

A third approach designed to improve agreement and reproducibility of scoring, often employed by vendors of complex biomarker IHC tests (such as PD L-1), is to initiate a formal training program for pathologists in the use of the scoring method (discussed in Part III). In this process a pathologist experienced in the use of the method trains a group of new users how to score the test (e.g. a specific PD L-1 test), using a representative set of 30 (more or less) training slides round a multiheaded microscope, followed by qualification of each pathologist for independent use by passing a test on a similar representative set (again usually 30 slides). The authors have had considerable direct experience of this training/qualification approach at multiple venues around the world and can attest that performance is enhanced (Jasani et al. 2020).

The challenge, however, is for the newly trained pathologists to establish a process of ongoing mutual monitoring of performance, in the absence of which concordance within the group may drop markedly.

13.4.4 Consensus or Ring Studies

An additional approach favored by joint study groups has been to seek consensus scoring among several different observers, using a standard scoring method (with or without additional pathologist training). Sometimes termed a 'ring study, or a ring trial' (e.g. De Winne et al. 2020), multiple observers score the same slides, submitting their results for central review and in some cases for an iterative process to reach a consensus score.

Conceptually this process essentially borrows from those external QC programs, exemplified by NordiQC and UKNEQAS, that require return of stained slides for central review. Laboratory performance is certainly improved by this method as discussed previously. In addition pathologist interpretation and scoring may be greatly improved in studies designed for that purpose; for HER2 in Japan (Umemura et al. 2008), for ER, PR and Ki67 in China (Pu et al. 2019).

13.5 Addition of Immune Cell Assessment

Follow up studies to the conjoint clinical trials of biomarkers and associated companion diagnostics (as reviewed in Part I) led to the realization that in order to maximize the clinical relevance of biomarker test results it was necessary to evaluate (score) the biomarker (e.g. PD L-1) in the context of the immunological background of the tumor, most simply expressed as the nature and extent of any immune infiltrate.

13.5.1 Immune Scoring; Immunoscore

The corollary was that rather than attempting to describe the immune infiltrate in a narrative report, some form of agreed scoring system should be devised to categorize its extent, type and location with respect to tumor. While much of the initial work was focused on colon cancer it is now generally accepted that the concept applies to cancer in general (Galon et al. 2006; Fridman et al. 2012; review, Bruni et al. 2020). From a diversity of proposals one, Immunoscore, has emerged as the forerunner with the tacit support of the international American Joint Committee on Cancer/Union for International Cancer Control (AJCC/UICC), The European Academy of Tumour Immunology (EATI) and many other supporting organization and institutions. More information may be found at the commercially sponsored website (http://www.immunoscore.org/history.shtml).

13.5.2 Composite or Proportion Scores

When the difficulty of separating tumor cells from other cell types expressing the biomarker (e.g. PD L-1 positive macrophages) is extreme, then some clinical trials have bypassed the issue by adopting a 'blended' or 'composite' scoring method, whereby the numerator is taken as all cells showing a positive signal (tumor cells and macrophages and lymphocytes) and the denominator is all the tumor cells; this approach gives something called Tumor Proportion Score (TPS) a Combined Positive Score (CPS), not a true percentage. While something of a scientific anathema, again a threshold is established (in clinical trials) allowing reporting simply as positive or negative, while worrying less about specific cell identification! This approach has given useful correlations in clinical trials, but it is not science. The distinction of tumor cells from immune cells is still of course critically important for determining the denominator in the TPS method, as referenced in the preceding paragraph.

13.5.3 Field of View (FOV) Selection Errors

FOV (ROI) selection is an integral part of most existing scoring methods. Selection bias for which FOVs are chosen can be improved by rules for selection, but not eliminated. The ultimate solution is likely to eliminate the bias of FOV (ROI) selection and to require computer based scoring of a digital whole slide image (WSI), an approach already rendered feasible by the increased scanning and analysis speed of modern systems. For reasons already described whole slide scoring is not possible by eye (Fig. 13.2).

13.6 Phenotypic Cell Identification and Scoring: Multiplex Methods

The above notwithstanding, it is the view of the present authors that a precise assessment of the immune infiltrate extends beyond the compass of H&E morphology alone. Precision scoring of immune cells clearly requires identification by phenotype, as for example by CD3, CD8, CD45 (RO) (lymphocytes and subsets thereof) and CD68 (histiocytes), correlated with precise location of the immune cells, either within the tumor core or at the margins. The Immunoscore website includes illustrations of basic examples of regions and the scoring process (Fig. 13.3).

Multiplex immune-staining, either bright field or by IF (Chap. 14), is capable of much more sophisticated analysis than is possible by any manual observer, including enumeration of cell types by phenotypic identification and by localization, extending to accurate data on cell relationships, such as mean distance of tumor cells from immune cells, elegantly shown by Bernard Fox's group (Feng et al. 2015). These approaches are discussed in more detail in Chap. 14, with reference to multiplex staining methodology and the requirement for digital analysis in order to achieve reproducible results, and are the main theme of Part IV of this book. Multiplex phenotypic methods necessarily incorporate computer-based interpretation and scoring.

13.7 Digital Computerized Scoring Algorithms

Digital algorithms have been developed with a goal of enhanced reproducibility and speed of scoring methods. Initial approaches are illustrated by the digital analysis of ER using the Allred score and a derivative of optical density for intensity of nuclear staining (Ilić et al. 2019). The authors also emphasized what has become the theme for this book, namely the critical need for standardization of the Total Test, particularly fixation and defined criteria for interpretation in order to maximize the value of digital analysis.

The first generation of these computer scoring algorithms for biomarkers (by IHC and IF) suffered from many of the same problems discussed in the preceding paragraphs:

(a) many current algorithms for IHC scoring rely upon manual selection of FOVs by a pathologist prior to scoring (counting). While the actual counts may be reproducible per FOV, the process of FOV selection is not. As noted above, this deficiency can be repaired by whole slide scoring (counting)

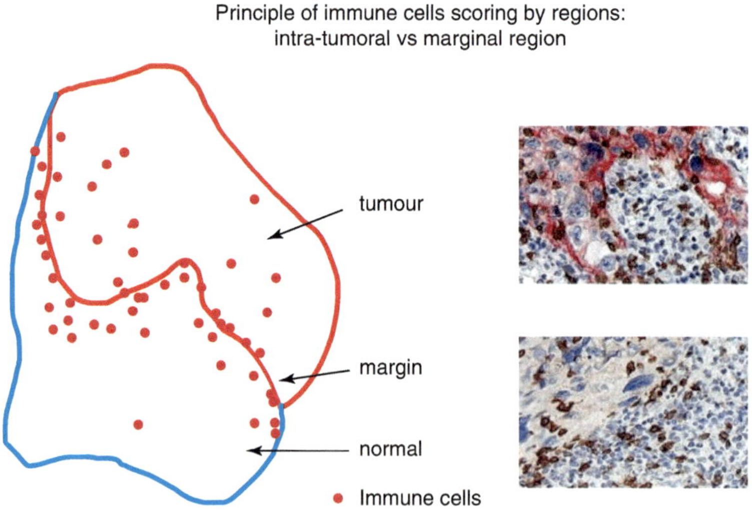

Fig. 13.3 Shows allocation of regions with bright field IHC scoring immune cells by phenotype (CD8, with PD L-1 double stain in red on tumor and immune cells. For further details and examples see the Immunoscore website. http://www.immunoscore.org/research.shtml

(Fig. 13.5), which requires digital whole slide imaging (WSI) as discussed in Part IV.

(b) the problem of separating positive (and negative) tumor cells from normal tissue cells, and from immune cells where necessary, is also inherent in many existing algorithms. This issue is being addressed by two approaches, that can be complementary.

The first is to add phenotypic cell recognition for tumor cells and immune cells in multiplex IHC and IF methods (Figs. 13.3, 13.4, 13.5 and Chap. 14).

The second is by integrating AI and machine learning for enhanced cell identification, often by using phenotypic cell identification in the training phase of the morphometric deep learning recognition process (Fassler et al. 2020; Rivenson et al. 2019; Tan et al. 2020). (Part IV).

(c) in many instances the gold standard to which algorithms have been designed and compared is the eye of the pathologist (or the consensus eye of several pathologists). The intrinsic flaw of this approach is that the derived algorithms can only be as good as the gold stan-

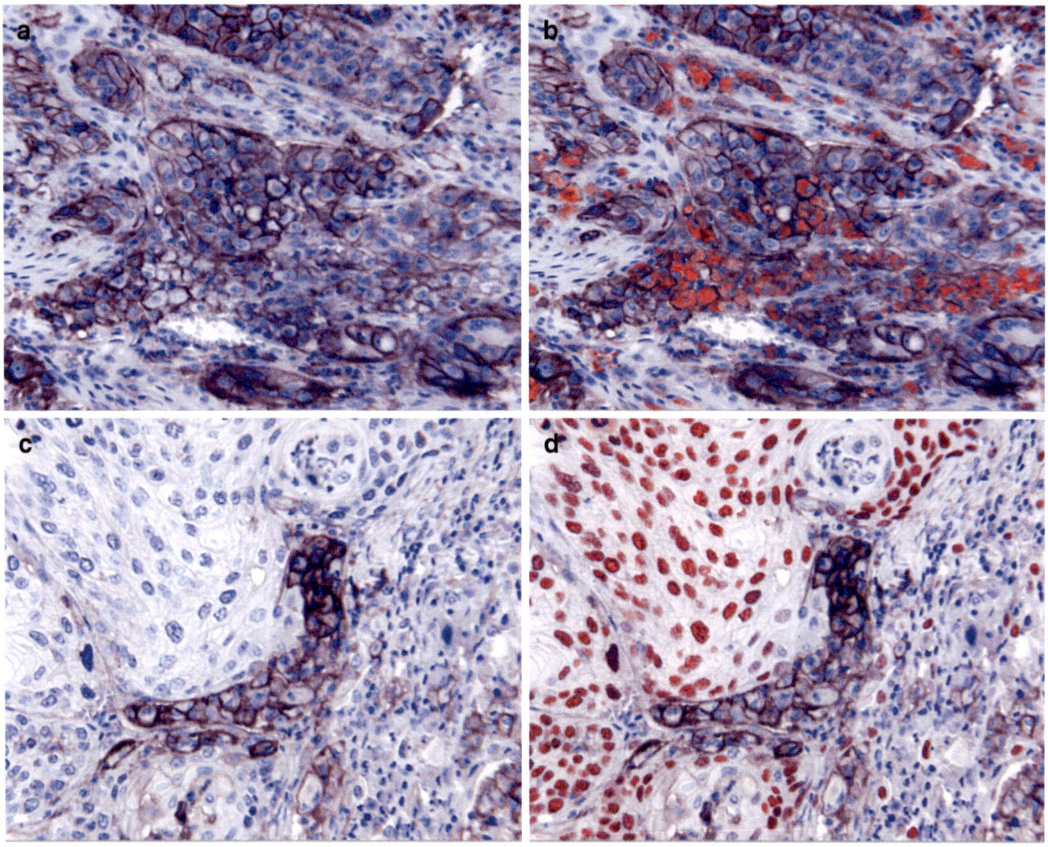

Fig. 13.4 (**a** and **b**) Bright field duplex phenotype by IHC (for multiplex IHC see Chap. 14). Image **a** (left) is an adenocarcinoma of lung showing PD-L1 staining (brown). **b** (right) shows PD-L1 plus CD68 (for histiocytes/macrophages—red). Distinguishing positive tumor cells from positive macrophages in image **a** by morphology alone is impossible. Comparing to image **b**, both the numerator and the denominator would be wrong, although in this strongly positive case they err in the same direction, and the derived score (in this single FOV) might be close to reality, by accident! (**c** and **d**) Bright field duplex phenotype by IHC (for multiplex IHC see Chap. 14). Image **c** (left) is a squamous carcinoma of lung; PD-L1 is brown. A minority of cells are positive and a score of 15% might be hazarded! Image **d** shows IHC staining of tumor (squamous) cell nuclei red by p63. Examination of the brown PD-L1 positive cells, show that none have a red nucleus and none are tumor cells. The PD-L1 score here is zero (Oops!) (Figure from Taylor 2020, by permission of Springer Nature)

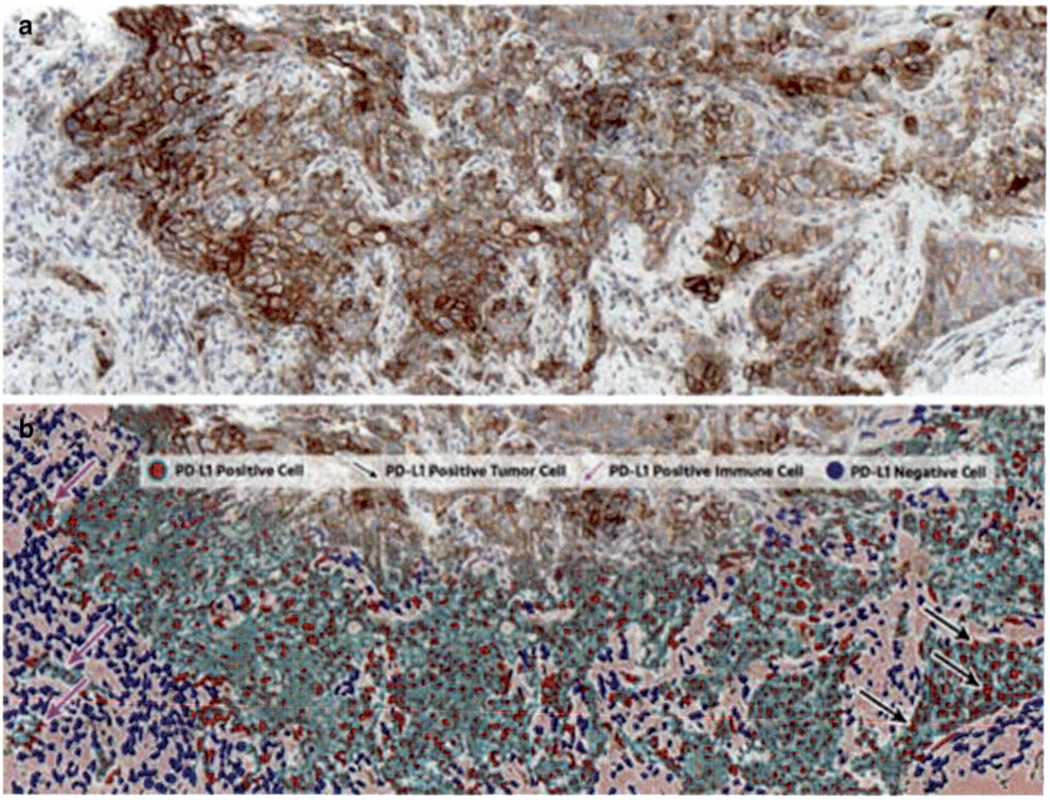

Fig. 13.5 Images show output of an algorithm that incorporates WSI image acquisition, visualization and scoring of biomarker (PD-L1) and machine learning/training for ID of immune cells in a study of 230 Non-small cell lung cancer cases. (**a**) is the raw PD -L1 image; (**b**) the pseudo-colored markup by the algorithm (Case from Dr. David Rimm's laboratory at Yale. Algorithm, OptraScan, California. Taylor et al. 2019, by permission of Wolters Kluwer Health Inc.)

dard pathologist(s); at worse, or better, the algorithm will not be concordant and will be judged to have failed. The standard for judgement in constructing an AI algorithm should be a defined value other than the subjective judgement of pathologists, for example clinical outcome as will be further discussed in Part IV.

References

Aisenberg AC. Comment on lymphoma classification. New Engl J Med. 1977;297:206.

Allred DC, Harvey JM, Berardo M, et al. Prognostic and predictive fctors in breast cancer by IHC analysis. Mod Pathol. 1998;11:115–24.

Bruni D, Angell HK, Galon J. The immune contexture and Immunoscore in cancer prognosis and therapeutic efficacy. Nat Rev Cancer. 2020. https://doi.org/10.1038/s41568-020-0285-7

Daltoé RD, Madeira KP, de Carvalho AA, de Rezende LCD, Silva IV, Rangel LBA. Evaluation of the progesterone receptor status in breast cancer using three different antibodies: a comparison by Allred score system. Int J Clin Exp Pathol. 2013;15:331–9. [Medline]

De Winne K, Sorber L, Lambin S, et al. Immunohistochemistry as a screening tool for NTRK gene fusions: results of a first Belgian ring trial. Virchows Arch. 2020. https://doi.org/10.1007/s00428-020-02921-6

Fassler DJ, Abousamra S, Gupta R, et al. Deep learning-based image analysis methods for brightfield-acquired multiplex immunohistochemistry images. Diagn Pathol. 2020;15:100. https://doi.org/10.1186/s13000-020-01003-0. https://www.leicabiosystems.com/resources/4-tips-for-digital-pathology-slide-scanning/

Fedchenko N, Reifenrath J. Different approaches for interpretation and reporting of immunohistochemistry analysis results in the bone tissue—a review.

Diagn Pathol. 2014;9:221. https://doi.org/10.1186/s13000-014-0221-9.

Feng Z, Puri S, Moudgil T, wood W, Hoyt CC, Wang C, Urba BD, Bifulico CB, Fox BA. Multispectral imaging of formalin-fixed tissue predicts ability to generate tumor-infiltrating lymphocytes from melanoma. J Immunother Cancer. 2015;3:47. https://doi.org/10.1186/s40425-015-0091-z.

Fitzgibbons PL, Dillon DA, Alsabeh R, Berman MA, Hayes DF, Hicks DG, Hughes KS, Nofech-Mozes S. Template for reporting results of biomarker testing of specimens from patients with carcinoma of the breast. Arch Pathol Lab Med. 2014;138:595–601. [Medline]

Fridman WH, Pagès F, Sautès-Fridman C, Galon J. The immune contexture in human tumours: impact on clinical outcome. Nat Rev Cancer. 2012;12:298–306. https://doi.org/10.1038/nrc3245.

Galon J, Costes A, Sanchez-Cabo F, et al. Type, density, and location of immune cells within human colorectal tumors predict clinical outcome. Science. 2006;313(5795):1960–4. https://doi.org/10.1126/science.1129139.

Hammond ME, Hayes DF, Dowsett M, et al. American Society of Clinical Oncology; College of American Pathologists. American Society of Clinical Oncology/College of American Pathologists guideline recommendations for immunohistochemical testing of estrogen and progesterone receptors in breast cancer (unabridged version). Arch Pathol Lab. 2010;134(7):e48–72. [Medline]

Hewitt SM, Robinowitz M, Bogen SA, Gown AM, Kalra KL, Otis CN, Spaulding B, Taylor CR. Quality assurance for design control and implementation of immunohistochemistry assays: approved guidelines, vol. 31. 2nd ed. Wayne, PA: Clinical Lab Standards Institute; 2011. p. 4.

Hirsch FR, Varella-Garcia M, Bunn PA Jr, Di Maria MV, Veve R, Bremmes RM, Baron AE, Zeng C. Franklin w (2003) epidermal growth factor receptor in non-small-cell lung carcinomas: correlation between gene copy number and protein expression and impact on prognosis. J Clin Oncol. 2003;21:3798–807.

Ilić IR, Stojanović NM, Radulović NS, Zivkovic VV, Randelovic PJ, Petrovic AS, Bozic M, Ilic RS. The quantitative ER immunohistochemical analysis in breast cancer: detecting the 3 + 0, 4 + 0, and 5 + 0 allred score cases. Medicina (Kaunas). 2019;55(8):461. https://doi.org/10.3390/medicina55080461.

Immunoscore. n.d. Accessed October 2020. http://www.immunoscore.org/history.shtml

Jasani B, Bänfer G, Fish R, Waelput W, Sucaet Y, Barker C, Whiteley JL, Walker J, Hovelinck R, Diezko R. Evaluation of an online training tool for scoring programmed cell death ligand-1 (PD-L1) diagnostic tests for lung cancer. Diagn Pathol. 2020;15(1):37. https://doi.org/10.1186/s13000-020-00953-9. PMID: 32303234; PMCID: PMC7164334.

Jensen TW, Ray T, Wang J, Li X, Naritoku WY, Han B, Bellafiore F, Bagaria SP, Cui X, Taylor CR, Ray PS. Diagnostic and prognostic value of FOXC1 expression in basal-like breast cancer: an omics-derived subtype-specific biomarker. JNCI. 2015;107(8):djv148. https://doi.org/10.1093/jnci/djv148.

Phillips T, Millett MM, Zhang X, Jansson M, Cleveland R, Simmons P, Cherryholmes G, Carnahan J, William J, Spaulding B, Satnick IR, Inzuna HD, Taylor CR, Cogswell J, Novotny J, Oroudjev E, Winther H. Development of a diagnostic programmed cell death 1-ligand 1 immunohistochemistry assay for Nivolumab therapy in melanoma. Appl Immunohistochem Mol Morph. 2018;26:6–12.

Phillips T, Simmons P, Inzunza HD, Cogswell J, Novotny J, Taylor CR, Zhang X. Development of an automated PD-L1 immunohistochemistry (IHC) assay for non small cell lung cancer. Appl Immunohistochem Mol Morph. 2015;23:541–9. https://doi.org/10.1097/PAI.0000000000000256.

Powsner SM, Costa J, Homer RJ. Clinicians are from mars and pathologists are from venus. Clinician interpretation of pathology reports. Arch Pathol Lab Med. 2000;124:1040–6.

Pu T, Shui R, Shi J, Liang Z, Yang W, Bu H, Li Q, Zhang Z. External quality assessment (EQA) program for the immunohistochemical detection of ER, PR and Ki-67 in breast cancer: results of an interlaboratory reproducibility ring study in China. BMC Cancer. 2019;19:978. https://doi.org/10.1186/s12885-019-6210-3.

Rivenson Y, Wang H, Wei Z, et al. Virtual histological staining of unlabelled tissue-autofluorescence images via deep learning. Nat Biomed Eng. 2019; https://doi.org/10.1038/s41551-019-0362-y. https://bioengineeringcommunity.nature.com/posts/44757-deep-learning-based-virtual-histology-staining-using-autofluorescence-of-label-free-tissue

Tan WCC, Nerurkar SN, Cai HY, Ng HHM, Wu D, Wee YTF, Lim JCT, Yeong J, Lim TKH. Overview of multiplex immunohistochemistry/immunofluorescence techniques in the era of cancer immunotherapy. Cancer Commun (Lond). 2020;40(4):135–53. https://doi.org/10.1002/cac2.12023. https://www.ncbi.nlm.nih.gov/pmc/articles/PMC7170662/

Taylor CR. Predictive biomarkers and companion diagnostics. The future of immunohistochemistry—'in situ proteomics', or just a 'stain'? Appl Immunohistochem Mol Morph. 2014;22:555–61.

Taylor CR. Milestones in immunohistochemistry and molecular morphology. Appl Immunohistochem Mol Morph. 2020;28:83–94.

Taylor CR, Cote RJ, editors. Immunomicroscopy: a diagnostic tool for the surgical pathologist. 3rd ed. Saunders, PA: Elsevier; 2005. (1st edition, Taylor was 1986; 2nd edition, Taylor and Cote was 1994)

Taylor CR, Jadhav AP, Gholap A, Kamble G, Huang J, Gown A, Rimm DL, Doshi I. A multi-institutional study to evaluate automated whole slide scoring of immunohistochemistry for assessment of programmed death-ligand 1 (PD-L1) expression in non-small cell lung cancer. Appl Immunohistochem Mol

Morphol. 2019;27(4):263–9. https://doi.org/10.1097/PAI.0000000000000737.

Umemura S, Osamura RY, Akiyama F, Honma K, Kurosumi M, Sasano H, Toyoshima S, Tsuda H, Ruschoff J, Sakamoto G. What causes discrepancies in HER2 testing for breast cancer? A Japanese ring study in conjunction with the global standard. Am J Clin Pathol. 2008;130:883–91. https://doi.org/10.1309/AJCP5UUMFMA5ZKII.

Willis RA. Pathology of tumours. London: Butterworths; 1948.

14 Immunofluorescence, In Situ Hybridization and Alternative Forms of 'Labeled' Microscopy

14.1 Labeled Microscopy Methods

Biomarker testing has proved a very fertile field for innovation, the development and application of multiple alternative methods for identifying and assessing biomarker expression, in certain cases overlaid with detection and evaluation of any associated immune response. Different methods have differing advantages and disadvantages, including perceived accuracy, performance issues, cost and logistics. Many of these issues have been discussed in preceding chapters, and the choice of test method may simply be governed by what is possible, and affordable. Data relating comparing the pros and cons of the various methods have been well reviewed in a meta-analysis by Lu et al. (2019).

14.2 Immunofluorescence—IF

As discussed earlier in Chap. 1, the immunofluorescence method has its origin some 80 years ago. The immunofluorescence-labeled antibody method exploits the specific binding between antibody and antigen, utilizing antibody labeled with a visible marker, in an exact parallel with IHC. In the first instance the label chosen was fluorescein isothiocyanate (FITC), which with suitable excitation and filters appears as a visible probe in darkfield illumination of tissue sections or cell preparations. The immunofluorescence technique was introduced in the 1940s by the work of Albert Coons, Astrid Fagraeus and others and rapidly developed into powerful research tool. However, the fact that IF was deemed only to work on frozen sections and required darkfield microscopy (Fig. 14.1) meant that the IF technique had little impact on diagnostic pathology, which as practiced by the surgical pathologist was, and is, heavily reliant upon use of "routinely" processed FFPE materials (review; Taylor 2020).

After decades with only limited application IF has quite suddenly undergone a spectacular revival, both as a research tool, exemplified by the tracking of sub-cellular organelles (Valm et al. 2017), but also in cancer pathology for performing multiplex staining of biomarkers and immune cells in cancer. This revival is contingent upon integration of several technical advances including a palette of new brighter fluorophores, improved methods of antibody engineering and labeling, and the advent of sophisticated computer-based digital image analysis that facilitated analysis of the IF stain and application to FFPE sections. These aspects will be reviewed later in this chapter in the subsection 'Emerging Methods.'

B. Jasani et al., *Precision Cancer Medicine*, https://doi.org/10.1007/978-3-030-84087-7_14

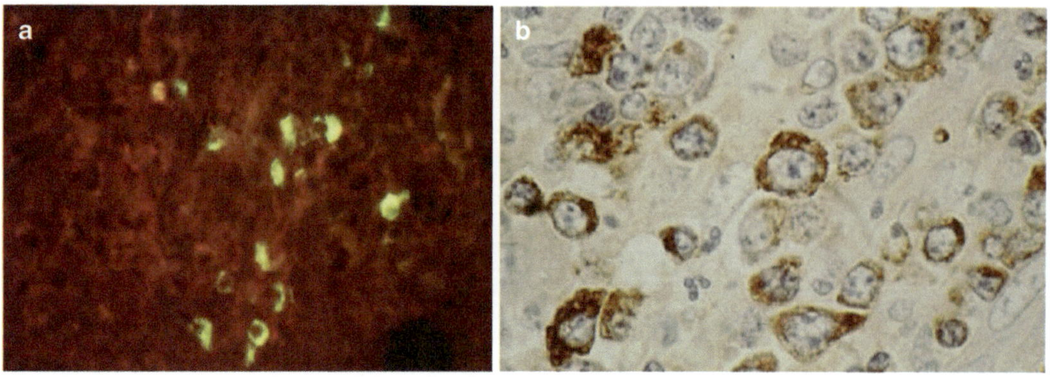

Fig. 14.1 Immunofluorescence (**a**) versus immunoperoxidase (IHC) (**b**) for IgG in plasma cell series. The lack of morphologic detail in the IF frozen section (**a**) as compared to the immunoperoxidase (IHC) stain of an FFPE section (**b**) illustrates the principal reasons for limited use of IF by surgical pathologists until its recent revival using digital imaging methods (vide infra). (Adapted from Taylor and Cote 2005. Fig. 1.3). (This figure was published in Immunomicroscopy, A Diagnostic Tool for the Surgical Pathologist. Eds. Taylor and Cote 2005; by permissions Elsevier)

14.3 In Situ Hybridization—ISH

In-situ-hybridization as a method has many parallels with IHC, in terms of overall principle of employing a system of probes and labels to visualize a specific target within a tissue section (Fig. 14.2). The nature of the probe and target differ; antibody and corresponding antigen for IHC; synthetic nucleotide probe and corresponding complementary RNA or DNA sequence for ISH. Both methods are subject to similar preanalytic and analytic issues, as described at length earlier in this section, including verification, validation and controls apply almost in their entirety and will not be repeated here. Both approaches may use either chromogenic (bright field) labels or fluorescent labels.

Molecular probes used in *in situ* hybridization (ISH) may be double stranded DNA, RNA ('antisense'), or synthetic oligonucleotide sequences, and binding may be DNA-DNA, DNA-RNA, or RNA-RNA; an example of a DNA probe simply diagrammed in Fig. 14.3. Double stranded DNA probes must be rendered single stranded by heating prior to hybridization. ISH can generally be employed in the same cell or tissue environment as IHC; including cytologic preparations, and frozen or formalin paraffin sections, with additional consideration being given to the preservation of the target DNA or RNA.

FISH (fluorescent ISH), the original in situ hybridization method applied to tissue sections, utilizes a fluorescent label, requiring dark field microscopy (see Fig. 14.4a); it is sensitive and reagents are widely available. CISH (chromogenic ISH) employs enzymatic labels and a variety of chromogens to convert the basic method to light microscopy, analogous to IHC (Fig. 14.4b). In CISH the nucleic acid probes are labeled either with digoxigenin or biotin, and then demonstrated after specific localization in the tissue sections with anti-digoxigenin or anti-biotin antibodies respectively, followed by signal amplification much as for IHC. With the advent of these highly 'sensitive' detection methods the overall sensitivity of CISH is comparable to FISH, and may be employed in double stains with IHC.

In general, nucleic acids (like proteins) are better preserved in fresh frozen sections, fixed for up to 1 h (e.g., in 4% formaldehyde or 1% glutaraldehyde) prior to hybridization. If FFPE sections are employed, the procedures used for AR in IHC (e.g. 10 minutes at 100 °C by microwave, in pH 6.0 citrate buffer) produce both increased sensitivity (here meaning detection of low levels of target) and better reproducibility for ISH methods. With biotinylated probes and chromogenic labels the same concerns exist for endogenous biotin, endogenous peroxidase, and alkaline

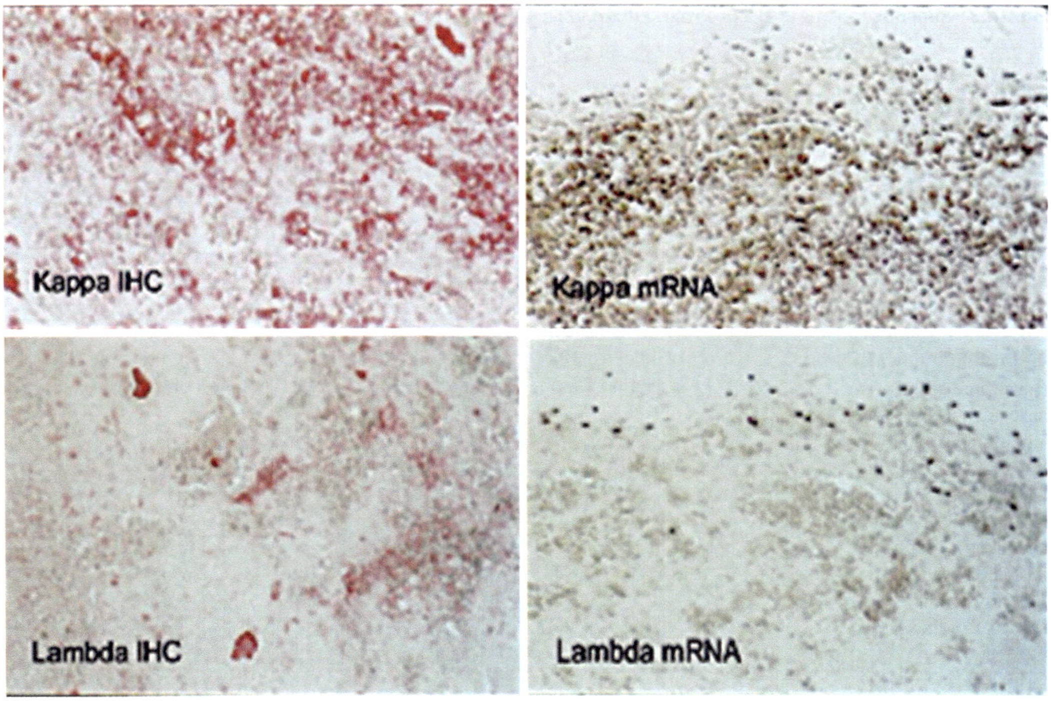

Fig. 14.2 IHC and CISH for kappa and lambda light chains; the stain results appear similar*, IHC demonstrating plasma cells by use of antibodies to target kappa and lambda proteins; ISH demonstrating plasma cells by use of nucleotide probes to target kappa and lambda RNA. Both methods use DAB as the chromogen on FFPE sections. (Adapted from Taylor and Cote 2005). *Note one difference in appearance is that the IHC method stains serum in vessels by labeling kappa and lambda protein in circulating immunoglobulins; while ISH (labeling RNA) does not stain vessels. (This figure was published in Immunomicroscopy, A Diagnostic Tool for the Surgical Pathologist. Eds. Taylor and Cote 2005; by permissions Elsevier)

phosphatase as in IHC and the blocking methods to inhibit such are the same (Chap. 8).

A further complication exists with regard to RNA, namely the rapid degradation of RNA by tissue RNAases, which may occur during warm and cold ischemia and must be effectively inhibited immediately the tissue is removed (e.g. by formamide). Note that RNA probes, as well as intrinsic tissue RNA (target) may be digested by any residual active tissue RNAases. While RNAases are inactivated by formalin fixation, it is worth noting that the use of AR to 'recover' the integrity of RNA target, may also restore the activity of the RNAase enzyme, re-establishing the RNA digestion process and leading to unexpected false negative results.

Controls are analogous to those used in IHC (Chaps. 10 and 11), with the potential addition of another negative control, namely eradication of the target DNA or RNA by pretreatment with DNAases or RNAases.

ISH reagents and methods are well developed commercially, especially for virus specific sequences of EBV, HPV, HSV and CMV, but have been rapidly expanded into the field of biomarkers (Her 2, N-myc, C-myc). ISH methods may be employed simultaneously, or sequentially, with IHC methods to yield a variety of double staining results, some of which have been exploited commercially in combined ISH/IHC biomarker tests (review American Society of Clinical Oncology (ASCO)/College of American Pathologists (CAP) guideline status, Ahn et al. 2020).

In addition, just as IHC stains may be combined to produce double or triple stains (multiplexed), so ISH probes may be combined to produce double or triple ISH stains. This offers

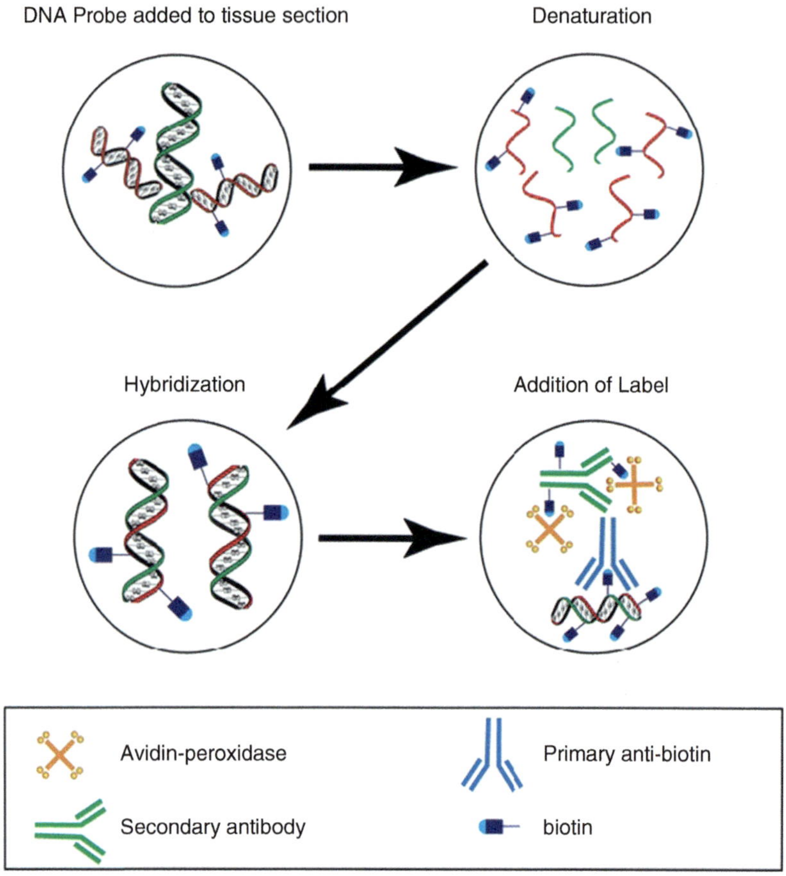

Fig. 14.3 Simplified diagram of the chromogenic ISH (CISH) method employing a DNA probe with ABC amplification. Today fluorescent labels are more widely employed, particularly with the advent of digital imaging for scoring and analysis. For IHC compare with Fig. 9.1. Amplification and detection methods also have advanced. (From Taylor and Cote 2005, Fig. 1.20) (This figure was published in Immunomicroscopy, A Diagnostic Tool for the Surgical Pathologist. Eds. Taylor and Cote 2005; by permissions Elsevier)

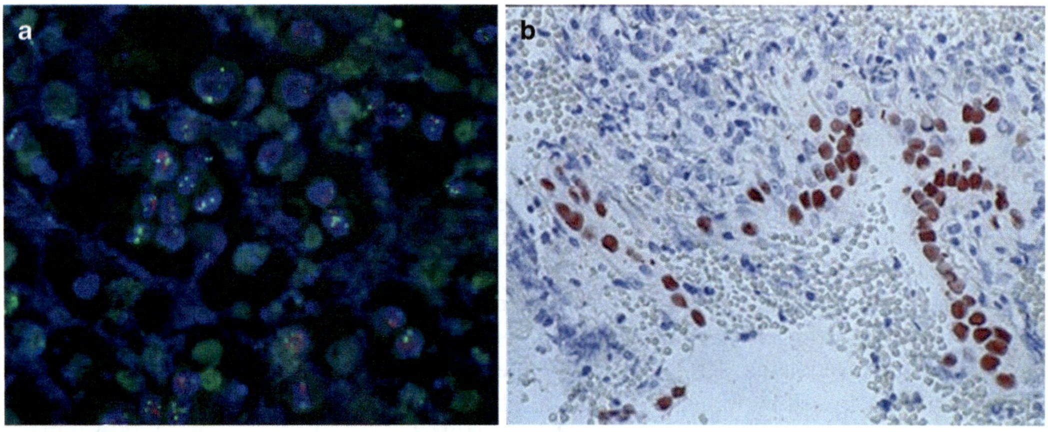

Fig. 14.4 (**a**) Shows FISH for HER2 (red) and CEP chr 17 (green) viewed directly by the usual darkfield illumination. Digital image analysis increasingly is used for viewing and scoring FISH (vide infra). (**b**) Shows CISH for human papilloma virus types 16, 18, 33 and 35. Both are FFPE sections following appropriate 'antigen retrieval.' (Adapted from Taylor and Cote 2005, Fig. 1.22). (This figure was published in Immunomicroscopy, A Diagnostic Tool for the Surgical Pathologist. Eds. Taylor and Cote 2005; by permissions Elsevier)

a variety of possibilities in sequential or simultaneous staining methods providing that the reagents are properly optimized at both probe and detection steps. The combining of two sequence specific probes, one labeled with digoxigenin, the other with biotin allows the demonstration of translocations, such as 8; 14 (8; 22, 2; 8) in Burkitt lymphoma, or 11; 22 in Ewing's tumor, by double staining methods. Multiplex ISH is expanding rapidly facilitated by the RNAscope approach, described later in this chapter (vide infra).

In general, when an ISH stain for an RNA target is part of the multiple ISH (of IHC combination) stain, then it is performed first in an attempt to reduce the possibility of digestion of the target RNA by RNAases following antigen retrieval. Chromogenic and radioisotope labeled probes may also be employed in multiple label methods and just as with IHC gold particles may serve as labels, which extends the applicability of ISH to electron microscopic examination.

Extending the parallels with IHC, methods have been developed to extend the sensitivity of ISH methods as in the demonstration of HER-2 amplification. Whereas IHC demonstrates the end product, namely HER-2 protein, ISH methods may demonstrate both messenger RNA expression and the extent of HER-2 gene amplification. A variety of ISH amplification methods are available (*vide infra*), the most effective of which enhance sensitivity by amplification at the signal end of the process, using methods analogous to those applied in IHC, such as tyramide amplification and polymeric label systems (Chap. 9). Chromogenic methods (CISH) under extreme levels of amplification (sensitivity) may show local 'diffusion' of the colored reaction product, as a result, of which it may be difficult to count precisely the number of labeled moieties present (i.e. the number of amplified copies of HER-2). In this regard fluorescent *in situ* hybridization (FISH), which is the usual method for detecting HER-2 is superior. Methods using colloidal gold labels (whimsically termed GOLDFISH—Ray Tubbs et al. 2013 personal communication and see Tubbs et al. 2013) do provide a non-fluorescent method of amplified ISH that maintains discreet target labeling, so permitting accurate counting of the amplification copies. The text edited by Hauptmann (2015) provides an excellent resource for those readers wishing further to pursue technical aspects of ISH.

Reporting of ISH based biomarker tests follows the same guidelines as for IHC, including provision in Synoptic report formats.

14.4 RNA Scope

As with IHC, there have been ongoing attempts to enhance the detection sensitivity of ISH (Wang et al. 2012; Tubbs et al. 2013; Hauptmann 2015). RNAscope® (https://acdbio.com/rnascope®-basescope™-and-mirnascope™assay) was launched as a proprietary, highly sensitive, enhanced ISH method that employs specially designed nucleotide probes together with a signal amplification cascade. Signal detection can be by brightfield microscopy using chromogenic labels, or more commonly by IF (epifluorescence) with a variety of fluorophores available for multiplexing. Detection sensitivity at the level of a single molecule is claimed under ideal conditions. Specificity is enhanced by a design that requires two separate specific probes to bind to the target molecule for signal amplification to occur, an approach that at the same time reduces non-specific background.

The pre-analytic issues described above for IHC (Chaps. 5, 6 and 7) apply equally to the RNAscope method, with the noted additional concerns regarding preservation of RNA. The design of the probe is, however, calculated to target relatively short RNA nucleotide sequences (40–50) such that partially degraded RNA also can be detected specifically. The RNAscope method has been applied successfully both to frozen sections and to FFPE sections, and the stained slides can be visualized under either a standard bright-field microscope (with chromogenic labels) or an epifluorescent microscope (with fluorescent labels). The RNAscope approach allows multiplex detection of four or more target genes (limited only by the number of spectrally discernible fluorescent dyes). The ability to ana-

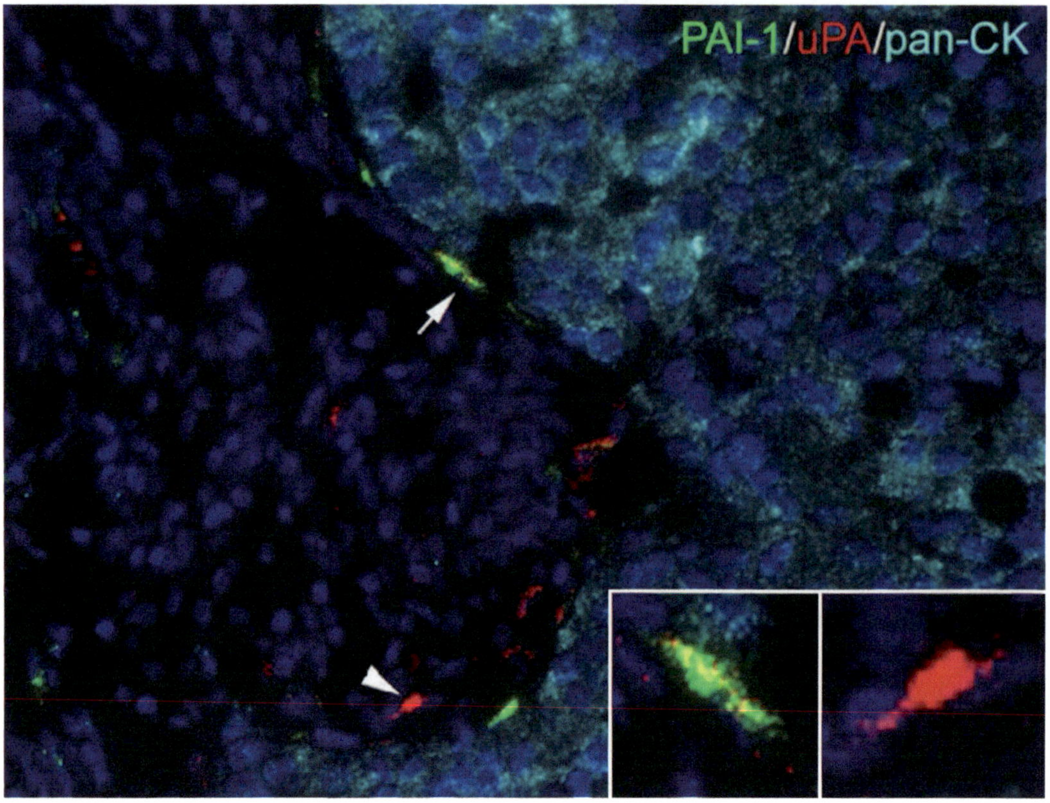

Fig. 14.5 RNAscope image showing the potential of the method; fluorescent labels, showing PAI-1 (Alexa fluor 488), uPA (Alexa fluor 546) and Pan Keratins (Alexa fluor 647) mRNAs in breast cancer. (From Wang et al. 2012, permission of Springer Nature)

lyze gene expression *in situ* in routine clinical specimen types, as well as high sensitivity and specificity, makes RNAscope a promising platform for translating many RNA biomarkers into clinical use (Fig. 14.5).

14.5 Advanced Multiplex Microscopy and Other Emerging Methods

14.5.1 Brightfield (IHC) Versus Immunofluorescence (IF) Methods

Multiplex testing of biomarkers and immune cells has proved its value in cancer immunotherapy research and is finding its way into routine practice, for two principal reasons.

Firstly, the method permits assessment of multiple antigens at the same time in the same section, including biomarkers of predictive interest, side by side with phenotypic markers to improve cell identification, including analysis of the extent and location of the immune response. Data suggest that multiplex IF methods are more effective in this respect than either IHC alone, of gene expression profiling (Lu et al. 2019).

Secondly multiplex methods allow evaluation of quantifiable controls alongside biomarker of interest that are present in unknown amounts, as part of true quantification ('in-situ-proteomics') (Chap. 11).

The identification of two or more markers (antigens) in FFPE tissues may of course be accomplished by IHC staining of adjacent serial sections from the same tissue block, then comparing the serial sections, but for intimately mixed cell populations and instances of co-localization of biomarkers markers on individual cells, multiplex staining of a single section is much more powerful. Also, as biopsies become ever smaller, and demands for testing ever greater, then multiplex methods allow more efficient use of limited tissue.

For several decades, traditional IHC-ISH immunoenzymatic techniques have permitted the demonstration of two or more targets concurrently within a single section (Fig. 14.6) (review; Taylor and Cote 2005). Many good quality commercial reagents are available to meet this purpose, exploiting primary antibodies of differing species and appropriate polymer linking reagents conjugated with peroxidase or alkaline phosphatase labels. Also multiple differently colored chromogens now are available and the method can be extended to three or four plex, beyond which cross reactivity intrudes and the resultant smorgasbord of colors become impossible to interpret by the pathologist's eye. Technologic advantages in spectral imaging have been employed to assist interpretation, where the eye, unaided, cannot. The major advantage over multiplex IF staining is that the morphologic details are better preserved in the and the colored reaction products are permanent for repeat examination.

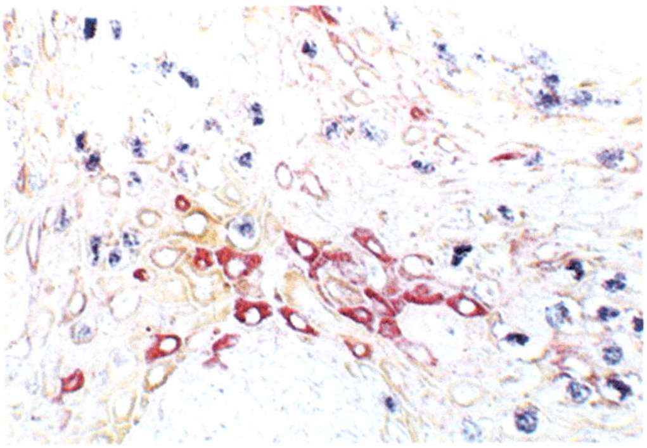

Fig. 14.6 Triple IHC-ISH stain. Double IHC stain for high and low molecular weight keratins (brown-DAB and red—AEC respectively) combined with ISH for HPV (blue -alkaline phosphatase—BBN). (Adapted from Taylor and Cote 2005, Fig. 2.17). (This figure was published in Immunomicroscopy, A Diagnostic Tool for the Surgical Pathologist. Eds. Taylor and Cote 2005; by permissions Elsevier)

However, technologic advances of digital image analysis have provided huge benefit to the IF method, allowing creation of virtual bright field imagery from the IF data, such that it is now the most commonly applied technology for multiplex studies, beyond the practical limits of a two or three plex achievable by bright field IHC.

In addition, there are emerging new approaches to multiplex labeling of biomarkers in FFPE tissue sections that do not depend upon use of fluorescent (or chromogenic IHC) labels. Two methods warrant brief description here, MIBI microscopy (multiplex ion beam imaging) and RMS (Raman Micro-spectroscopy). For both methods there is a growing background of research data that support their potential value. For both methods there are obstacles that presently inhibit emergence into routine use, partly technical, and partly related to cost, logistics and regulatory issues.

A plethora of other methods that seek to exploit and expand digital microscopy (microimaging), such as light sheets, 3D microscopy, MALDI-MS microscopy, near infra-red microscopy, lens-less microscopy and STM (scanning tunnel electron microscopy), for which practical diagnostic application is more remote in time and less certain, will be touched on in Part IV.

Bright field (light microscope) images, as in IHC, have advantages over IF methods in terms of correlating labeling with the conventional morphologic criteria that form the basis of anatomic pathology diagnosis (see Fig. 13.4a–d).

14.5.2 Multiplex Digital IF

Immunofluorescence (IF) as a practical method for surgical pathology has been resurrected by the development of epifluorescence techniques, a broad palette of new brighter fluorophores, effective amplification methods and the advent of integrated computer-based digital image analysis, which together have facilitated multiplex IF staining of FFPE sections. In particular digital technics of spectral unmixing and color segregation facilitate multiplex display and the creation of virtual bright field H&E or IHC brightfield-like images that restore morphologic interpretation (albeit of a manipulated image) (Fig. 14.8). These remarkable capabilities shared with one of the authors (CRT) a decade ago (Personal communication -Clifford Hoyt) have been followed by extension of computerized imaging and analysis into many fields, such as generating an H&E by transillumination epi-fluorescence without ever cutting a tissue section (Giacomelli et al. 2016), or extending to the reverse process of converting an H&E stained slide to a simulated fluorescent image (Burlingame et al. 2019).

The intensity of the fluorescent signal also has more of a direct linear relationship with level of target expression (than does IHC/DAB intensity) which lends to accurate quantification by digital analysis when using appropriate controls (as discussed in Chap. 11). Technical reviews of multiplex IF may be found elsewhere (Lin et al. 2018; Taube et al. 2020), the latter being an excellent 'best practices' review for both multiplex IHC and IF. The purpose of the present book is to retain focus on the advantages and limitations of the use of these methods for cancer biomarkers, diagnostically, with emphasis on prognostic and predictive applications.

There are two main approaches to multiplex IF, one of which applies the reagents sequentially, the other where multiple primary antibodies are added simultaneously, with a second step being the addition of the multiple labelling reagents. Each of these approaches had advantages and disadvantages that will be discussed briefly.

14.5.2.1 The Sequential Method

The sequential method has been in use for a decade or more (Figs. 14.7 and 14.8). Primary antibodies derived from different species and directed against a different biomarker are selected and validated. Each primary antibody is then applied separately to the section and each then is labeled with the appropriate secondary link antibody and amplification system before a final washing. The second primary antibody and its corresponding (differently colored) label are then added, and so forth, for the third and fourth (or more) pairs of primary antibodies and labels. For each primary antibody and secondary label, the completed protocol (Total Test) must be separately validated, exactly as described in Chaps. 9 and 10.

In practice it is not this simple. The multiple validated protocols are run sequentially, but then must be validated again after the multiplex staining is completed to provide assurance that there is no cross reactivity and no loss of sensitivity for target detection, when compared to each step run separately. Practical experience shows that the sequence in which the various primary antibody/fluorophore label pairs are applied has an impact on relative intensity of staining observed for each step in the final multiplex stain; once optimized therefore the sequence should not be changed. In order to boost the fluorescent signal for digital scanning and for viewing, powerful amplification

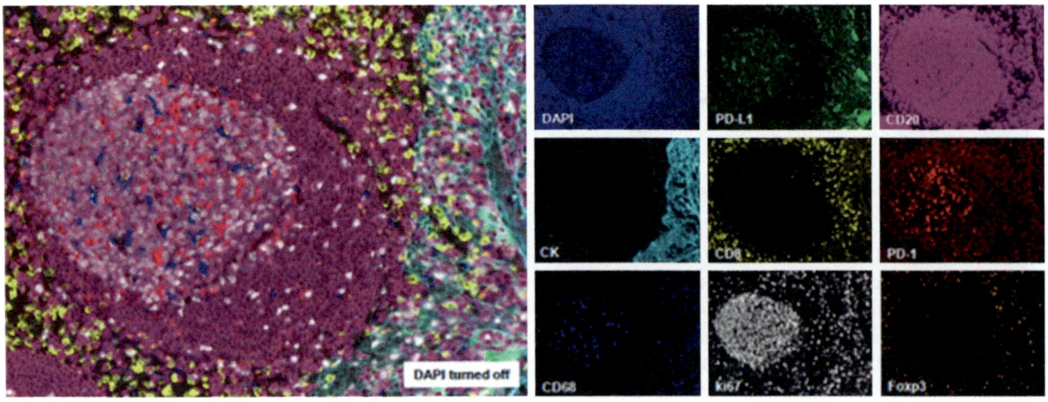

Fig. 14.7 Multiplex 9 color IF; mixed sequential and simultaneous labeling method (Courtesy of Cliff Hoyt, Akoya Biosciences)

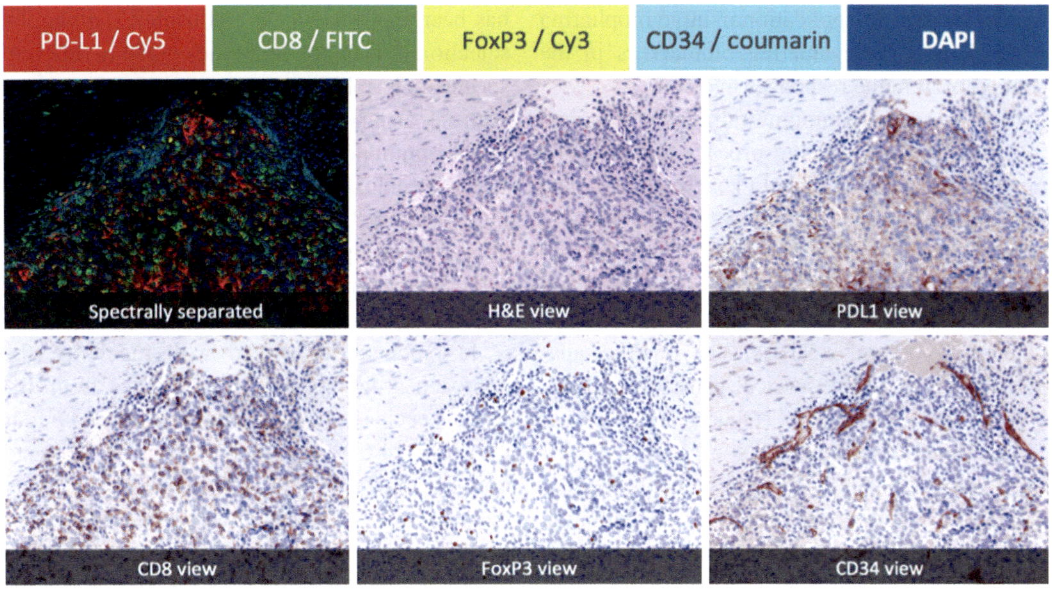

Fig. 14.8 Multiplex IF showing spectral separation and conversion to 'simulated H&E', plus simulated brightfield IHC as separate stains as shown in the work of Bernard Fox and colleagues, Portland, Oregon in studies with PerkinElmer using the Vectra system with Inform software. https://www.perkinelmer.com/PDFs/downloads/PRD-Quantify-Biomarkers-in-Tissue-Sections.pdf (Courtesy of Cliff Hoyt, Akoya Biosciences)

methods are used, such as tyramide or catalytic signal amplification, (Chap. 9), which can be difficult to control and reproduce and demand still higher levels of performance controls.

A sequential 5 (or 6) plex stain requires the performance of 5 (or 6) successive complete protocols, one for each primary antibody (although in some systems two steps can be combined into one as described below; see also Fig. 14.8). The staining process is, therefore, very labor intensive and time consuming, and is only likely to be reproducible if performed on an automated staining platform. It requires two or more working days for completion. To this must be added the time necessary for scanning the fluorescent staining product(s), which is itself very variable according to the type of scanner employed (speed and resolution), whether the whole slide is scanned (WSI) or only selected fields of view, and whether scanning is conducted only once when the multiplex is completed, or multiple times, once after each stain protocol. In the latter instance the product of the preceding stain is imaged, then stripped and bleached; multiplexing then is performed at the level of the software integrating the successive digital images.

Just how far this approach can be stretched is illustrated by the 60 plex staining of FFPE sections conducted by Lin et al. (2018) using successive cycles (three antigens in each cycle, with hydrogen peroxide bleaching), imaging after each cycle and ending with an H&E stain, prior to assembly of the multiple images into a composite for segmentation and analysis. After the first few antibodies all the remaining primary reagents were directly conjugated to avoid cross reactivity. The authors noted that each cycle took 6–8 h implying that completion required 2 weeks or more, not including time, effort and cost of direct conjugation of multiple primary antibodies. Also, by the end of the process the cell quality was deteriorating, so clearly there are limits, and the method has no practical service application.

The above discussion serves to emphasize that the IF sequential multiplex method is extremely powerful in exploring biomarkers and immune response in cancer and five or six plex stains may have a more routine place in clinical management (Lee et al. 2019) supplementing bright filed methods which are easier to visualize directly (e.g. Tumeh et al. 2014). Multiplex IF also is finding increasing application in large biopharma research labs for evaluating biomarkers in the context of immune responses in cancer.

However, at a minimum multiplex IF requires integration of the staining process for each primary antibody and its label (The Total Test), the scanning hardware and software, the spectral imaging and analysis software and the digital display, plus sophisticated QA of the completed multiplex protocol. Meeting these requirements, in terms of cost and expertise, is beyond the capability of all but a few surgical pathology service laboratories and also most research labs.

A number of commercial sources have developed and integrated the key components for successful performance of multiplex IF staining, including reagents, protocol, scanning hardware and software. Some also have combined IHC brightfield protocols (using HRP) with the IF method and with ISH, relying upon spectral unmixing to separate and display signals (Fig. 14.8) (review; Foldesi 2020). The authors collectively have experience of several of these commercial multiplex systems. It is not the intent here to recommend any one over the others. However, it is strongly recommended that one of these commercial integrated systems be selected, trialed in house and validated for the intended use, in preference to attempts to develop any de novo in house system, for which validation is exhaustive and exhausting.

14.5.2.2 The Simultaneous Method

The simultaneous method, in which a cocktail of multiple primary antibodies is added as a single step, followed by a single multi-specific detection step, greatly reduces the technical complexity of multiplex staining, essentially yielding a single protocol, with the major advantage of reducing technical staining time to within a single day. Success of this approach is heavily dependent upon the quality and availability of reagents; particularly specially paired primary and secondary labeling reagents. The secondary labeling (or linker) antibody that is selected for each primary antibody must have zero cross reactivity for any of the other primary antibodies. As noted above, for several decades this requirement has been met for duplex and triplex staining, by selection of primary antibodies made in different species (e.g. rabbit and mouse) and pairing each with secondary antibody specific for rabbit or mouse immunoglobulin respectively (see Figs. 13.4a–d and 14.6). This approach can also be integrated into the sequential IF process described above, reducing the total number of sequential protocols by combining two otherwise sequential steps into one.

In practical terms and with ingenuity, the approach utilizing primary antibodies from different species can be extended to three or four plex (Fig. 14.6), but beyond that is difficult due to limited choice of primary/secondary antibody pairs from species that show no cross reactivity for detection (review; Taylor and Cote 2005). For IF this problem has largely been resolved by the chemical conjugation of unique 'tags' (haptens or DNA tags) to different primary antibodies, coupled with generation of secondary antibodies specific to the 'tags' (regardless of the species type of the primary antibody), each of which is then linked to a differently colored fluorophore. Using this method, it has been possible successfully to perform six or even ten plex IF staining (see Fig. 3.5 and 14.10). A limited number of commercial sources are available for these reagents, which for successful application require sophisticated arrays of filters, plus digital scanning and spectral analysis software. As with the sequential method meeting these requirements, particularly the generation of an array of validated hapten or DNA tagged antibodies, is beyond the capability of all but a few surgical pathology service laboratories, and recourse to one of the proven vendors is recommended.

Another adaptation of this approach, similar in concept, is to use molecular engineering techniques to generate a range of primary antibodies each of which incorporates a unique epitope (signature epitope- SigerMabs) that does not occur in nature. Each of these antibodies can be constructed to be antigenically unique and has no cross-reacting epitopes in nature. The corresponding secondary antibodies can then be prepared with very high specificity. Sigermabs provide an example of this approach (Fig. 14.9).

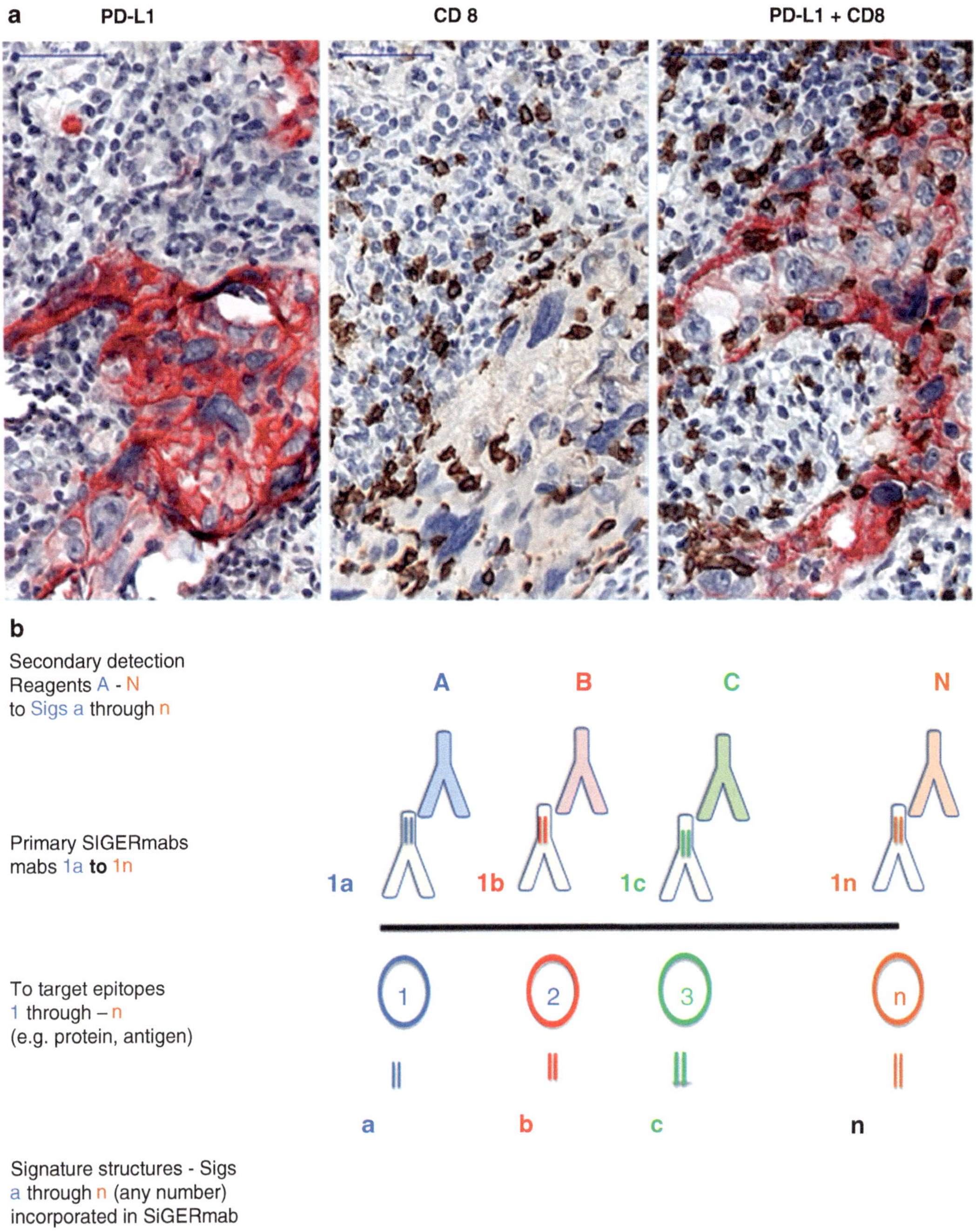

Fig. 14.9 (**a**) An example of the simultaneous approach, both primary antibodies are added at the same time; similarly, the labeling reagents are added together, giving a rapid multiplex procedure. (**b**) Illustrates the principle by which each primary antibody is bioengineered to contain a unique sequence targeted by the specially prepared secondary reagents. The 'signature' sequences are unique in nature, greatly reducing cross reactivity or unanticipated bonding of the labeling antibodies (Study result of collaboration—Jacinto Villaneuva, Calico Labs (now Abcam) and Taylor labs, 2017)

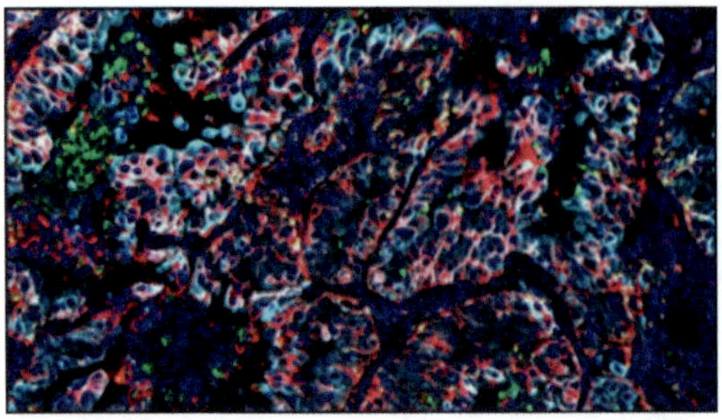

Fig. 14.10 Multiplex image with Ultivue system—non-small cell lung cancer: PD-L1 (red), Pan-CK (cyan), CD68 (yellow), CD8 (green), nuclear counterstain (blue). (Permission of Mark Rees, Vice President, Ultivue, Cambridge, MA). https://ultivue.showpad.com/share/5Qgdm3MPmo4y2cFNCYKbf/0)

DNA labeling (or barcoding) methods are commercially available (e.g. Ultivue, Cambridge, MA, www.ultivue.com) and show similar capabilities to 10 and 12 plex panels, coupled with whole slide imaging techniques and computer based image analysis and quantification (Fig. 14.10).

The authors collectively have experience of several of these multiplex systems, previewed here as an appetizer for more comprehensive treatment in Part IV of this book. No one system of method is advocated over the others, but it is strongly recommended that one of these commercial products be selected, inclusive of scanning hardware and analysis software, trialed in house and then validated for the intended use.

Validation is demanding but essential, and follows the same guidelines already set forth in Chaps. 9, 10, 11, 12 and in Part III. In the specific context of multiplex staining, the necessary steps in setting up the test and validating individual reagents, protocols and the final Total Test result are reviewed by Parra et al. (2017) and Taube et al. (2020). The latter review is comprehensive and includes both IHC and IF, with a comparison of the relative merits of each method.

14.6 MIBI Microscopy (Multiplex Ion Beam Imaging)

MIBI microscopy does not use either chromogenic or fluorescence labels, but instead relies upon metal label probes with ion beam excitation and detection by adapted mass spectrometry methods. Using a derivative MIBI method Levenson and colleagues (2015) illustrated a ten-plex panel of breast markers in bright field with a resolution claimed to be comparable to orthodox light microscopy (Fig. 14.11). All labels were applied in a single step and detected in a single imaging procedure. The potential exists for multiplexes of 40 or more markers, with high sensitivity and specificity and stable product was discussed.

The enormous potential of this technology was made manifest by Keren and colleagues who demonstrated a 36 plex method (Keren et al. 2019). The huge amount of data generated by this method when coupled with sophisticated digital analysis for PD-L1 and immune cell labeling is well illustrated in the published manuscript.

There are of course caveats and obstacles to be surmounted. The MIBI labeling method is not immune from the pre-analytic issues that apply to IHC and IF (Chaps. 4, 5, 6, 7, and 8) and the rigors of analytic validation and control, including reagents and protocol, apply equally or more so; in fact they are multiplexed! (Chaps. 9, 10, 11, and 12). Issues for future resolution include establishing that each the multiple labeling reagents and protocols is optimal (or at least sufficient) for the target molecule in question. A single labeling step is wonderful in terms of time and effort, but it means that a single AR procedure is used for all targets, with no warranty that AR is optimal for any one protein, or all. Instrumentation remains complex and very expensive, which alone precludes routine deployment at present.

14.7 Raman Microscopy (Vibrational) Spectroscopy (RMS)

Raman microscopy has the potential for development into a routinely useful label free method of antigen detection that may be adapted to FFPE tissues, but also is effective with more minimal approaches to tissue sample preparation (frozen sections). The Raman microscope integrates a light or confocal microscope with a laser excita-

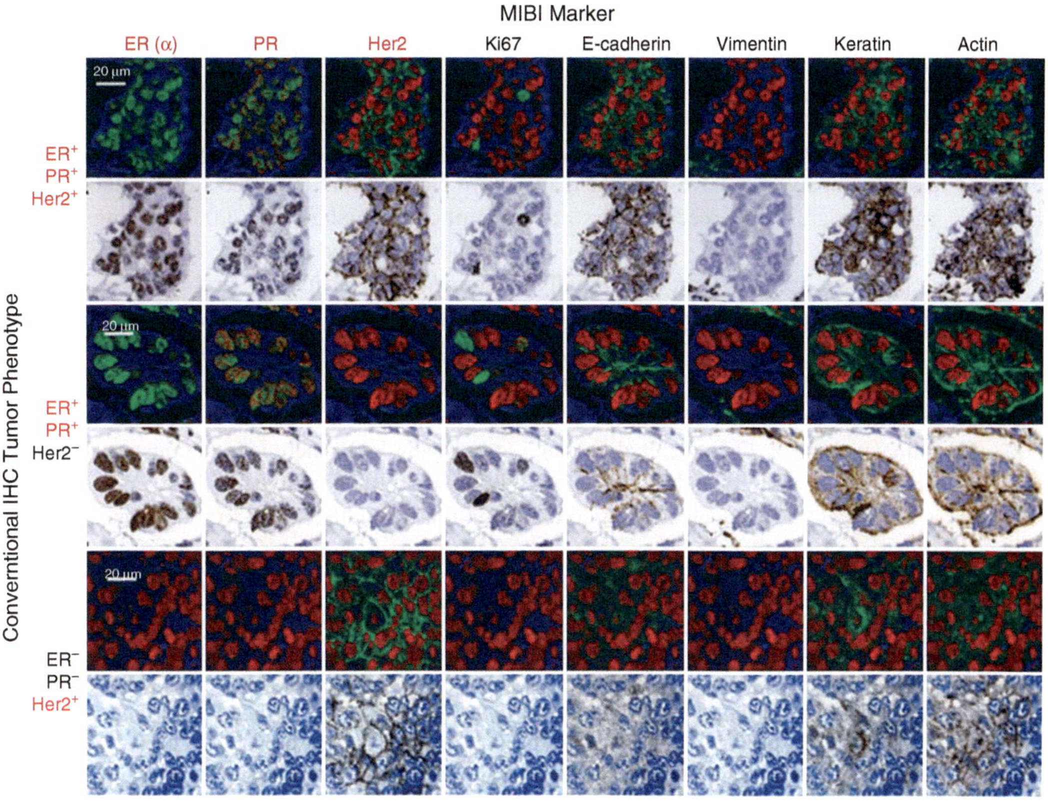

Fig. 14.11 MIBI multiplex imaging showing eight markers: HER2, ER, PR, Ki67, E-cadherin, vimentin, keratin and actin, each displayed in the appropriate subcellular location. Field of view.80 mm^2 (From Levenson et al. 2015) (Figure by permission of Springer Nature)

tion system, a series of filters, a spectrometer and a computer for signal detection, analysis and display.

As with MIBI (multiplex ion beam imaging), RMS has the potential for simultaneous detection and display of multiple antigens (and other molecules) beyond the compass of bright field IHC, rivalling or exceeding multiplex immunofluorescence methods. RMS is able to generate molecular and biochemical maps of tissue sections, both spatial and by quantity of component molecules with high levels of specificity and sensitivity. Objective cellular examination at a molecular level (Molecular Morphology) is a holy grail for anatomic pathology. RMS is claimed to have that potential, while at the same time offering the option of avoiding many pre-analytic issues (such as fixation and sectioning) and obviating subjective interpretation by pathologists. Integrated with a suitable spectroscopic digital display RMS can also generate realistic virtual H&E images for reference to the surgical pathology Gold Standard (the glass slide H&E).

The basis for the method itself is not new (Raman and Krishnan 1928). The spectroscopic scattering effects in tissues were documented in the 1960s (review; Kong et al. 2015). Application in biology was initially complicated by numerous variables, with slow acquisition and display of signal a particular problem. Entry into the clinical mainstream was also hampered by high technical demands in terms of types of lasers that could be readily deployed in surgical pathology laboratories, a problem which for many years translated into high cost, limited availability and very limited clinical experience.

However, the availability of new near-infrared fiber lasers, coupled with strategies for integrating spectroscopic data, accelerated development of computer hardware and software, and the advent of digital technology, image analysis and machine learning capabilities have combined to facilitate rapid progress in recent years, as reviewed in Part IV.

Over the past two decades there is a rapidly expanding literature for RMS across many fields, extending into biology, pathology and biomarkers (Kong et al. 2015 [Fig. 14.12]). Forays into the field of cancer diagnosis (Chowdary et al. 2007; Gaifulina et al. 2014; Orringer et al. 2017), have led to claims of sensitivity and specificity of diagnosis at well over 90% for detection of colon cancer. Comparisons also have been made with IHC, as by Lewis et al. (2018), who showed excellent correlation (again greater than 90%) for desmin, KI67 and MUC2 in specimens of human colon without the need for staining or for antibodies. Quantification of biomarkers (e.g. HER2, Heier et al. 2021) also has been demonstrated.

The advantages claimed for Raman Spectroscopy include applicability to relatively thick tissue slices as well as orthodox frozen and FFPE sections, together with an interesting capability for tracking the chemical modification of proteins that occurs in fixation. While there are reports that RMS is less affected by fixation in terms of detection and display of proteins, others have claimed that the effects of formalin can be significant (Huang et al. 2003), leading to a recommendation for use of fresh tissues. This recommendation is itself a problem in biomarker analysis, because fresh tissues generally are not available and are subject to the same major logistical issues that for decades hampered growth of IF methods. In the many published studies employing RMS there is little consensus as to an optimal protocol for a method of sample preparation that would be suited to routine use, whether for fresh non-processed or FFPE tissues (Huang et al. 2003). Importantly there is little comparative validation among the various approaches. Similarly, there is no uniformity in how the sample is presented to the Raman device for spectroscopic analysis (thickness, size, practical application to slide etc.).

Raman micro-spectroscopy devices themselves, continue to undergo rapid technical development, becoming more compact, easier to use

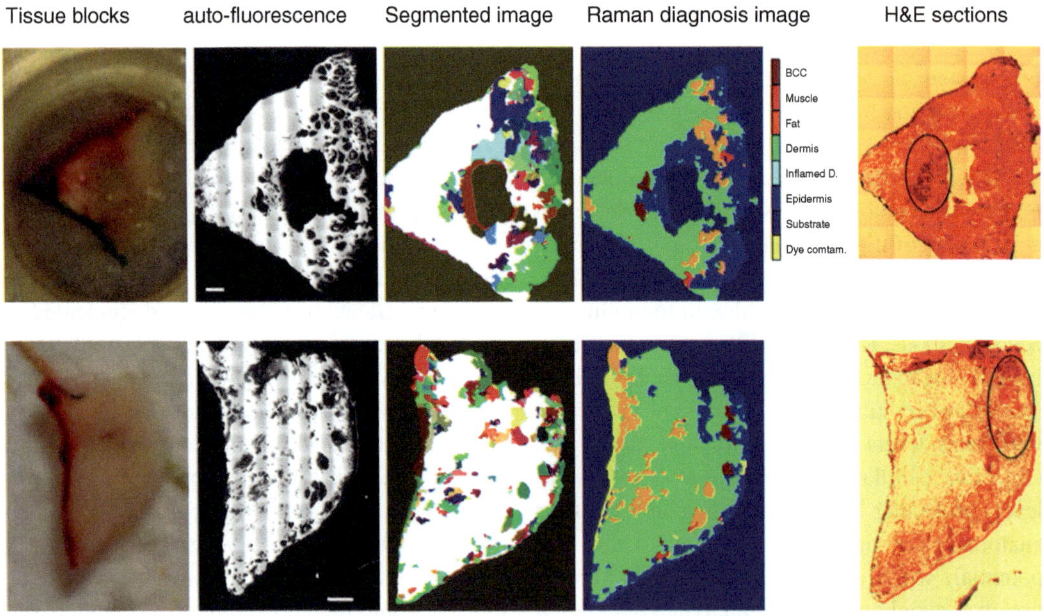

Fig. 14.12 Raman microspectroscopy applied to basal carcinoma of skin, generating pseudo-H&E image. Scale bar: 2 mm (From Kong et al. 2015) (Reprinted under Creative Commons CC-BY, with thanks to Elsevier and the authors)

and less expensive. Recently a number of leading manufacturers have begun to produce integrated Raman microscopes at lower cost, more suited to application in surgical pathology laboratories. However, there is no standardization or validation of RMS devices, or even agreement as to validation criteria. True, there is no such thing as a 'standard light microscope' (the microscope pre-dates FDA regulatory authority in the US), nor likely will there be. However, as noted below, Raman devices are in the digital arena and as such are subject to regulation for effectiveness and safety.

Reported clinical applications incorporate image construction and machine learning approaches into algorithms for a direct tissue-based diagnosis (Kong et al. 2015; Lewis et al. 2018), exemplified by diagnosis of cancer, of tumor margins, and display of IHC-like antigen localization. However, the issue of validation with respect to existing long-established technologies (H&E, IHC, IF) looms large. The Raman microscope image is by definition in digital format and regulatory authorities have placed high demands for approval of digital imaging devices in diagnostic practice, albeit varying in different countries. It is a near certainty that validation will at some point require clinical trials, comparable to those for digital WSI scanning devices (e.g. for primary H&E diagnosis by digital imaging—Mukhopadhyay et al. 2018).

Until such a time as approval is negotiated this very promising approach seems likely to be limited to experimental and research use.

14.8 Part II—Summary

Precision Medicine requires Precision Pathology (Part III), which in turn requires that traditional subjective approaches to a tissue diagnosis are supplemented by more objective approaches that involve the use of digital methods and AI (Part IV).

Multiplex tissue labeling methods are essential for evaluating complex biomarkers, such as PD-L1, where it is necessary to identify and score biomarker expression on diverse cell types that can only be positively identified by use of simultaneous phenotypic labels. Simultaneous rapid multiplex procedures that are compatible with digital analysis have the potential to convert a qualitative stain into a quantitative tissue based assay, in situ proteomics with accurate measurement and quantification that is an absolute essential for Precision Pathology.

As a final frontier AI machine learning methods already hint at the potential for extracting far more clinically actionable information from high quality H&E sections than can be appreciated by the eye of the pathologist. Information includes correlation with biomarker expression (eg. HER2, ER, PR), and a leap still further to correlate directly with prognosis and treatment selection, all derived from unsupervised machine learning approaches whereby the AI process develops its own internal parameters that unknown to, and largely cannot be directly appreciated by pathologists.

These aspects will be discussed more fully in Part IV.

References

Ahn S, Woo JW, Lee K, Park SY. HER2 status in breast cancer: changes in guidelines and complicating factors for interpretation. J Pathol Transl Med. 2020;54(1):34–44. https://doi.org/10.4132/jptm.2019.11.03.

Burlingame EA, McDonnell M, Schau GF, Thibault G, Lanciault C, Morgan T, Johnson BE, Corless C, Gray JW, Chang YH. SHIFT: speedy histological—to—immunofluorescent translation of whole slide images enabled by deep learning. bioRxiv. 2019. https://doi.org/10.1101/730309.; https://www.biorxiv.org/content/10.1101/730309v1.full.pdf

Chowdary MVP, Kumar KK, Thakur K, Anand J, Krishna CM, Mathew S. Discrimination of normal and malignant mucosal tissues of the colon by Raman spectroscopy. Photomed Laser Surg. 2007;25:269–74.

Foldesi B. Overview of multiplex immunohistochemistry. Biomol. 2020. https://www.biomol.com/resources/biomol-blog/overview-of-multiplex-immunohistochemistry

Gaifulina R, Lau K, Rodriquez-Justo M, Kendall CA. Light at the end of the tunnel: application of Raman spectroscopy in colon cancer diagnostics. Editorial. Austin J Clin Pathol. 2014;1:1021.

Giacomelli MG, Husvogt L, Vardeh H, Faulkner-Jones BE, Hornegger J, Connolly JL, Fujimoto JG. Virtual hematoxylin and eosin transillumination microscopy using epi-fluorescence imaging. PLoS One. 2016;11(8):e0159337. https://doi.org/10.1371/journal.pone.0159337.

Hauptmann G. In situ hybridization methods. New York, NY: Humana Press; 2015. https://doi.org/10.1007/978-1-4939-2303-8.

Heier S, Muralitharan S, Freeland J, von Bueren E, Gobetti A. Comparing IHC, IR and Raman spectroscopy for classification of tissue and cell lines containing different levels of HER2 expression. Abstract poster presentation. ThermoScientific. 2021. https://static.thermoscientific.com/images/D20334~.pdf. Accessed Feb 2021.

Huang Z, McWilliams A, Lam S, English J, McLean DI, Lui H, Zeng H. Effect of formalin fixation on the near-infrared Raman spectroscopy of normal and cancerous human bronchial tissues. Int J Oncol. 2003;23(3):649–55.

Keren L, Bosse M, Thompson S, et al. MIBI-TOF: a multiplexed imaging platform relates cellular phenotypes and tissue structure. Sci Adv. 2019;5(10):eaax5851. https://doi.org/10.1126/sciadv.aax5851.

Kong K, Kendall C, Stone N, Notingher I. Raman spectroscopy for medical diagnostics—from in-vitro biofluid assays to in-vivo cancer detection. Adv Drug Deliv Rev. 2015;89:121–34.

Lee C-W, Ren YJ, Marella M, Wang M, Hartke J, Couto SS. Multiplex immunofluorescence staining and image analysis assay for diffuse large B cell lymphoma. J Immunol Methods. 2019;478:112714. https://doi.org/10.1016/j.jim.2019.112714.

Levenson RM, Borowsky AD, Angelo M. Immunohistochemistry and mass spectrometry for highly multiplexed cellular molecular imaging. Lab Investig. 2015;95:397–405. https://doi.org/10.1038/labinvest.2015.2.

Lewis AT, Gaifulina R, Guppy NJ, Isabelle M, Dorney J, Lloyd GR, Rodriguez-Justo M, Kendall C, Stone N, Thomas GM. Developing Raman spectroscopy as a diagnostic tool for label-free antigen detection. J Biophotonics. 2018;2:11. https://doi.org/10.1002/jbio.201700028.

Lin JR, Izar B, Wang S, Yapp C, Mei S, shah PM, Santagata S, Sorger PK. Highly multiplexed immunofluorescence imaging of human tissues and tumors using t-CyCIF and conventional optical microscopes. elife. 2018;7:e31657. https://doi.org/10.7554/eLife.31657.

Lu S, Stein JE, Rimm DL, et al. Comparison of biomarker modalities for predicting response to PD-1/PD-L1 checkpoint blockade a systematic review and meta-analysis. JAMA Oncol. 2019; https://doi.org/10.1001/jamaoncol.2019.1549.

Mukhopadhyay S, Feldman MD, Abels E, et al. Whole slide imaging versus microscopy for primary diagnosis in surgical pathology: a multicenter blinded randomized non-inferiority study of 1992 cases (pivotal study). Am J Surg Pathol. 2018;42:39–52. https://doi.org/10.1097/PAS.0000000000000948.

Orringer DA, Pandian B, Niknafs YS, et al. Rapid interoperative histology of unprocessed biopsy specimens via fibre-laser-based stimulated Raman scattering microscopy. Nat Biomed End. 2017;1:0027. https://doi.org/10.1038/s41551-106-0027.

Parra ER, Uraoka N, Jiang M, Cook P, Gibbons D, Forget M-A, Bernatchez C, Haymaker C, Wistuba II, Rodriguez-Canales J. Validation of multiplex immunofluorescence panels using multispectral microscopy for immune-profiling of formalin-fixed and paraffin-embedded human tumor tissues. Sci Rep. 2017;7:13380. https://doi.org/10.1038/s41598-017-13942-8.

Raman CV, Krishnan KS. A new type of secondary radiation. Nature. 1928;121:3048.

Taube JM, Akturk G, Angelo M, et al. The Society for Immunotherapy of cancer statement on the best practices for multiplex immunohistochemistry (IHC) and immunofluorescence (IF) staining and validation. J ImmunoTherapy Cancer. 2020;8 https://doi.org/10.1136/jitc-2019-000155.

Taylor CR. Milestones in immunohistochemistry and molecular morphology. Appl Immunohistochem Mol Morph. 2020;28:83–94.

Taylor CR, Cote RJ, editors. Immunomicroscopy: a diagnostic tool for the surgical pathologist. 3rd ed. Saunders, PA: Elsevier; 2005. (1st edition, Taylor was 1986; 2nd edition, Taylor and Cote was 1994)

Tubbs RR, Wang H, Wang Z Minca EC, Portier BP, Am G, Lanigan C, Luo Y, Cook JR, Ma X-J. Ultrasensitive RNA in situ hybridization for detection of restricted clonal expression of low abundance immunoglobulin light chain mRNA in B-cell lymphoproliferative disorders. Am J Clin Pathol. 2013;140:736–46.

Tumeh PC, Harview CL, Yearly JH, Shinaku IP, EMJ T, et al. PD-1 blockade induces responses by inhibiting adaptive immune resistance. Nature. 2014;515:568–71. https://doi.org/10.1038/nature13954.

Valm A, Cohen S, Legant W, Melunis J, Hershberg U, Wait E, Cohen AR, Davidson MW, Betzig E, Lippincott-Schwartz J. Applying systems-level spectral imaging and analysis to reveal the organelle interactome. Nature. 2017;546:162–7. https://doi.org/10.1038/nature22369.

Wang F, Flanagan J, Su N, Wang L-C, Bui S, Nielson A, Wu X, Vo H-T, Ma X-J, Luo Y. RNAscope: a novel in situ RNA analysis platform for formalin-fixed, paraffin-embedded tissues. J Mol Diagn. 2012;14(1):22–9. https://doi.org/10.1016/j.jmoldx.2011.08.002.

Part III

Role of the Pathologist in Predictive Biomarker Analysis

15 Implementation of Precision Cancer Diagnostic Test

15.1 Introduction to Role of the Pathologist in Predictive Biomarker Analysis

Precision cancer medicine is founded and has evolved largely on the basis of tumour biomarker-directed predictive cancer therapy. The strength of this association has grown to such an extent that the use of predictive biomarker tests to guide the therapy for individual cancer patients has become the cornerstone of personalised medicine (Kato et al. 2017).

Tumour biomarkers represent a wide variety of molecules such as proteins, DNA, or RNA that are detectable either

(a) in free solution as released or extracted from the tumour cells; or
(b) in situ as integral parts of the tumour tissue, circulating tumour cells or sub-cellular organelles such as exosomes.

Cancer biomarkers have been found to be useful in:

(a) Early tumour detection (screening)
(b) Identification of tumour origin and type or subtype (diagnosis);
(c) Cytological grading and invasion staging (prognosis);
(d) Assessment of likely response and/or resistance to cancer therapy; (prediction); and
(e) Assessment of tumour response (therapeutic monitoring)
(f) Translational Medicine led development of new cancer therapies

Figure 15.1 illustrates the multifarious role of the pathologist in the management of cancer biomarking.

The success and the clinical value of cancer biomarkers have been largely founded on the pathologist's skills, knowledge and experience of using histological and protein biomarker stained tumour sections to make individual tumour specific diagnosis, prognosis and prediction.

In the era of precision medicine the role of the pathologist is evolving to provide integration of the diagnostic process at multiple points along the cancer care pathway (Plotkin et al. 2019), as illustrated in Fig. 15.2. This includes interaction with the radiologist and the surgeon, conduction of histopathological analysis and biomarker testing, followed by active participation as a member of the cancer care team to ensure standardized reflexive biomarker testing to reduce waste & turnaround time, and guide the most effective patient treatment plan as explained in Chap. 16 and illustrated in Fig. 16.1.

With the advent of the genomic (DNA) and transcriptomic (RNA) methods of tumour tissue analyses, it has also become possible to study patterns of tumour associated DNA and RNA expression. These however, have revealed that tumour types or subtypes defined to be apparently identical

B. Jasani et al., *Precision Cancer Medicine*, https://doi.org/10.1007/978-3-030-84087-7_15

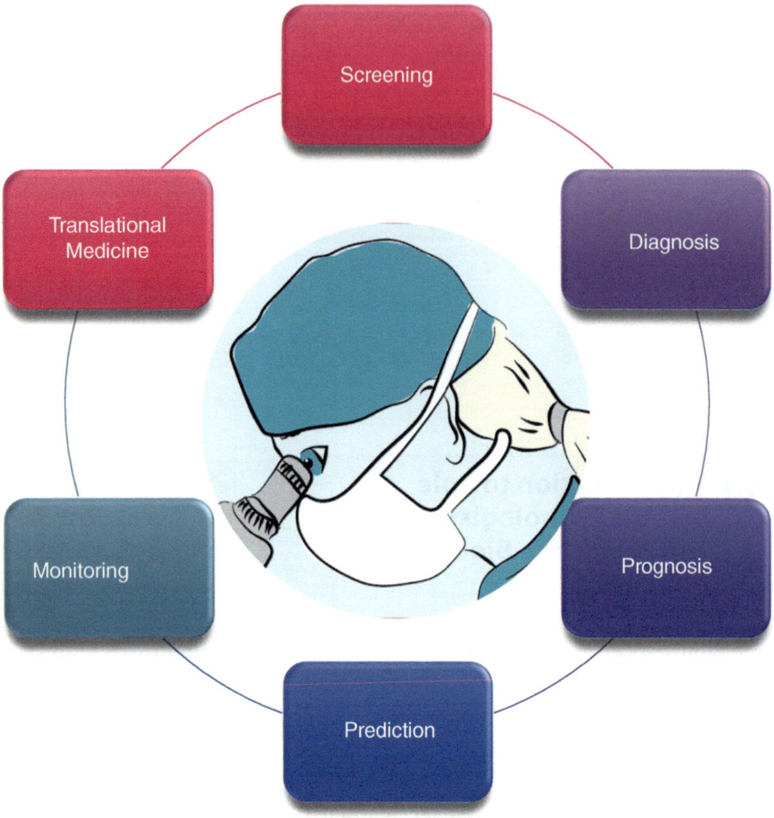

Fig. 15.1 Multifarious role of the pathologist in cancer biomarking

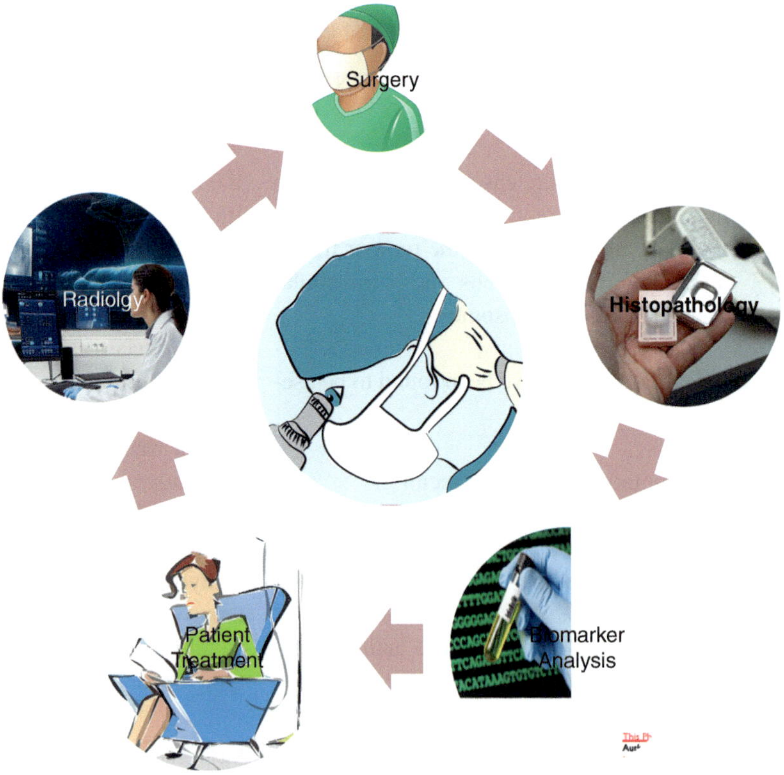

Fig. 15.2 Integrative role of pathologist in diagnostic management of the patient

by morphological and protein biomarker analyses, may have distinct molecular profiles which may be associated with distinct prognostic and/or predictive outcomes. This realisation has created a new challenge for the pathologist to learn to classify prognostic and predictive behaviour of tumours according to their molecular profiles. The accompanying development of molecularly targeted cancer therapies based on this finding has introduced an additional challenge for the pathologist to evaluate individual tumours with semi-quantitative as well as quantitative methods for more precise and accurate prediction of response or resistance of a given tumour to a particular biomarker targeted therapy.

This progress has led to the emergence of "Biomarker-led Precision Cancer Medicine", with an extension of the established role of the pathologist as described by the Role of the Pathologist, The Royal College of Pathologists of Australasia (https://www.rcpa.edu.au/getattachment/9831e1ab-c7aa-4a7d-93e9-7d77bf7df23f/The-Role-of-the-Pathologist.aspx), to include development and implementation of high precision cancer biomarker assays, based on the use of novel molecular profiling and digital and computational methods (Perez 2020).

Biomarker assays for their safe and effective application require evaluation for analytical performance (ability of assay to measure the biomarker quantity) and clinical performance (ability of assay result to inform of the clinical condition of interest). Additionally, they need to be assessed for their clinical utility to check if they ultimately improve patient outcomes when used as intended (Pennello 2013).

The aim of Part III of the Book, is to present the pivotal role of the pathologist in the implementation (this Chapter), routine application (Chap. 16), and guidance of precision predictive cancer diagnostic testing (Chap. 17).

15.2 Implementation of Predictive Biomarker Tests

The precision of predictive biomarker analysis is ultimately dependent on the strength of association between the amount of biomarker presence or expression and the degree of tumour's sensitivity (or resistance) to the biomarker targeted treatment. The purpose of Precision Cancer Medicine is to evaluate the strength of this association using accurate and reproducible tests capable of determining with high precision individual patient's response or resistance to the biomarker targeted therapy. For this it is essential to ensure that the required high precision assays are implemented properly and reliably. As discussed in this Section and described in more detail by Dobbin et al. (2016), this requires participation of the pathologist in the three key stages of the implementation process as schematically depicted in Fig. 15.3.

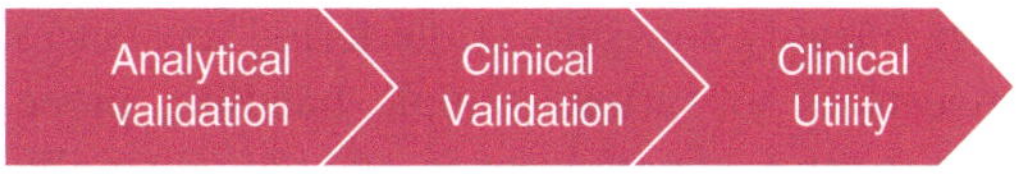

Fig. 15.3 Current role of the pathologist in implementation of a biomarker test

These include as described next:

(a) Analytical validation to check whether the test accurately and reliably measures the analyte of interest in the appropriate patient specimen and confirm run-to-run, batch-to-batch and lab-to-lab reproducibility of the assay.
(b) Clinical validation to assess the assay's accuracy and reliability in identifying patients with the target pathological state and separate one population into two or more groups with distinct clinical or biological outcomes or differences.
(c) Clinical Utility to evaluate evidence that use of the tumor biomarker test to guide clinical decisions results in improved measurable clinical outcomes compared with those if the biomarker test results were not applied.

15.3 Analytical Validation

Analytical validity is an assessment of how well the assay detects the desired analyte the context of its intended clinical use. This involves assessment of accuracy, precision, lower limit of detection, linearity, robustness (interfering substances, robustness to various sample handling procedures), range of performance, and reproducibility across instruments, by different laboratory staff and by different laboratories if more than one laboratory is involved in performing the assay in a clinical setting (Mandle 2015).

The analytical validation will also assess whether the assay can meet performance metrics that have been defined or intended to be necessary for clinical use of that assay. For example, if an assay to detect minimal residual disease needs to detect one malignant cell in one million circulating tumour cells, the assay validation must assess its performance to achieve this. The assessment in this respect includes how well the assay detects an analyte when it is present (sensitivity), and how often the assay result is negative when in fact the analyte is not present (specificity). The analytical validation plan must also ascertain how often the assay is "positive" when the analyte is not present (false positive) and how often the assay is negative when in fact the analyte is present (false negative). The developer must decide on the acceptable rates (or limits) of false positive and false negative results, according to the assay intended accuracy. The assay must then be developed to "fit" these demands. Once the analytical validation is complete, assay procedures, reagents, software, etc. should be "locked down" to ensure no further changes are introduced to the methodology which can alter its characteristics.

The analytical validation process involves a comprehensive set of experiments that evaluate and document the quantitative performance of an assay, including sensitivity, specificity, accuracy, precision, detection limit, range and limits of quantitation.

These parameters need to be assessed in terms of reproducibility of the assay performed under a variety of normal, but also variable, test conditions. Variable conditions might include different machines, operators, and reagent lots. Ruggedness provides an estimate of experimental reproducibility with unavoidable error.

The overall assessment amounts to a measure of the precision of an analytical procedure which is defined as the closeness of agreement (degree of scatter) between a series of measurements obtained from multiple sampling of the homogeneous sample under the prescribed conditions.

Precision may be considered at three levels:

(a) repeatability,
(b) intermediate precision: and
(c) reproducibility.

Repeatability expresses the precision under the same operating conditions over a short interval of time. This is also referred to as intra-assay precision.

Intermediate precision on the other hand relates to within-laboratories variations on different days equivalent to run-to-run reproducibility. It also includes a measure of reproducibility between different analysts and use of different equipment or assay platforms within the same laboratory.

Formally the term 'Reproducibility' is reserved for the measurement of precision of the assay when compared between laboratories either for the purpose standardisation of the methodology for application in routine or for collaborative research studies as discussed later.

In predictive biomarkers studies involving immunohistochemistry, the precision of the assay is dependent ultimately on the pathologist conducting the following functions:

1. Selection of the test tissue material according to its quality and representativeness of the lesion;
2. Interpretation and scoring of the results according to the various thresholds of positivity.

Precision is investigated using homogeneous, ideally on an authentic (full scale) samples, or alternatively more practically on a pilot-scale or a bench-top scale sample or sample solution. The precision of an analytical procedure is expressed as the variance, standard deviation or coefficient of variation of a series of measurements.

15.3.1 Repeatability

Repeatability relates to an estimate of slide-to-slide (or intra-run) and batch-to-batch (inter-run) precision.

Repeatability is an estimate of precision of a biomarker assay performance and usually involves requires the following approach to measure it:

- A minimum of five formalin-fixed paraffin-embedded (FFPE) tissue blocks of archived surgical resection tumour tissue with adequate amount of viable tumour tissue showing a range of biomarker expression (negative, low, moderate and high) are first identified by the pathologist. From these serial sections are cut for comparison of their staining characteristics as described below.
- For the intra-run analysis, a number of serial sections (usually 3) are freshly cut and stained simultaneously with the test assay platform under scrutiny.

15.3.2 Intermediate Precision

For the inter-run comparison usually five serial sections are cut from each one of usually five independent tumour blocks. These are stored at the room temperature under the same ambient conditions.

On day 1 representative of Run One, one section from each of the five blocks is randomly selected and placed in assay platform racks, and taken through the assay procedure. The process is repeated on four consecutive days to complete the staining required for the validation process. Biomarker analysis is performed on each of the 5 days using the same assay platform. In each of these runs positive and negative controls ae included to exclude any untoward variability in the assay performance.

Together, these data are produced to demonstrate operator independent assay reproducibility, and the stability of the performance over consecutive days of operation, independent of the rack positions.

15.3.3 Role of the Pathologist in Repeatability and Intermediate Studies

The role of the pathologist is to read the results of each of the above assay runs under the microscope or on a digital image platform to record the consistency of performance both qualitatively and semi-quantitatively as follows:

Qualitative assessment is usually done on a four point scale to record both the intensity and distribution of the staining. For intensity readout the following categoric scale of 4 levels is usually used:

1. Negative
2. Weak
3. Moderate
4. Strong

The semi-quantitative approach involves the same categoric scale as the one given above for recording the intensity of staining, except these are represented numerically to allow calculation of a semi-quantitative score:

1. 0: no staining
2. 1: weak intensity
3. 2: moderate intensity; and
4. 3: strong intensity.

In addition the following a categoric scale of 4 is used to provide numerical estimates of the distribution of the staining as follows:

1. 1: 0% to represent no staining:
2. 2: 1–25% focal distribution:
3. 3: 25–75% to represent heterogeneous distribution
4. 4: >75% representative of homogeneous staining

These figures are used to provide estimates of intensity-distribution based on the following two most commonly scoring systems:

(a) Allred Score; or
(b) H-Score

For Allred score the intensity grading and distribution grading of the staining analysed are simply added together to give a possible range of scores from a minimum of 0 to a maximum of 8.

For the H-Score method the intensity gradings 0, 1, 2 and 3, respectively, are multiplied by the raw percentage score obtained for the distribution of staining, resulting in an H-score ranging from a minimum of 0 to a maximum of 300.

15.3.4 Reproducibility

This relates to laboratory-to-laboratory comparison of reproducibility of biomarker assay performance. It is a more complex process which relates to a comparison of different assay platforms in different laboratories run by different laboratory personnel to check how reproducible and therefore comparable the results of different assays performed on the same set of tissue samples are.

For such a study, it is essential that a set of centrally stained tissue microarray slides are used to minimise the variability due to the pre-analytical quality of the tissue sample. In addition it is necessary to have a common easy to follow scoring method to score the staining resulting from each individual assay application. For this provision of a simple set of instructions combined with web-based 'training' and 'test' images is useful to evaluate reproducibly the extent of tumour staining at a given threshold of intensity of staining, for example, to determine the percentage of stained tumor cells in each of the tissue microarray sections.

Using such an the approach, it has been possible to examine the inter-laboratory reproducibility and comparability of clinical trial assays as well as validated laboratory developed tests, for example, for estimating tumour associated Ki-67 (Polley et al. 2015), PD-L1 expression in non-small cell lung cancer (Scheel et al. 2018) and more extensively for evaluating PD-L1 expression in samples of lung and head and neck cancer representative of multiple histologies, as well as in melanoma, using multiple assay platforms at multiple diagnostic cut-points (Koppel et al. 2018).

15.3.5 Total Test Reproducibility

For supporting clinical trial sample analyses at separate laboratory sites, it is necessary to test the reproducibility based on the entire procedure or the Total Test (as defined in Part II) from pre-analytical, analytical to post-analytical steps. The pre-trial study by conducted by one of the author's group (Richman et al. 2016) for a molecularly stratified clinical trial for patients with advanced colorectal cancer, provides a good example. Thus Laboratories in Leeds and Cardiff were set to perform the molecular testing and underwent a rigorous pre-trial inter-laboratory analytical validation of several assays including pTEN and mismatch repair (MMR) protein expression assessed by immunohistochemistry (IHC), and mutation status at KRAS codons12/13/61/146, NRAS codons12/13/61, BRAF codon600 and PIK3CA codons542/545/546/1047, using pyrosequencing analysis. Both mutation testing and immunohistochemical assays were found to be reproducible at the two sites and the only unresolvable issue found to be related to tumour heterogeneity which was the likely cause of observed for a minority of pyrosequencing discrepancies.

15.3.6 Role of the Pathologist in Assay Reproducibility Studies

The recent systematic review by Koomen et al. (2020) provides useful insight into the role of the pathologist in studies conducted to examine the comparability of standardised validated immunohistochemical assays and laboratory-developed tests (LDTs) (Koomen et al. 2020).

Accordingly, pathologists are centrally involved and responsible for the following four important stages of conducting such studies:

(a) Careful selection of appropriate tumour samples from a bank of archived surgically resected tumour material;
(b) Establishment of a standardised reproducible method for scoring the tumour associated biomarker staining;
(c) Deriving a reliable consensus score for each of the tumour samples; and
(d) Reproducible scoring of all the samples resulting from the study.

The pathologists involved in this process need to have received expert competency based training (Jasani et al. 2020) and are experienced in interpretation and scoring of the tumour associated biomarker expression in the particular tumour type and indication for therapy.

For the selection of the study samples large resection specimens are preferred in order to capture a greater spectrum of tumour heterogeneity in terms of variations in staining intensity and immune cell infiltration as well as to afford enough tissue material for distribution to the several respective laboratories involved the reproducibility and comparability study.

Representation of spectrum of the most common tumour types and subtypes as well as the expected range of tumour biomarker expression levels. For example, 1% and 50% tumour cell staining, to account for companion diagnostic testing for pembrolizumab in pre-treated and non-pretreated NSCLC, respectively. The cases may also be elected to represent equally the three main categories of PD-L1 expression in NSCLC (e.g. <1%, 1%–49% and >50%) but bearing mind that in real clinical practice, the prevalence for each category may not be similar, especially when studying biopsies, where the negative cases (<1%) may be more frequent because of tumor sampling bias.

For the establishing the consensus score for each sample, it is important the slides are scored by a panel of several (usually three) independent expert pathologists to avoid any systematic bias in interpretation and scoring [Adam et al. 2018], and also provide a measure of interobserver variability amongst the experts as a reference range.

For scoring the slides are anonymised with respect to the IHC platforms. Furthermore to reduce intra-observer variability in evaluating the staining, the stained sections are scored consecutively by the pathologist on the same day.

Finally, several studies have shown that it is possible to set up laboratory developed tests (LDTs) that match the staining results of the PD-L1 IHC assays. However, careful calibration and validation is essential. It seems to be easy to miss the appropriate measurement range and set up a LDT that does not show similar staining patterns and therefore is likely not to have the same predictive value. These results are reflected data of external quality assessment programs such as NordiQC which indicate that LDTs may be successful but have higher failure rates (Büttner et al. 2017).

15.4 Clinical Validation

After the analytical validity of a biomarker assay is established, as described above, the test must be evaluated to assess its clinical performance both in predicting the clinical outcome of interest, i.e., clinical validation.

Clinical validity refers to how well the assay result, the biomarker, relates to the clinical outcome of interest, such as frequency of relapse, response to therapy, or survival. Here consideration must be given to how the assay will be used to be sure the assessment of its clinical validity is carried out in the appropriate patient population. Assessment of clinical validity relates to the both analytical performance and to the intended clinical use. The assessment of clinical validity can be an iterative process. If the analytical performance of the assay has been designed well, the analytical validation will not likely have to be repeated unless there are changes or upgrades to the assay or pre-analytic requirements. Of course, if the measurement of the analyte or signature no longer correlates at all with clinical outcome when used in a new dataset, the assay itself may need to be redeveloped (Lively et al. 2015).

15.4.1 The Role of the Pathologist

Pathologist in the capacity of the Medical Director of the laboratory holds the ultimate responsibility for planning and conduction of the clinical validation studies (Fitzgibbons et al. 2014).

The guidelines issued by the College of American Pathologists recommend the need for demonstration of the analytic validity of the predictive biomarker assay before it is judged to be safe for clinical application. This latter recommendation has led to a positive impact on the overall laboratory performance according to a subsequent survey performed by Fitzgibbons et al. (2017).

Including the involvement of the laboratory medical director in virtually all diagnostic laboratories in the United States to determine for example:

(a) how many validation tissue samples are required for clinical validation of a given predictive biomarker test, as well as the number of positive and negative tissue samples to be included for reliable evaluation;
(b) whether the use whole sections is necessary instead of economically more manageable TMAs and/or MTBs. This is a particularly important decision where the fixation and processing of TMAs/ MTBs cannot be confirmed to be similar to clinical specimens.

The role of the pathologist is also clearly required for assessment of the clinical performance of a test relating to ability of its results to inform of the clinical condition of interest.

A critical component of determining the relative level of evidence to support clinical validity of a tumor biomarker test is the quality of the reporting of the studies that are used to evaluate the marker assay. Several efforts have been proposed to standardize reporting of tumor biomarker test studies, analogous to those required for therapeutic investigations (Hayes 2015). These have included descriptive analysis of the pre-analytical factors that could substantially influence reproducibility of the assay; the so-called Biospecimen reporting for improved study quality (BRISQ) criteria (Moore et al. 2011).

The Biospecimen Reporting for Improved Study Quality (BRISQ) recommendations are intended to apply to any study in which human biospecimens are used. The purpose of reporting these details is to supply others, from researchers to regulators, with more consistent and standardized information to better evaluate, interpret, compare, and reproduce the experimental results.

Clinical validity refers to how well the assay result, the biomarker, relates to the clinical outcome of interest, such as frequency of relapse, response to therapy, or survival. Here consideration must be given to how the assay will be used to be sure the assessment of its clinical validity is carried out in the appropriate patient population. Assessment of clinical validity relates to the both analytical performance and to the intended clinical use. The assessment of clinical validity, particularly, can be an iterative process. If the analytical performance of the assay has been designed well, the analytical validation will not likely have to be repeated unless there are changes or upgrades to the assay or pre-analytic requirements. Of course, if the measurement of the analyte or signature no longer correlates at all with clinical outcome when used in a new dataset, the assay itself may need to be redeveloped.

Prospective-retrospective clinical validations refer to the type of study that assesses the performance of the assay on clinical samples from patients who participated in a (completed) clinical trial, and for whom the outcome of the treatment in the clinical trial is known. Prospective-retrospective assessments are sometimes ideal for clinical validation, if they can be performed rigorously in a sample from a well-defined patient population.

In any retrospective trial, tissue or other samples may not have been collected and stored in an ideal way for the biomarker assay, and so assessment of their fitness for the assay must be performed.

In the planning of a retrospective study, careful consideration should be given to the study power and sample size as precious archived specimens should not be wasted on a retrospective study that is not likely to evaluate the clinical validity of an assay.

It is important to emphasise that assessment of clinical validity for an assay that measures multiple analytes, such as "omics" assays, are much more complex than single biomarker based clinical validation studies. Though beyond the scope of the Chapter it is important to point out briefly certain pitfalls associated with the development of such predictors. Likewise, continuous-valued biomarkers that require a "cutpoint" that defines "positive" and "negative" may require several sets of clinical data to refine and lock down the "cutpoint" before use in the clinic.

15.5 Clinical Utility

The final stage in the development of a biomarker predictive of clinical outcome is the assessment of its clinical utility through the application of the analytically validated assay within a clinical trial, with multiple design options depending on the intended use of the test and availability of specimens from previous clinical trials.

In Cancer Medicine, clinical utility is often equated with determining which therapy to use. Clinical utility depends on clinical validity in the same way as clinical validity depends analytical validity. The use of a clinically valid—i.e. the test result correctly predicts response to a drug—then acting on the clinically valid marker can lead to a change in clinical outcome and hence clinical utility, at any stage of diagnostic process from tumour diagnosis to prognosis to prediction.

15.5.1 The Role of the Pathologist

Clinical utility is the determination of whether use of the biomarker assay for decision-making leads to improved clinical results for patients. Does the biomarker add value to techniques already in use? Will the use of the biomarker result in a different, beneficial treatment for the patient? If a "biomarker positive" assay result predicts a group of patients that benefit more from a treatment than the biomarker-negative group, but the biomarker-negative group still derives as much or more benefit from the treatment as they would with any other treatment, there would be no reason to perform the assay for such a treatment decision. On the other hand, if a biomarker predicts benefit of a treatment for one or more subgroups of patients, while defining a group that will not benefit or may even have a worse outcome, that biomarker would be truly useful for guiding treatment decisions.

The pathologist's contribution is towards improving patient outcome efficacy through accurate prognostic analysis to determine the aggressiveness of treatment required and predictive analysis to select with high precision the most effective therapy for the patient and avoid treatment unlikely to work or do harm to the patient. The overall aim is to achieve a balance of outcomes where the expected health benefits exceed the expected negative consequences.

The pathologist can also contribute to prospective-retrospective studies by providing highly reproducible and accurate evidence supporting the clinical utility of the predictive biomarker. This strategy allowed, for example, the validation of the clinical utility of detecting KRAS mutation in patients with metastatic colorectal cancer. Prospective-retrospective analysis of tissues from patients with metastatic colorectal cancer who participated in several randomized studies of the efficacy of EGFR monoclonal antibodies (cetuximab or panitumumab) showed that such patients were not likely to benefit from treatment with EGFR monoclonal antibodies if their tumor had a KRAS mutation status (Maughan et al. 2011).

Another example in which prospective-retrospective studies were used to address clinical utility relates to the development of the breast cancer classifier OncotypeDx™. This assay uses reverse transcription polymerase chain reaction (RT-PCR) to assess the expression of 16 cancer-related genes and five reference genes in paraffin embedded early stage, node negative, estrogen receptor-positive tumors to predict the likelihood of distant recurrence. A locked down assay and prespecified study plan were used to evaluate tamoxifen-treated patients from a completed trial of adjuvant tamoxifen versus placebo in node negative, estrogen receptor-positive breast cancer patients. The assay was able to separate patients into low, intermediate, and high risk for distant recurrence-free survival at 10 years. A subsequent prospective-retrospective study evaluated whether high-risk patients, as evaluated by the assay, derived benefit from adjuvant chemotherapy. In this study, samples that had been banked from node negative, estrogen receptor-positive breast cancer patients who participated in a randomized adjuvant clinical trial to evaluate the worth of adding chemotherapy to tamoxifen treatment were used. The study showed that the patients classified as high risk by the assay derived benefit from adding chemotherapy to tamoxifen. Finally, a prospective study (Clinicaltrials.gov Identifier NCT00310180) was conducted to evaluate whether patients classified as intermediate risk by the assay had better distant disease-free survival by adding chemotherapy to hormone therapy in the adjuvant setting. This trial has completed accrual and final results are pending.

A further example relates to the authors' own work (BJ) to testing of clinical utility of the use of trastuzumab approved in the United Kingdom for adjuvant treatment of human epidermal growth factor receptor 2 (HER2)+ breast cancer in 2006 at significant economic cost and with limited evidence in smaller T1N0 tumours. The South East Wales Cancer Network which covers a population of 1,420,000 and has maintained a reliable database of treatments used. This database was used to check the outcome of Trastuzumab use was efficacious as expected, especially in patients with T1N0 cancers. Case notes of patients with HER2+ disease eligible for adjuvant Trastuzumab over 2005–2008 were reviewed. Disease-free survival (DFS) and overall survival (OS) were calculated with the Kaplan–Meier method using SPSS (version 16.0.01 for Windows, SPSS, Chicago, IL, USA). A total of 239 of 338 (70.7%) eligible HER2+ patients received treatment. At 3 years, the DFS of the treated group was 90.3% vs 73.3% and the OS was 98.5% vs 87.6%. In all, 47 of 92 stage I patients received Trastuzumab. Despite a trend towards worse prognostic factors in the treated group the DFS was 100% vs 84.1% and the OS was 100% vs 93.3%. The results were found be comparable to those from landmark Trastuzumab trials. The evidence indicated that smaller HER2+ cancers may behave aggressively in stage I tumours adding further support to the use of Trastuzumab in these patients (Webster et al. 2012). This study was followed through by analysis of possible impact of HER2 copy number in IHC2+/FISH-amplified breast cancer on outcome of adjuvant trastuzumab treatment (Borley et al. 2014) emphasising the importance of including HER2 gene copy number as an additional indicator for stratifying both the management and the follow-up of breast cancer patients.

Neoadjuvant therapy appears to represent an effective approach to testing the clinical utility of a biomarker led targeted therapy as demonstrated by a recent study by Katayama et al. (2021). The data indicate that the maximum benefit of neoadjuvant anti-HER2 therapy is observed in the subgroup of patients with tumours that are HER2 IHC 3+, histological grade 3 or IHC 2+/*HER2* amplification co-existing with ER-negativity, emphasising the important role of the pathologist in providing accurate and comprehensive information on every patient to the oncologist.

Molecular diagnostics can have broad impacts for patient care. Molecular results need to be integrated with additional clinical findings into the medical team's global patient assessment and management, especially in the context of patient-centered care. The decision to perform molecular testing is made by the treating clinician on the basis of the patient's symptoms, history, and clinical findings, often after consultation with a molecular pathology/medical genetics professional. The reasons for testing are commonly classified as diagnosis, prognosis, and prediction (Joseph and Lyon 2003).

15.6 Summary & Future Needs & Trends

The second stage is directed towards evaluation for clinical utility and use of the tumor biomarker test, either in a prospective-retrospective study using archived specimens or in prospective clinical trials designed to 'test the test' for its intended clinical use.

Careful planning and execution is needed to assure that the assay is analytically validated, meaning that it measures the biomarker with accuracy and reproducibility. Once analytically validated, it is of importance to show that assay results correlate with the outcome of interest; that it has clinical validity. Throughout the whole process, it is necessary to keep in mind the clinical need that they intend to address. This is the central role played by the pathologist. Beyond this it is essential to show the clinical utility of the biomarker test, i.e. the feasibility of its use in the routine clinical practice and that the assay use is able to bring a benefit to the patient (Pennello 2013; Khoury et al. 2018).

The role of the pathologist in the practical steps required for establishing clinical utility from rigorous analytical validation of an assay through to its equally stringent clinical validation, are crucial to subsequent decisions for reimbursement of the cancer patient care. Without this the high precision diagnostics could have limited availability to cancer patients at their most vulnerable times and at the same time risk the failure to translate scientific advances into high quality and cost-effective care (Parkinson et al. 2014).

As we fully enter the era of precision cancer medicine, it is critical that we continue to apply the scientific method to the consideration of what tumor biomarker tests to use to guide patient management. Maintaining this level of rigor may become even more difficult, yet will remain even more important, as the fields of genomic and computational pathology based therapies continue to evolve. Applying diagnostic or therapeutic strategies because they make sense, or because they are appealing, is a seductive but dangerous approach. It is essential that any tumor biomarker test used to guide treatment management have both analytical validity and clinical utility assured by central involvement of the pathologist. As we move into this brave new world, we have to keep in mind that "A Bad Tumor Biomarker Test Is as Bad as a Bad Drug." (Hayes 2015), or a similarly "Garbage in Garbage Out" observation noted by O'Hurley et al. (2014) linked to the risk of using inadequately well validated immunohistochemical biomarkers. In this context it is also worth quoting following set of adages from Westgard and Westgard (2018):

- The Truth requires that a test be related to the disease process of interest and that the interpretative guidelines be understood in terms of the quality (or limits of variation) required for the test.
- For the Whole Truth to be known, the test must be measured by a reliable method having the proper specifications for precision and accuracy.
- To provide Nothing but the Truth, a test result should not be confounded by unknown or undisclosed factors, such as changes in the subject due to biological variation or changes in the method due to lack of stability and quality control.
- In this context it has become increasingly necessary to extend the role of the pathologist to involve biomarker discovery and pre-clinical development and optimisation of biomarker tests as well as diagnostic competency training and testing, especially with respect to analysis of predictive biomarker such as PD-L1 (Cheung et al. 2019) as summarised in Fig. 15.4

In the next two chapters (Chaps. 16 and 17, respectively), the role of the pathologist in ensuring precision in interpretation and reporting of the biomarker test results as well as his critical guidance and quality checks in conducting of molecular and computational analyses with high precision are described and discussed.

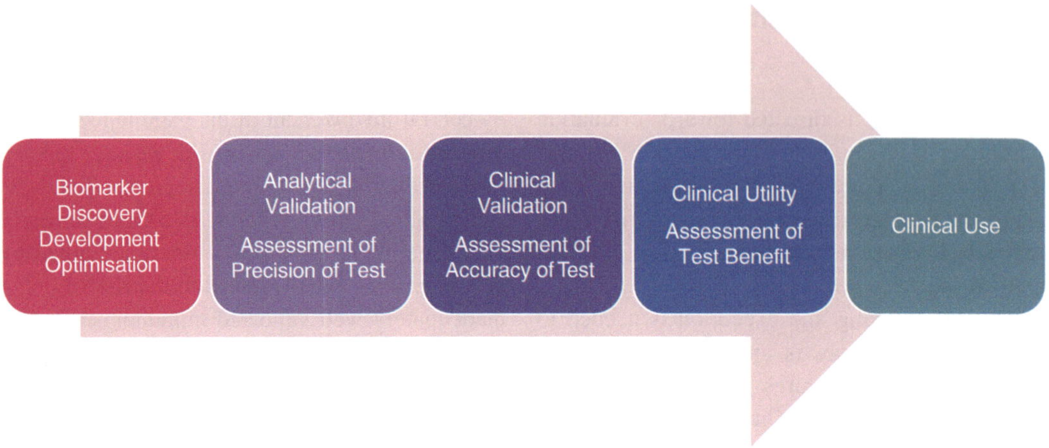

Fig. 15.4 Extension role of pathologist to biomarker discovery phase of predictive biomarker test development

References

Adam J, Le Stang N, Rouquette I, Cazes A, Badoual C, Pinot-Roussel H, Tixier L, Danel C, Damiola F, Damotte D, Penault-Llorca F, Lantuéjoul S. Multicenter harmonization study for PD-L1 IHC testing in non-small-cell lung cancer. Ann Oncol. 2018;29(4):953–8. https://doi.org/10.1093/annonc.

Borley A, Mercer T, Morgan M, Dutton P, Barrett-Lee P, Brunelli M, Jasani B. Impact of HER2 copy number in IHC2+/FISH-amplified breast cancer on outcome of adjuvant trastuzumab treatment in a large UK cancer network. Br J Cancer. 2014;110(8):2139–43. https://doi.org/10.1038/bjc.2014.147.

Büttner R, Gosney JR, Skov BG, Adam J, Motoi N, Bloom KJ, Dietel M, Longshore JW, López-Ríos F, Penault-Llorca F, Viale G, Wotherspoon AC, Kerr KM, Tsao MS. Programmed death-ligand 1 immunohistochemistry testing: a review of analytical assays and clinical implementation in non-small-cell lung cancer. J Clin Oncol. 2017;35(34):3867–76. https://doi.org/10.1200/JCO.2017.74.7642.

Cheung CC, Barnes P, Bigras G, Boerner S, Butany J, Calabrese F, Couture C, Deschenes J, El-Zimaity H, Fischer G, Fiset PO, Garratt J, Geldenhuys L, Gilks CB, Ilie M, Ionescu D, Lim HJ, Manning L, Mansoor A, Riddell R, Ross C, Roy-Chowdhuri S, Spatz A, Swanson PE, Tron VA, Tsao MS, Wang H, Xu Z, Torlakovic EE, Canadian Association of Pathologists-Association Canadienne Des Pathologistes' National Standards Committee for High Complexity Testing (CAP-ACP NSCHCT). Fit-for-purpose PD-L1 biomarker testing for patient selection in immuno-oncology: guidelines for clinical laboratories from the Canadian Association of Pathologists-Association Canadienne Des Pathologistes (CAP-ACP). Appl Immunohistochem Mol Morphol. 2019;27(10):699–714. https://doi.org/10.1097/PAI.0000000000000800.

Dobbin KK, Cesano A, Alvarez J, et al. Validation of biomarkers to predict response to immunotherapy in cancer: volume II — clinical validation and regulatory considerations. J Immunother Cancer. 2016;4:77. https://doi.org/10.1186/s40425-016-0179-0.

Fitzgibbons PL, Bradley LA, Fatheree LA, et al. Principles of analytic validation of immunohistochemical assays: guideline from the College of American Pathologists Pathology and Laboratory Quality Center. Arch Pathol Lab Med. 2014;138(11):1432–43.

Fitzgibbons PL, Goldsmith JD, Souers RJ, Fatheree LA, Volmar KE, Stuart LN, Nowak JA, Astles JR, Nakhleh RE. Analytic validation of immunohistochemical assays: a comparison of laboratory practices before and after introduction of an evidence-based guideline. Arch Pathol Lab Med. 2017;141(9):1247–54.

Hayes DF. Biomarker validation and testing. Mol Oncol. 2015;9(5):960–6. https://www.ncbi.nlm.nih.gov/pmc/articles/PMC5528748/

Jasani B, Bänfer G, Fish R, Waelput W, Sucaet Y, Barker C, Whiteley JL, Walker J, Hovelinck R, Diezko R. Evaluation of an online training tool for scoring programmed cell death ligand-1 (PD-L1) diagnostic tests for lung cancer. Diagn Pathol. 2020;15(1):37. https://doi.org/10.1186/s13000-020-00953-9.

Joseph L, Lyon E. The Spectrum of clinical utilities in molecular pathology testing procedures for inherited conditions and cancer a report of the Association for Molecular Pathology from the framework for the evidence needed to demonstrate clinical utility task force co-chairs: Loren Joseph and Elaine Lyon. AMP; 2003. http://amp.org/AMP/assets/File/education/webinar/Handout_FEND_Overview_Sept28_003.pdf?pass=88

Katayama A, Miligy IM, Shiino S, et al. Predictors of pathological complete response to neoadjuvant treatment and changes to post-neoadjuvant HER2 status in HER2-positive invasive breast cancer. Mod Pathol. 2021;34(7):1271–81. https://doi.org/10.1038/s41379-021-00738-5.

Kato S, Subbiah V, Kurzrock R. Counterpoint: successes in the pursuit of precision medicine: biomarkers take credit. J Natl Compr Cancer Netw. 2017;15(7):863–6. https://doi.org/10.6004/jnccn.2017.0127.

Khoury JD, Wang WL, Prieto VG, Medeiros LJ, Kalhor N, Hameed M, Broaddus R, Hamilton SR. Validation of Immunohistochemical Assays for Integral Biomarkers in the NCI-MATCH EAY131 Clinical Trial. Clin Cancer Res. 2018 Feb 1;24(3):521–31. https://doi.org/10.1158/1078-0432.CCR-17-1597. Epub 2017 Aug 24. PMID: 28839110; PMCID: PMC5796858.

Koomen BM, Badrising SK, van den Heuvel MM, Willems SM. Comparability of PD-L1 immunohistochemistry assays for non-small-cell lung cancer: a systematic review. Histopathology. 2020;76(6):793–802. https://doi.org/10.1111/his.14040.

Koppel C, Schwellenbach H, Zielinski D, Eckstein S, Martin-Ortega M, D'Arrigo C, Schildhaus HU, Rüschoff J, Jasani B. Optimization and validation of PD-L1 immunohistochemistry staining protocols using the antibody clone 28-8 on different staining platforms. Mod Pathol. 2018;31(11):1630–44. https://doi.org/10.1038/s41379-018-0071-1.

Lively T, Sachs MC, Conley B. Translating promising biomarkers into oncology clinical practice. Oncol Hematol Rev. 2015;11:14–8.

Mandle R. Assay validation methods - definitions and terms. 2015. www.cbrlabs.com/assayvalidation.html; https://www.fws.gov/aah/PDF/QI-Terms%20and%20Defs.pdf.

Maughan TS, Adams RA, Smith CG, Meade AM, Seymour MT, Wilson RH, Idziaszczyk S, Harris R, Fisher D, Kenny SL, Kay E, Mitchell JK, Madi A, Jasani B, James MD, Bridgewater J, Kennedy MJ, Claes B, Lambrechts D, Kaplan R, Cheadle JP, MRC COIN Trial Investigators. Addition of cetuximab to oxaliplatin-based first-line combination chemotherapy for treatment of advanced colorectal cancer: results of the randomised phase 3 MRC COIN trial. Lancet. 2011;377(9783):2103–14. https://doi.org/10.1016/S0140-6736(11)60613-2.

Moore HM, Kelly AB, Jewell SD, McShane LM, Clark DP, Greenspan R, Hayes DF, Hainaut P, Kim P, Mansfield EA, Potapova O, Riegman P, Rubinstein Y, Seijo E, Somiari S, Watson P, Weier HU, Zhu C, Vaught J. Biospecimen reporting for improved study quality (BRISQ). Cancer Cytopathol. 2011;119(2):92–101. https://doi.org/10.1002/cncy.20147.

O'Hurley G, Sjöstedt E, Rahman A, Li B, Kampf C, Pontén F, Gallagher WM, Lindskog C. Garbage in, garbage out: a critical evaluation of strategies used for validation of immunohistochemical biomarkers. Mol Oncol. 2014;8(4):783–98. https://doi.org/10.1016/j.molonc.2014.03.008.

Parkinson DR, McCormack RT, Keating SM, Gutman SI, Hamilton SR, Mansfield EA, Piper MA, Deverka P, Frueh FW, Jessup JM, McShane LM, Tunis SR, Sigman CC, Kelloff GJ. Evidence of clinical utility: an unmet need in molecular diagnostics for patients with cancer. Clin Cancer Res. 2014;20(6):1428–44. https://doi.org/10.1158/1078-0432.CCR-13-2961.

Pennello GA. Analytical and clinical evaluation of biomarkers assays: when are biomarkers ready for prime time? Clin Trials. 2013;10(5):666–76. https://doi.org/10.1177/1740774513497541.

Perez EA. Biomarkers and precision medicine in oncology practice and clinical trials. In: Ramirez A, Trapido E, editors. Advancing the science of cancer in latinos. Cham: Springer; 2020. https://doi.org/10.1007/978-3-030-29286-7_11.

Plotkin E, Allen TC, Brown S, Gutman P, Herndon D, Nowak JA. Integration of pathology within the multidisciplinary cancer care team. J Clin Oncol. 2019;37(27):suppl 49.

Polley MY, Leung SC, Gao D, Mastropasqua MG, Zabaglo LA, Bartlett JM, McShane LM, Enos RA, Badve SS, Bane AL, Borgquist S, Fineberg S, Lin MG, Gown AM, Grabau D, Gutierrez C, Hugh JC, Moriya T, Ohi Y, Osborne CK, Penault-Llorca FM, Piper T, Porter PL, Sakatani T, Salgado R, Starczynski J, Lænkholm AV, Viale G, Dowsett M, Hayes DF, Nielsen TO. An international study to increase concordance in Ki67 scoring. Mod Pathol. 2015;28(6):778–86. https://doi.org/10.1038/modpathol.2015.38.

Richman SD, Adams R, Quirke P, Butler R, Hemmings G, Chambers P, Roberts H, James MD, Wozniak S, Bathia R, Pugh C, Maughan T, Jasani B. FOCUS4 Trial Management Group. Pre-trial inter-laboratory analytical validation of the FOCUS4 personalised therapy trial. J Clin Pathol. 2016;69(1):35–41. https://doi.org/10.1136/jclinpath-2015-203097. Epub 2015 Sep 7. PMID: 26350752; PMCID: PMC4717430.

Scheel AH, Baenfer G, Baretton G, Dietel M, Diezko R, Henkel T, Heukamp LC, Jasani B, Jöhrens K, Kirchner T, Lasitschka F, Petersen I, Reu S, Schildhaus HU, Schirmacher P, Schwamborn K, Sommer U, Stoss O, Tiemann M, Warth A, Weichert W, Wolf J, Büttner R, Rüschoff J. Interlaboratory concordance of PD-L1 immunohistochemistry for non-small-cell lung cancer. Histopathology. 2018;72(3):449–59. https://doi.org/10.1111/his.13375.

Webster RM, Abraham J, Palaniappan N, Caley A, Jasani B, Barrett-Lee P. Exploring the use and impact of adjuvant trastuzumab for HER2-positive breast cancer patients in a large UK cancer network. Do the results of international clinical trials translate into a similar benefit for patients in South East Wales? Br J Cancer. 2012;106(1):32–8.

Westgard JO, Westgard S. QC in 2018: a stark reminder about the truth standard for laboratory testing. 2018. https://www.westgard.com/truth-standard-qc.htm

16 Role of Pathologist in Precision Cancer Diagnosis

16.1 Introduction

Immunohistochemistry (IHC) currently represents the most widely used approach for cancer biomarker analysis in routine pathology practice. It is applied as a descriptive, qualitative, tissue-based, in situ protein immunoassay, for which the readout of the results is principally performed by pathologists using a light microscope or whole slide digital image system.

Since the result of a predictive cancer biomarker test is likely to have a direct impact on the treatment choice as well as its outcome for an individual cancer patient, predictive biomarker analyses has been classified by FDA as moderate to high risk Class II tests (https://www.fda.gov/medical-devices/overview-device-regulation/regulatory-controls). This has led to the classification of the readouts or results of IHC tests into two categories according to their likely impact on the patient management outcome:

1. Class I Test results which are produced by the pathologists mainly for their own use for establishing and stipulating the tumour diagnosis.
2. Class II results which are meant for the cancer physicians or oncologists to take critical patient management decisions on the choice of treatment, for the need for additional testing, or follow-up.

Reporting of Class II results requires for its safety and success the use of a biomarker assay implemented with the help and guidance of the pathologist in charge of the diagnostic process, to ensure its analytical and clinical validity, accuracy and precision. The tests used for prognostic and predictive analysis of tumours which fall under this category are therefore first required to be validated analytically and clinically as described in Chap. 15, under the close supervision and collaboration of a pathologist. Furthermore, it is important for the pathologist to ensure that the validated test is performed and applied to the required standard on each and every sample, and that results are also interpretated, scored and reported with the same high precision and accuracy to the oncologist. In this context the role of a pathologist normally concerned mainly with the third or the post-analysis phase of the Total Test described in Part II, is extended to include checking and recording of the quality of the performance of pre-analytical and analytical phases of analysis. The use of formalin fixed paraffin embedded solid tissue samples for the vast majority of cancer biomarker testing represents a significant pre-analytical source of variability in the quality of testing, and pathologist's expertise and experience are needed record it as well as take an account of it in their diagnostic analysis and reporting.

Adequate appropriate training and competence testing are necessary for the pathologist to

B. Jasani et al., *Precision Cancer Medicine*, https://doi.org/10.1007/978-3-030-84087-7_16

undertake for them to have the qualification and capacity to minimise variability in interpretation, scoring and reporting of the biomarker results.

Depending on the laboratory test used, several independent factors are likely to be the pre-analytical source of error. For example, background signal and morphologic clarity of IHC/IF can be influenced by sample fixation time, quality of embedding, or time from extraction to preservation (McKean et al. 2020).

Secondly, there is need for the pathologist to have a working knowledge of analytical sensitivity of the assay determined by the fraction of responders that are marker-positive (or positive predictive value (PPV)); as well as specificity determined by the fraction of non-responders that are marker-negative (or negative predictive value, NPV) based on a cut-off point for positivity determined by the ROC analysis on the clinical trial data set. The ultimate aim of the predictive biomarker specific test applied to any given patient tissue specimen is to achieve the same level of precision as achieved for the clinical trial samples. The role of the pathologist is to assess the performance of Total Test from the pre-analysis to the post-analysis phase in order to ensure that the required level of precision has been achieved to report the case safely to the oncologist, as well as to point out any shortcomings or failure of the analysis.

For the Class II category tests general controls alone are not sufficient to provide reasonable assurance of the safety and effectiveness of the test. There is a need to include special quality measures to provide a stepwise quality check and assurance of their analytic validity (the accuracy of a test in detecting the specific entity that it was designed to detect) and clinical validity (the accuracy of a test for a specific clinical purpose). They in fact require rigorous quality management using internationally recognized standards, since errors in testing can be costly not only to the patient but could also have a significant financial burden on the healthcare system. For example, the erroneous determination the ER status in approximately 12,025 patients in the U.S. during 2012, led to a cost of nearly $1 billion (Garrison Jr et al. 2015) Around the same time, 15–20 per cent of CLIA-certified laboratories were found to incorrectly perform HER2 analyses adding further to the cost burden.

For this reason, predictive biomarker testing for personalised treatment predictive of chemotherapy, immunotherapy, or targeted therapy or a combination are now regulated by a co-ordinated and harmonised quality assurance (QA) system based on and/or complying with the relevant (inter)national standards issued by the International Organization for Standardization (ISO), the College of American Pathologists (CAP), or the Clinical Laboratory Improvement Amendments (CLIA).

The purpose of this chapter is to describe the role of pathologist for assurance of good diagnostic practice with guidance from regulatory body and expert opinion based recommendations, to achieve these objectives safely and effectively in a diagnostic or clinical trial setting, for targeted therapies listed in Targeted Therapies, National Cancer Institute (2020—https://www.cancer.gov/about-cancer/treatment/types/targeted-therapies/targeted-therapies-fact-sheet); and described in a chapter led by one of the authors (BJ) in Heinmoller et al (2018), Badve and Kumar (2019).

16.2 Regulatory Body and Expert Opinion Based Recommendations

The Clinical Laboratory Improvement Amendments (CLIA) recommendations are helpful to cover pre-analytic requirements governing specimen submission and handling and those ensuring the analytic validity of the test performance. It does not offer regulation of the clinical validity of laboratory developed predictive assays. For this it is important to follow FDA's regulation of companion diagnostic tests. However since for the laboratory-developed tests, this requirement is not enforceable, the laboratory has to establish its own performance specifications for analytical sensitivity, specificity, and other performance characteristics required for test performance. Hence the test is approved to be of adequate standard only at the discretion of the laboratory director working in close collaboration with the lead pathologist.

16.3 Role of Pathologist in Assurance of Good Diagnostic Practice

In addition, CLIA and FDA led processes even when combined together are not sufficient to offer a full regulatory control over all the factors pertaining to clinical validation. In addition though the FDA remit includes analytic validity (the accuracy of a test in detecting the specific entity that it was designed to detect) and clinical validity (the accuracy of a test for a specific clinical purpose), it does not cover issues relating to clinical utility (the clinical and psychological benefits and risks of positive and negative results of a given technique or test). This means that even a companion diagnostic test is unable to sufficiently guarantee the accuracy needed for clinical decision making for individual patients in routine practice at the community level.

The promise of personalized medicine offered through predictive testing of the tumours is therefore difficult to deliver with adequate precision, certainty and transparency due to gaps in the regulatory quality control of the Total Test. This is particularly true for all Class II tests whether they are companion diagnostic tests or even fully automatic machine driven cancer biomarker analysis. The situation has become even more critical with the advent of predictive biomarker analysis for immune checkpoint inhibitor directed cancer therapy due to the expected higher rates of errors associated with semi-quantitative scoring of PD-L1 staining by the pathologists (Humphries et al. 2020).

A higher risk of variability between observers has also been observed with semi-quantitative estimation of the percentage of neoplastic cells required for EGFR and other types of mutation analysis, where an accurate estimation in the FFPE samples is necessary prior to analysis (Lhermitte et al. 2017).

A recent world-wide External Quality Assurance survey of possible sources of errors in predictive biomarking, indicates a crucial role for the pathologist to perform a step wise internal quality check of the Total Test, to safe-guard against errors in predictive cancer biomarking. This notion is supported by the finding that laboratories with a larger capacity of professionally trained personnel are able to perform the analysis with fewer method-based errors and those in particular operated by departments of pathology also have fewer sample-related issues. Also such laboratories are significantly less likely to be error prone with respect to the pre-analytical phase related issues and are less likely to denote the received sample material to be the cause of assay failure.

Minimisation of errors in predictive biomarker analysis has been observed to be associated with involvement of the pathologist in College of Pathology proficiency testing on a 6-monthly basis for CLIA-certified laboratories across the USA. This combined with the regular External Quality Control assessment of the laboratory analytical performance, is probably responsible for the observed reduction of the risk of systematic analytical error from 30–40% down to around 10% level (Wasielewski et al. 2008).

The pathologist's extended role for providing the required standards of precision and accuracy of predictive biomarker tests in addition to that summarised in Fig. 15.4, Chap. 15, is also meant to include:

(a) Application of rigorous internal quality control checks on each case sample for recording of any deviation in the quality of tissue or staining arising due to likely error prone steps of pre-analytical and analytical phases, respectively, of the assay; and
(b) compliance with CLIA, FDA and expert opinion based recommendations and guidelines for accurate and reproducible interpretation and reporting of the patients results, for handling the post-analytic phase of the Total Test process.

A list of currently approved/recommended tests for predictive biomarker analysis of solid tumours is provided in Table 16.1. Detailed protocols for managing the interpretation, scoring and reporting of the results of these tests, are available individual cancer types from the websites of:

Table 16.1 List of approved/recommended tests for predictive biomarker analysis of solid tumours

Biomarker test	Detects	Assay type(s)	Cancer type/indication	Therapeutic prediction
ALK	Gene fusion; protein expression	FISH, NGS, RT-PCR; IHC	NSCLC: Adenocarcinoma, large cell, NOS	Sensitivity to ALK TKIs (alectinib; crizotinib)
EGFR	Mutations exons 19, 20 & 21	NGS, multiple mutation testing	NSCLC: Adenocarcinoma, large cell, NOS	Sensitivity or resistant to EGFR TKIs
ROS1	Fusion rearrangement	NGS, FISH, RT-PCR	NSCLC: Adenocarcinoma, large cell, NOS	Sensitivity to ROS1 TKIs
PD-L1	Low (>1%) or high (50%) protein expression	IHC	Adenocarcinoma, large cell, NSCLC, squamous cell NOS	Responsiveness to pembrolizumab in first-line or second-line
KRAS/NRAS (exons 2, 3, and 4 in both)	Mutation	NGS	Metastatic colorectal adenocarcinoma	Indication for avoidance cetuximab or panitumumab treatment
BRAF	Mutation V600E	NGS, pyrosequencing, AS-PCR	Metastatic synchronous or metachronous colorectal adenocarcinoma of any stage	Potential sensitivity irinotecan plus cetuximab or panitumumab combination with BRAF inhibitor (e.g. vemurafenib)
HER2	Protein overexpression and/or HER2 gene amplification	IHC/FISH	Gastric, esophageal, and gastroesophageal junction cancers	Sensitivity to trastuzumab therapy
PD-L1 (CD274) and HER2 protein	Protein overexpression/ HER2 gene amplification	IHC/FISH	HER2-ve & PD-L1+ & MMR+ gastric, esophageal, and gastroesophageal junction cancers	Sensitivity to anti–PD-L1 or PD-1 therapy
ESR1 (ER)	ER protein expression	IHC	Stage III, IV, and recurrent uterine/ endometrial carcinoma	Sensitivity to endocrine therapy
BRCA1, BRCA2, PALB2, BRIP1, RAD51C, and RAD51D	Mutations	NGS	Ovarian cancer	Sensitivity to PARP inhibitors
ER/PR	Protein expression	IHC	Non-invasive and invasive breast cancer, stage I-IV	Sensitivity to endocrine therapy
HER2	Protein expression/ gene amplification	IHC/FISH	Invasive breast cancer, stage I-IV	Sensitivity to HER2 targeted therapy trastuzumab, pertuzumab, lapatinib, or trastuzumab emtansine
BRCA1 and BRCA2	Germ line mutation	NGS	Invasive breast cancer, stage IV	Sensitivity to PARP inhibitors
Oncotype Dx	Gene expression	RT-PCR	Stage I, II ER-positive/ PR-positive, HER2-negative breast cancer	Predictor of chemotherapy benefit

Table 16.1 (continued)

Biomarker test	Detects	Assay type(s)	Cancer type/indication	Therapeutic prediction
MDM2, CDK4	Gene amplification	NGS	Well & de-differentiated liposarcoma	Potential sensitivity to CDK4/CDK6 inhibitor
IDH1/IDH2	Mutation	NGS	Chondrosarcoma	Potential sensitivity to IDH1 inhibitor
PD-L1	Protein expression	IHC	Recurrent, unresectable, or metastatic nasopharynx carcinoma	Sensitivity to Pembrolizumab
BRAF V600	Mutation	NGS	Resected, stage III, BRAF V600E/ V600K–mutant melanoma	Sensitivity to BRAF/MEK inhibitor combination (dabrafenib plus trametinib)

Table 16.2 Examples of professional society based consensus guidelines on predictive biomarker testing of solid cancers

Cancer specific biomarker test	Professional body	Recommendations/guidelines weblink
HER2 testing in breast cancer	ASCO/CAP	https://pubmed.ncbi.nlm.nih.gov/32346807/ Zhang et al. (2020)
ER & PR testing in breast cancer	ASCO/CAP	https://pubmed.ncbi.nlm.nih.gov/31928404/ Allison et al. (2020)
HER2 testing in gastric cancer	ESMO	https://oncologypro.esmo.org/education-library/factsheets-on-biomarkers/her2-in-gastric-cancer
Lung cancer PD-L1 testing in	CAP	https://www.cap.org/protocols-and-guidelines/upcoming-cap-guidelines/pd-l1-testing-of-patients-with-lung-cancer-for-immunooncology-therapies College of American Pathologists
Lung cancer predictive biomarker testing	SSMO/SSP	https://link.springer.com/article/10.1007/s12094-019-02218-4#citeas Garrido et al. (2020)
Colorectal cancer biomarker testing	SSMO/SSP	https://link.springer.com/article/10.1007/s12094-020-02357-z Garcia-Alfonso et al. (2020)
Ovarian cancer BRCA mutation	ESMO	https://www.annalsofoncology.org/action/showPdf?pii=S0923-7534%2820%2942164-7 Miller et al. (2020)
Lung cancer Immune check point PD-L1 testing	SITC	https://jitc.bmj.com/content/6/1/75 Brahmer et al. 2018

ASCO/CAP The American Society of Clinical Oncology/College of American Pathologists, *ESMO* European Society of Medical Oncology, *SMOS/SSP* Spanish Medical Oncology Society/Spanish Society for Pathology, *SITC* The Society for Immunotherapy of Cancer

(a) College of American Pathologists 'Cancer Reporting and Biomarker Reporting Protocols'—https://www.cap.org/protocols-and-guidelines/cancer-reporting-tools/cancer-protocol-templates
(b) European Society for Medical Oncology Factsheets of Validated Biomarkers—https://oncologypro.esmo.org/education-library/factsheets-on-biomarkers
(c) The Society for Immunotherapy of Cancer Practice Guidelines https://www.sitcancer.org/research/cancer-immunotherapy-guidelines#:~:text=The%20SITC%20Cancer%20Immunotherapy%20Guidelines,develop%20evidence%2D%20and%20consensus%2Dbased

In addition, the reader is recommended to follow journal articles published by various pathological societies or consortiums, to provide the latest updates on consensus guidelines for pathologist led management of cancer specific predictive biomarking. Some of the recent updates are listed in Table 16.2.

The next part of the Chapter considers the role of the pathologist involved in application of the consensus guidelines/recommendations, for ensuring:

(a) internal quality assessment and evaluation of the case results in terms of factors likely to adversely influence the pre-analytical and analytical phases of test; and
(b) accurate and reproducible interpretation, scoring and reporting of the test result.

16.4 Internal Quality Assurance of Pre-Analysis Phase

The key sources of errors in pre-analytical phase relate to the quality of the tumour sample with respect to its adequacy of:

(a) tissue preservation and presentation
(b) amount and representativeness

16.4.1 Potential Errors Due to Inadequate Tissue Preservation

For optimal immunohistochemical detection of prognostic and predictive biomarkers it is recommended that tissue be fixed in buffered 10% formalin for at least 6–8 h and no more than 72 h, unless another fixative that has been validated is used: https://www.cap.org/protocols-and-guidelines/cancer-reporting-tools/cancer-protocol-templates

16.4.1.1 Potential Causes of False Negative or Weak Results

- Tumor cell damage by heat through cautery used for surgical resection of the tumour
- Prolonged (i.e. >1 h) cold ischemic time leading to autolytic antigenic degradation.
- Under (<6 h) or overfixation (>72 h) fixation
- Type of fixative: e.g., estrogen receptor protein (ER) degradation in acidic fixatives or acidification unbuffered formalin through accumulation of formic acid.
- Decalcification of bone containing biopsy

16.4.2 Adequacy and Representativeness of Biopsy Material

- Low tumor content, as defined by the molecular diagnostics laboratory. The cut-off for acceptable tumor content depends on the method used by the laboratory. Samples with tumor content below the recommended cutoff may be falsely negative and should be reported as indeterminate if no mutations are detected.

If more than one tissue block is available for a given tumor, the most representative sample should be tested. More than one block may be tested when the reporting pathologist determines that such additional testing is necessary to confirm the biomarker status of the tumor. If additional blocks from the same sample are tested, the results from all tested blocks should be combined as if it were present in a single paraffin block.

If more than one sample from two different sites e.g. primary and corresponding metastatic tumors biopsies, the most representative sample should be tested. More than one sample may be tested when the reporting pathologist determines that such additional testing is necessary.

If the initial sections taken from the available sample contains less than the minimum required number of tumor (or other target) cells as defined by the interpretive manual for a specific assay and purpose, testing of additional levels may be performed with extra tissue containing additional tumor cells to reach the required threshold. If additional levels are tested, the results of all tissue from all levels may be combined as if it were present in a single level, if it complies with the recommendations.

Identification of archived formalin fixed and paraffin embedded (FFPE) tissue blocks containing cancer and its associated surrounding tissue or tumour micro-environment (TME) present in adequate amount and in an acceptable state of morphological integrity and preservation.

Post-operative primary tissue samples containing tumor tissues and adjacent normal tissues, collected from the institutional tissue archives or tissue biobank all with informed written patients' consents and agreements to participate in the research. The study protocols to be approved by the Institutional Ethics Review Committee. Similarly all the experimental procedures and tissue collections performed in accordance with the approved guidelines.

Selection of indication specific unaffected normal tissue samples and 'normal appearing' normal tissue surrounding the cancer lesion, for a qualitative check of biomarker specific expression provide a measure of background level of expression.

Selection of sets of tissue blocks from different types and sub-types of the indication specific cancer as well as several other cancer types, to assess the analytical specificity and sensitivity of the biomarker assay, and establish an optimal assay protocol.

Selection of indication specific cancer tissue blocks of different types and subtypes, as well as of different grades and levels of progression (metaplasia, dysplasia, in situ, and well-to poorly-differentiated invasive cancer lesion), for qualitative and semi-quantitive evaluation of the range of biomarker expression associated with different grade and invasive levels of disease progression.

Primary tumour samples containing evidence of local invasion at the site of the tumour origin, with associated TME tissue. Where possible the representative block(s) should also include any associated pre-neoplastic lesions such as hyperplasia, metaplasia, and dysplasia, as well as in-situ cancer development.

The tumour sample should be verified to include the presence of indication specific tumour type and subtype using H & E stained sections freshly cut from the retrieved tissue blocks.

Examination of freshly cut sections stained with H & E for the confirmation and an estimate of the quality and amount tumour.

16.5 Internal Quality Assurance of Analysis Phase

The pathologist led quality assurance is based on achieving two distinct but overlapping goals

(a) assessment directed at judging the quality of the process; and
(b) evaluation which is orientated towards providing a judgment on the quality of the product resulting from the process.

The role of the pathologist is to systematically assess and evaluate the impact of pre-analytic, analytic and post-analytic procedures on quality of biomarker specific staining in order to interpret and score the results in a systematic and reproducible way. In the pre-analytical phase of the assay this involves assessment of the quality of tissue preservation and evaluation of the quantity, distribution and the characteristics of the viable tumour and non-tumour tissue included in the biopsy. The analytical phase assesses the tissue section quality and evaluates the biomarker staining in terms of its specificity and sensitivity based on a set of external and internal controls. The post-analytical phase then follows to assess the quality of biomarker staining of tumour and non-tumour tissue components and evaluate the extent, the distribution and intensity of the biomarker staining to provide a score defining the biomarker status of the tumour.

16.5.1 Pre-Analytic Phase Exclusion Factors

1. Tissue section:
   (a) disruption
   (b) overlap
   (c) washing out
   (d) thickness
2. Tissue integrity:
   (a) crushing and/or cautery damage;
   (b) retraction artifact
   (c) poor nuclear definition

16.5.2 Analytic Phase Exclusion Factors

- Nonoptimized antigen retrieval
- Type of antibody

- Dark hematoxylin counterstain obscuring faintly positive diaminobenzidine (DAB) staining
- Staining quality
  (a) Poor counter staining
  (b) Excessive background staining and/or endogenous pigment interference
  (c) Potential false negative staining
  (d) Uneven staining
- False-negative results: Failure to detect ER or PgR is the greatest problem with this assay because patients may not receive effective therapy. This may occur if specimen handling was inadequate, if artifacts (crush or edge artifacts) make interpretation difficult, or if the analytic testing failed. To avoid false-negative results, appropriate internal and external controls should be positive. When a tumor is negative (non-immunoreactive), it is essential that the internal control cells be assessed to ensure that they show positive staining (as expected). If the internal controls are also negative, the test should not be reported as negative but should be considered indeterminate ("Cannot be determined").[2] The test should be repeated on another block or specimen.
- When a tumor is negative but no internal control cells are present in the test section, the pathologist must exercise judgment as to whether the assay can be interpreted as a true negative. This should include consideration of histologic type and grade, cold ischemia and fixation times, and the status of external controls. If the pathologist decides that hormone receptor status cannot be determined, the test should be reported as such and repeated or performed on another block or specimen.
- Treatment of the tissue that could potentially alter immunoreactivity (eg, decalcification)[7]
- Status of controls:
  - Internal—normal epithelial cells positive or negative for ER and PgR
  - External—type and expected level of expression
- Adequacy of sample for evaluation

False-negative IHC results for HER2 may be due to:

- Prolonged cold ischemia time.
- Tumor heterogeneity. When a negative result is found, but only a small biopsy sample was tested, repeat testing on a subsequent specimen with a larger area of carcinoma should be considered, particularly if the tumor has characteristics associated with HER2 positivity (ie, tumor grade 2 or 3, weak or negative PgR expression, increased proliferation index).
- Improper antibody titration (concentration too low)

False-positive results: False-positive results occur less frequently. Rare reasons would be the use of an impure antibody that crossreacts with another antigen or misinterpretation of entrapped normal cells or an in situ component as invasive carcinoma. False-positive tests can also be generated by image analysis devices that mistakenly count overstained nuclei. It has been suggested that highly sensitive assays may detect very low levels of ER in cancers that will not respond to hormonal therapy, but that has not been proven by a clinical trial.

False-negative and false-positive results can be reduced by paying attention to the following:

- Staining of normal breast epithelial cells. Normal epithelial cells serve as a positive internal control and should always be assessed. If the normal cells are negative, repeat studies on the same specimen or on a different specimen should be considered. If normal cells are not present (eg, core biopsy) and the test results are negative, testing should be repeated on another block or subsequent specimen.
- External controls (must stain as expected). These controls help ensure that the reagents have been appropriately dispensed onto the slide with the clinical sample.
- Correlation with histologic type and grade of the cancer. The study should be repeated if the results are discordant (eg, ER-negative low-grade carcinoma).

False-positive IHC results for HER2 may be due to:

- Edge artifact. This is usually seen in core biopsies, where cells near the edges of the tissue stain stronger than in the center, possibly because antibody pools at the sides. Specimens with stronger staining at the edge of the tissue should be interpreted with caution.
- Cytoplasmic positivity, which can obscure membrane staining and make interpretation difficult.
- Overstaining (strong membrane staining of normal cells). May be due to improper antibody titration (concentration too high).
- Misinterpretation of ductal carcinoma in situ (DCIS). High-grade DCIS is often HER2 positive. In cases with extensive DCIS relative to invasive carcinoma (particularly microinvasive carcinoma), HER2 scoring may mistakenly be done on the DCIS component. Care must be taken to score only the invasive component.

False-negative and false-positive results can be reduced by paying attention to the following:

- Tissue controls. External controls must stain as expected. There are no normal internal controls for HER2 protein assessment by IHC.
- Correlation with histologic and other biomarker results. If the HER2 test is negative by IHC, but the tumor has characteristics associated with HER2 positivity (see above), repeating the test by ISH should be considered.

16.5.3 Evaluation of the Quality of Biopsy Material

1. Section quality
   (a) Overall
      - Good
      - Acceptable
      - Low
   (b) Integrity
      - Acceptable
        - Intact
        - Partially overlapping
        - Partially disrupted
        - Partially washed-off
      - Unacceptable
        - Largely washed-off
        - Largely disrupted
   (c) Thickness
      - Optimal
      - Too thick
      - Too thin
2. Fixation quality
   (a) Tissue preservation
      - Adequate
      - Poor
3. Tissue Integrity
   (a) Intact
   (b) Crushed
   (c) Cautery damage

16.5.4 Evaluation of Distribution and Quantity of Tumour Tissue

1. Tumour content
   (a) Present
      - Adequate
      - inadequate
   (b) Absent
2. Viable tumour presence
   (a) % of lesional area
   (b) % of whole section
3. Necrosis
   (a) % total amount in
   (b) %lesional area
4. Tumour stromal cell proportion and distribution
   (a) % overall TIL presence
   (b) Pattern of distribution
      - Intra-tumoural
      - Intra-tumoural stroma
      - Peritumoural

16.5.5 Assessment of Quality of Assay Performance

It is strongly recommended for the pathologist to examination of the quality of the propriety or in-house assay linked positive and negative controls. The minimum composition of external controls for FDA (or other regulatory body) approved clinical assay IHC Kits must be compliant with the Kit manufacturer's instructions. In addition to these the quality of staining in indication specific positive and negative tissue controls should be checked to ensure whether whole range of staining intensity and distribution expected are exhibited. Lastly, there is a need to assess the expected intensity and distribution of staining associated any relevant internal control tissue.

16.5.6 Selection and Use of Control

It is strongly recommended that external on-slide controls are used for every slide.

The composition of these for FDA (or other regulatory body) approved IHC Kits must be in compliance with the Kit manufacturer's instructions. The minimum composition of external on-slide controls for LDTs should mirror the requirements of the corresponding fit-for-purpose FDA (or other regulatory body)-approved kit.

According to expert opinion based guidelines the required minimum composition of the external on-slide controls for example for PD-L1 testing may include indication specific tumour tissue:

1. showing low to moderate positivity for PD-L1 in the specified cell population(s), and
2. negativity for PD-L1 again in a specified cell population.

The laboratory should ideally assess the external on-slide control by light microscopy before a slide being released from the laboratory. However, when examined by the pathologist, if the external on-slide controls demonstrate either unacceptable background or lack of signal in any positive control tissue, such IHC slides should be failed and the results reported to the laboratory for a repeat analysis, as well as the root cause for the failure investigated to avoid similar mishap in the future.

16.6 Quality Assurance of Post-Analytic Phase

16.6.1 Post Analysis Factors Influencing Quality of Biomarker Assessment

1. Tissue sample adequacy
   (a) No relevant tissue
   (b) Not enough relevant tissue
2. Staining
   (a) Tissue distribution
      - Tumour cells
        – Carcinoma-in-situ
        – Invasive cells
      - Stromal cells
        – Inflammatory cells
        – Connective tissue cells
          1. Endothelial cells
          2. Fibroblasts
   (b) Cellular distribution
      - Membrane
      - Cytoplasmic
      - nuclear
   (c) Cellular intensity
      - Strong
      - Moderate
      - Weak
      - Negative

16.6.2 Indication Specific Interpretation, Scoring and Reporting

For reporting with high accuracy for targeted therapy of solid tumours (El-Deiry et al. 2019), the pathologist should:

(a) follow recommendations and guidelines based on clinical trials evidence;
(b) conduct analysis with high precision using a analytically and clinically validated protocol;

(c) report results based on the therapy specific reporting protocols and threshold(s)
(d) received expert training and certification in indication specific biomarker analysis
(e) maintain standards with regular proficiency testing and refresher training

16.6.3 Assessment of Appropriateness and Completeness of Biomarker Analysis

Use of H & E stained tissue section for assessment of the type and the source of biopsy

1. Type of procedure used to obtain the tumour biopsy sample
   (a) Fine needle aspiration biopsy
   (b) Needle core biopsy
   (c) Excision biopsy
   (d) Resection biopsy
2. Site of biopsy
   (a) Primary
   (b) Metastatic
   (c) Indetermined
3. Site of lesion
   (a) Organ of origin
   (b) Tissue of origin
   (c) Indetermined

16.6.4 Evaluation of Accuracy of the Results

1. Tumour Grade
   (a) High
   (b) Moderate
   (c) Low
2. Macroscopic description
   (a) Type of biopsy and number of biopsy fragments
   (b) Lesion location
      - Primary
      - Metastatic
      - Recurrent
   (c) Lesion origin
      - Organ of origin
      - Tissue of origin
3. Microscopic description
   (a) Confirmation or exclusion of location of the lesion and organ and tissue of origin
   (b) Identification of cellular origin of the lesion
4. Diagnostic analysis
   (a) Morphological
      - Confirmation or exclusion of cancer
      - Type and subtype of cancer
   (b) Immunohistochemical
      - Further confirmation or exclusion of cancer
      - Refined typing and subtyping of cancer
   (c) Molecular
      - Definitive confirmation or exclusion of cancer
      - Definitive typing and subtyping of cancer
5. Prognostic Analysis
   (a) Morphological
      - Grading of the tumour process
      - Staging of the tumour process
   (b) Immunohistochemical
      - Confirmation of morphological grading of the tumour process
      - Confirmation of morphological staging of the tumour process
   (c) Molecular
      - Definitive grading of the tumour process
      - Definitive staging of the tumour process
6. Predictive analysis
   (d) Immunohistochemical
      - Tumour associated drug specific target protein overexpression
      - Tumour associated drug specific target protein under expression
   (e) Molecular
      - Tumour associated drug specific target activated gene mutation or amplification
      - Tumour associated drug specific target gene inactivation or absence

16.7 Summary and Future Needs & Trends

Diagnostic testing appears to influence 60–70% of all decision making in Precision Cancer Medicine (Dzau et al. 2016) supporting the belief that "Good care starts with good diagnosis" (Nass et al. 2019).

As discussed in this chapter pre- and post-analytical steps of the total testing process (TTP) are more error-prone than the analytical phase. Most errors (almost 90%) are identified in pre-analytic and post-analytic steps outside of the laboratory control (Plebani 2010). Consistent with this observation overall accuracy of morphological interpretation on breast cancer specimens was found to be 75% amongst over 100 practising pathologists compared to 90% expected from the consensus scores achieved by 3 panel experts, given the task of making 240 categories of histology diagnoses derivable from 60 breast specimens (Elmore et al. 2015).

With advent of precision cancer medicine based on a biomarker test to guide selection of patient population for biomarker targeted treatments or drug trials, the accuracy of the biomarker test needs to be improved if treatment or the clinical trial is likely to be adequately successful (Park et al. 2019). For a predictive biomarker analysis categorised as a Class II diagnostic test which is similar to a point of care test (POCT), the tolerable error rate should be aimed to be in the range 2.7 to 12.7% (Plebani 2010). The pathologist central to accurate and reproducible interpretation and reporting of the biomarker test holds a pivotal position to achieve, to maintain as well as to improve the application of the total testing process (TTP) to this level of accuracy through:

(a) accounting for possible sources of pre-analytical variability (largely deriving from the quality of the tumour biopsy) using a series of protocolled rigorous and diligent internal quality checks; and
(b) improvement and maintenance of interpretation and reporting skills through competency linked expert training, as proposed and presented by a recent Position Paper of the European Society of Pathology (Matias-Guiu et al. 2020).

References

Allison KH, Hammond MEH, Dowsett M, McKernin SE, Carey LA, Fitzgibbons PL, Hayes DF, Lakhani SR, Chavez-MacGregor M, Perlmutter J, Perou CM, Regan MM, Rimm DL, Symmans WF, Torlakovic EE, Varella L, Viale G, Weisberg TF, McShane LM, Wolff AC. Estrogen and progesterone receptor testing in breast Cancer: ASCO/CAP guideline update. J Clin Oncol. 2020;38(12):1346–66. https://doi.org/10.1200/JCO.19.02309.

Badve S, Kumar G (eds.). Predictive Biomarkers in Oncology. Applications in Precision Medicine. Springer International Publishing 2019.

Brahmer JR, Govindan R, Anders RA, et al. The Society for Immunotherapy of Cancer consensus statement on immunotherapy for the treatment of non-small cell lung cancer (NSCLC). J Immunother Cancer. 2018;6:75. https://doi.org/10.1186/s40425-018-0382-2.

College of American Pathologists. PD-L1 testing of patients with lung cancer for immunooncology therapies. CAP; 2021.

Dzau VJ, Ginsburg GS, Chopra A, Goldman D, Green ED, Leonard DGB, McClellan M, Plump A, Terry SF, Yamamoto KR. Realizing the full potential of precision medicine in health and health care: a vital direction for health and health care. *NAM perspectives*. Discussion paper. Washington, DC: National Academy of Medicine; 2016. https://doi.org/10.31478/201609k.

El-Deiry WS, et al. The current state of molecular testing in the treatment of patients with solid tumors, 2019. CA Cancer J Clin. 2019;69(4):305–43. https://doi.org/10.3322/caac.21560.

Elmore JG, Longton GM, Carney PA, et al. Diagnostic concordance among pathologists interpreting breast biopsy specimens. JAMA. 2015;313(11):1122–32. https://doi.org/10.1001/jama.2015.1405.

García-Alfonso P, García-Carbonero R, García-Foncillas J, et al. Update of the recommendations for the determination of biomarkers in colorectal carcinoma: National Consensus of the Spanish Society of Medical Oncology and the Spanish Society of Pathology. Clin Transl Oncol. 2020;22:1976–91. https://doi.org/10.1007/s12094-020-02357-z.

Garrido P, Conde E, de Castro J, Gómez-Román JJ, Felip E, Pijuan L, Isla D, Sanz J, Paz-Ares L, López-Ríos F. Updated guidelines for predictive biomarker testing in advanced non-small-cell lung cancer: a National Consensus of the Spanish Society of Pathology and the Spanish Society of Medical Oncology. Clin Transl Oncol. 2020;22:989–1003.

Garrison LP Jr, Babigumira JB, Masaquel A, Wang BC, Lalla D, Brammer M. The lifetime economic burden of inaccurate HER2 testing: estimating the costs of false-positive and false-negative HER2 test results in US patients with early-stage breast Cancer. Value Health. 2015;18(4):541–6. https://doi.org/10.1016/j.jval.2015.01.012.

Heinmoller P, Baenfer G, Grzelinksi M, Alexander K, Jasani B. Quality control of immunohistochemical and in situ hybridization predictive for treatment: Experience from international guidelines and international quality control schemes. In: Sunil Badve, George Louis Kumar (Eds.), Predictive Biomarkers in Oncology, 525–37 - December 2018. https://doi.org/10.1007/978-3-319-95228-4_48.

Humphries MP, Bingham V, Abdullahi Sidi F, et al. Improving the diagnostic accuracy of the PD-L1 test with image analysis and multiplex hybridization. Cancers (Basel). 2020;12(5):1114. https://doi.org/10.3390/cancers12051114.

Lhermitte B, et al. Adequately defining tumor cell proportion in tissue samples for molecular testing improves interobserver reproducibility of its assessment. Virchows Arch. 2017;470(1):21–7.

Matias-Guiu X, Stanta G, Carneiro F, et al. The leading role of pathology in assessing the somatic molecular alterations of cancer: position paper of the European Society of Pathology. Virchows Archiv Int J Pathol. 2020;476(4):491–7. https://doi.org/10.1007/s00428-020-02757-0.

McKean WB, Moser JC, Rimm D, Hu-Lieskovan S. Biomarkers in precision cancer immunotherapy: promise and challenges. Am Soc Clin Oncol Educ Book. 2020;40:e275–91. https://doi.org/10.1200/EDBK_280571.

Miller RE, Leary A, Scott CL, Serra V, Lord CJ, Bowtell D, Chang DK, Garsed DW, Jonkers J, Ledermann JA, Nik-Zainal S. ESMO recommendations on predictive biomarker testing for homologous recombination deficiency and PARP inhibitor benefit in ovarian cancer. Ann Oncol. 2020;31(12):1606–22.

Nass SJ, Cohen MB, Nayar R, Zutter MM, Balogh EP, Schilsky RL, Hricak H, Elenitoba-Johnson KSJ. Improving cancer diagnosis and care: patient access to high-quality oncologic pathology. Oncologist. 2019;24(10):1287–90. https://doi.org/10.1634/theoncologist.2019-0261.

Park JJH, Siden E, Zoratti MJ, Dron L, Harari O, Singer J. Lester RT. Thorlund K, Mills EJ. Systematic review of basket trials, umbrella trials, and platform trials: A landscape analysis of master protocols. Trials 2019, 20, 572.

Plebani M. The detection and prevention of errors in laboratory medicine. Ann Clin Biochem. 2010;47(Pt 2):101–10. https://doi.org/10.1258/acb.2009.009222.

Wasielewski RV, Hasselmann S, Rüschoff J, Fisseler-Eckhoff A, Kreipe H. Proficiency testing of immunohistochemical biomarker assays in breast cancer. Virchows Arch. 2008;453(6):537–43. https://doi.org/10.1007/s00428-008-0688-4.

Zhang H, Moisini I, Ajabnoor RM, Turner BM, Hicks DG. Applying the new guidelines of HER2 testing in breast cancer. Curr Oncol Rep. 2020;22(5):51. https://doi.org/10.1007/s11912-020-0901-4.

Role of Pathologist in Precision Molecular and Digital Image Analyses

17

17.1 Introduction

Precision cancer diagnosis is aimed at detecting individual cancer associated genetic changes amenable to molecularly targeted treatments. This requires first of all a diagnostic identification of the presence of cancer cells in the biopsy taken from the tumour bearing tissue. It also includes the typing and the subtyping of the tumour cell origin and its grading in terms of its likely behaviour. The cancer specimen is then subjected to in situ (or morpho-molecular) or tissue extraction based molecular analysis (See Part II for information on the extraction method used) to identify qualitative or quantitative protein, RNA and/or DNA related changes potentially associated with the likely prognostic and the predictive behaviour of the cancer before and subsequent to molecularly targeted treatment.

The aim of this section is to describe the role of the pathologist in conducting and guiding morpho-molecular and molecular analyses for precision cancer diagnosis, and how the findings of such studies help to improve the precision of drug targeted treatment of the cancer patient. It also describes the demand on the pathologist to take up specialist training to have the knowledge and expertise to guide the development and validation of novel digital image based computational, (machine learning and artificial intelligence) analyses required for defining more complex features of the tumour potentially associated with its prognostic and predictive behaviour as well as resistance to treatment, such as:

(a) tumour heterogeneity; and
(b) tumour microenvironment

In the light of these developments there is a growing need to re-define as well as refine the role of an anatomic pathologist to match up with the new needs of Precision Cancer Medicine. There is already a demand for the pathologists to undertake additional specialist training in molecular and computational pathology. Though it is necessary to emphasise that at a solid foundation in anatomic pathology is needed to constitute the bedrock and the basis of virtually all cancer diagnostics as prophesised by Rosai (2007). This is particularly important to bear in mind since molecular pathology though gaining rapid momentum as the cornerstone of Personalised Cancer Medicine, is not yet mature enough to be applied as a stand-alone discipline in routine practice without pitfalls (Sun and Pfeifer 2019). A balanced solution appears to be in adjusting and evolving role of anatomic pathology to meet the changing perspectives and requirements of molecular medicine as it develops into a diagnostic discipline in its own right, as philosophically anticipated by LiVolsi and Upton (2012) and critically appraised by Dubbink et al. (2014).

As mentioned, to accommodate the demands of molecular cancer medicine, the pathologist's

B. Jasani et al., *Precision Cancer Medicine*, https://doi.org/10.1007/978-3-030-84087-7_17

role in some sense, has already undergone an evolution from morphological to morpho-molecular analysis of the type, the grade and the stage of the cancer based on a succession of advances made in immunohistochemistry and in situ molecular analysis. Pathologists have also adopted to become essential physicians on the oncology care team with their growing practice based specialized knowledge and skills to inform molecularly targeted therapies. However, with the more recent advent of the use of digital image based and computational methods, the pathologists are again in need to adopt to computational cancer diagnostics run on basis of a co-ordinated digital image architecture that supports and harmonises pathology, radiology, and informatics (Nass et al. 2019).

Here, the increasing use of whole slide digital images of tumour tissue biopsy sections is an example of changing the field of pathology to facilitate telemedicine, expert consultations as well as webinar based expert training and competency testing of pathologists. The new wave of change also holds the potential to improve the accuracy of overall diagnostic reporting aided by rapid second review required for selected difficult cases (Nakhleh et al. 2016). Added to is the promise of the emerging applications of artificial intelligence (AI) (described in detail in Part IV of this Book) which could help clinicians to overcome cognitive overload from diagnostic information. In this regards, AI offers the potential to highlight areas of interest in a specimen to allow pathologists focus their skills and attention to evaluate micro-invasive or micro-metastatic tumour components with an increased potential for distant metastasis (Bejnordi et al. 2017).

Digitization of microscopic images also offers a powerful facility to compile large digital pathology data sets that can be used to develop AI algorithms for computational machine led diagnostic methods (Volynskaya et al. 2018). This is fostering a growing collaboration between pathologists and biomedical informaticians for provision of more precise and accurate diagnostic information to guide high precision cancer treatment and monitoring as highlighted in Fig. 17.1.

The aim of this Chapter is to describe the emerging role of the pathologist in proper guidance of molecular and AI methods to achieve greater accuracy in predictive cancer diagnostics.

17.2 Role of Pathologist in Morpho-Molecular Diagnosis of Cancer

Cancer diagnosis depends on initial anatomic or morphological identification and typing and subtyping of the cancer cells included within the tissue sample or biopsy. This remains the base of all cancer diagnosis because the actual definition of cancer cells is ultimately based on their morphological characteristics visible under the light microscope in tissue sections stained with a dye such as Haematoxylin and Eosin (H & E). The cellular information revealed by H & E is sufficient in most cases to identify the lesion as a cancer as well as its cell and tissue origin. It also helps to assess the severity (the grade) and the degree of progression (the stage) of the cancerous disease process as defined by morphological alterations in the size and shape and the distribution of the cancer cells as well as tumour invasion associated changes in the surrounding stromal cells or the tumour micro-environment, TME.

The morphological analysis at the light microscopic level however relies upon a fundamental assumption that cancer cells forming the cancerous tissue or lesion are all derived from a single cell forming a clone of genetically identical cells i.e. a monoclonal tumour. On this basis all the tumour cells present within the same tumour biopsy are seen to be morphologically the same or 'mono-morphic' in terms of their size and shape which in turn are generally similar to the cells of their origin but distinct from the cells surrounding them and forming the stroma or the so-called tumour micro-environment (TME).

Morphological diagnosis in this sense is a process of visual pattern recognition which is necessarily subjective and depends heavily for its accuracy and reproducibility on the knowledge, skills and the experience of the pathologist to recognise morphological patterns typical of various

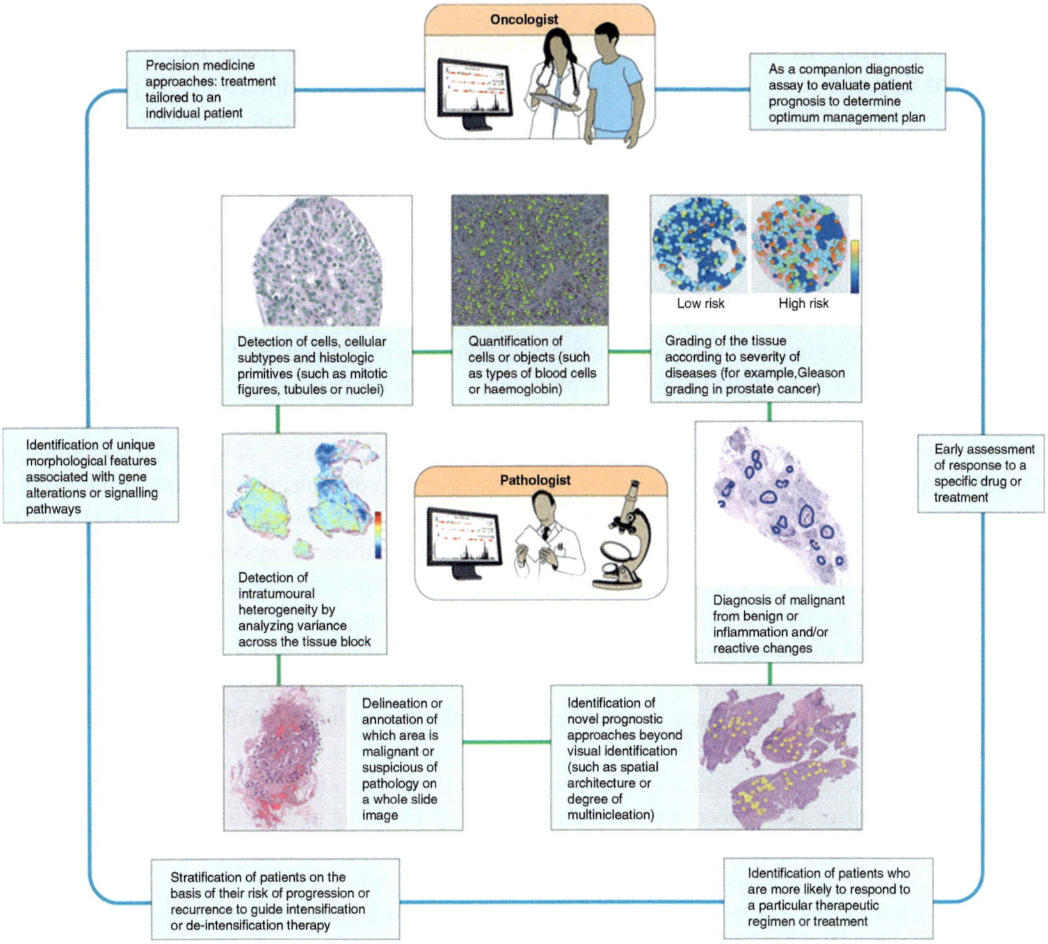

Fig. 17.1 Emerging role of the pathologist for provision of evidence-based integrated diagnostic report for planning for high precision treatment and disease monitoring (Bera et al. 2019)

cancer types and sub-types, an expertise, a process which requires many years of continual training and practice on part of the pathologist.

To alleviate the dependency on this type of subjective approach, it has proved necessary to develop molecular markers or biomarkers capable of identifying tumour cells according to the presence of molecules consistently if not uniquely associated with the structural and functional characteristics of individual types and subtypes of cancer cells. This has led to the development of immunohistochemistry (IHC) which utilises antibodies directed at cell and tissue specific protein molecules, applied in combination with a detection system capable of a simple but precise deposition of a signal—visualisable readily under the light microscope (see Part II for details).

Fortuitously, the use of the IHC method has been found to be applicable to the same kind of tissue biopsy material prepared for H & E based morphological analysis, thereby allowing a direct correlation of between protein composition and morphological characteristics of the cancer cells, resulting in a more precise (objective, accurate and reproducible) diagnostic analysis of the cancer.

17.3 Role of Pathologist in Molecular Analysis of Cancer

With our greater understanding of the biology of cancer cells at the molecular level, it has become apparent that although at the cellular level cancers generally do arise from a single cell of a given tissue type and subtype, a process which makes them resemble closely to each other, the actual process leading to the development and the growth of the cancer as a whole seems to involve genetic alterations diverse enough to make the individual cancer a mosaic of many molecularly or genetically unique subsets of cells or subclone. These genetic differences relate to the cancer predisposing genes inherited by the patient combined with a unique blend of somatic and epigenetic alterations associated with the process of cancer formation and progression pertaining to its development in a particular patient. The end result is a molecular profile which is more less unique to the particular patient's cancer.

Fortunately, the genetic changes associated with the behaviour of the cancer cells and their response or resistance to the treatment appear to be broadly shared by cancers arising from the same as well as different tissue types or subtypes. In addition, similar to IHC, it has been found possible to apply molecular techniques directly to routine diagnostic tissue biopsies material. This has allowed the pathologist to correlate the findings of H & E and IHC analyses with those obtained from molecular analysis performed on the same biopsy material, and thereby formulate an integrated more precise and accurate diagnostic prognostic, predictive and therapeutic analyses based on a combination of morphological, immunohistochemical and molecular methods.

17.4 Role of Pathologist in Guidance of Cancer Molecular Profiling

Tumor molecular profiling is generally performed on DNA extracted from formalin-fixed paraffin-embedded tumour tissue specimen sections. Prior to testing, an H & E stained tissue section taken from a tissue block representative of the tumour is examined by the pathologist to confirm the presence of the tumor, annotate the area and determine the tumor content in the whole specimen and the annotated region of interest (ROI).

The pathologist's review of haematoxylin & eosin (H&E) stained slides, is also to ensure sample quality, tumor DNA sufficiency by visually estimating the percentage tumor nuclei and tumor annotation for manual macrodissection. There is considerable variation in tumor nuclei percentage between pathologists, potentially undermining the precision of molecular evaluation and emphasising the need for more reliable quantitative tumor evaluation. A system called TissueMark for automated tumor annotation and percentage tumor nuclei measurement in NSCLC using computerized image analysis has been developed (Hamilton et al. 2015), for more reliable tissue samples for molecular profiling in discovery and diagnostics.

A study conducted on colorectal cancer samples by Dufraing et al. (2019) has recommended that only pathologists should be involved in the estimation of neoplastic cell content though molecular biologists/technicians may substitute, if specific training has been given to them and a pathologist is available for any feedback. The estimation should be directed to an area with the highest density of viable neoplastic cells and lowest density of inflammatory cells, using a protocol established to be reliable for the needs of micro- and macro-dissection, interpretation and reporting practices of a particular cancer type.

In general, the amount of cells and the concentration of the extracted DNA is a central issue to resolve in most mutational analysis using formalin fixed paraffin embedded tissue material (Kim and Tsao 2014). The cyto-block specimen, as well as small biopsy samples that yield a very low amount of DNA, can detect mutations only when using more sensitive detection methods. Samples with <300 viable tumour cells, run the risk of an insufficient result due to interference from artefactual mutations associated with formalin fixed specimens. A successful mutation test should be aimed to be based on a minimum 400 tumour cells/specimen has been suggested. The highest test success-rate has been found to be associated with ≥30% tumour cellularity within the macrodissection area, and a ≥2 mm tumour area marked for macrodissection.

The procedure of microdissection involves haematoxylin and eosin (H&E)–stained slide annotated by the pathologist, with the annotated slide guiding the technician to manually scrape the tissue with a scalpel or razor blade from a consecutive, unstained slide. This process is time-consuming and laborious when multiple slides need to be processed simultaneously to produce enough input material for downstream processes. To resolve this issue an accurate automated macro-dissection system has been innovated recently by Javey et al. (2021) AVENIO Millisect System. The automated method is illustrated in Fig. 17.2, and has the potential to extract DNA, RNA and protein from high- and low-tumor content FFPE tumor tissue specimens with high efficiency and a product quality comparable to the commercially available kits for nucleic acid and protein extraction from multiple vendors with very similar quantitation and quality assessment results.

Generic guidelines for the pathologist led management of molecular analysis of cancer samples have been provided by Cree et al. (2014) and more recently by Moore et al. (2018). In addition a tailor-made training of pathologists is recommended to provide them an understanding of:

- the clinical relevance of a particular molecular test result;
- the technologies used to generate the result;
- whether the test is technically satisfactory and how troubleshoot if a sub-optimal result is suspected;
- any biological variables affecting the test result;
- complex data (ie, bioinformatics) linked to the test result;

Table 17.1 provides a summary of the various molecular tests for cancer tissue analysis. Details of these tests are available from: Vnencak-Jones et al. (2016). A more recent appraisal of the molecular methods has been provided by

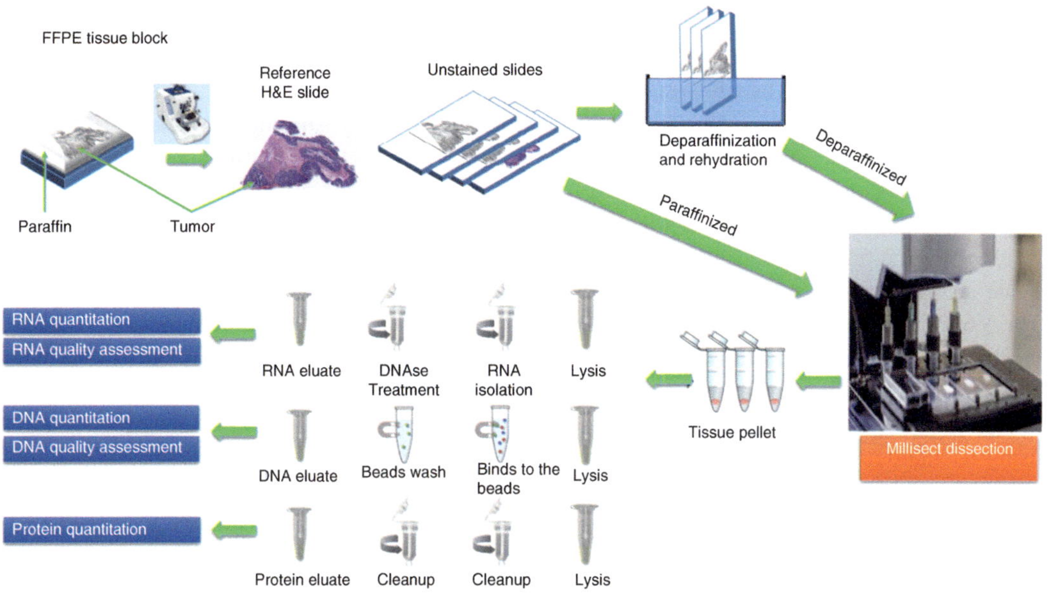

Fig. 17.2 Automated macro-dissection system

Table 17.1 Types of molecular tests and variants detected

Molecular methodology	Variant types: SNVs	Small duplications, insertions, deletions, indels	Exon duplications, deletions or gene copy number changes	SVs
Allele-specific PCR	✓			
PCR and sanger dideoxy sequencing	✓	✓		*a*
PCR and pyrosequencing	✓	•		
PCR and MS	✓	•		
PCR and single base extension	✓			
MLPA	✓		✓	
FISH			*B*	✓
NGS—Custom panels (amplicon capture)	✓	✓		
NGS—Custom panels (hybridization capture)	✓	✓	✓	*c*
NGS—Whole exome sequencing	✓	✓	✓	•
NGS—Whole genome sequencing	✓	✓	✓	✓
ddPCR	✓	✓		*c*
BEAMing	✓	✓		*c*

Pathologists in charge of molecular tumor testing hold the responsibility to have a competent knowledge of the validity and sensitivities and specificities of each of testing platforms used by them or available for use to them. This is especially important if they are using laboratory-developed assays.

Tests for molecular profiling of tumors range from simple to complex. The simplest tests detect only one type of mutation in one gene, such as a single nucleotide variation (SNV). An example of the result and significance of such test is T to A substitution mutation at position c.1799 of BRAF, resulting in the amino acid substitution of glutamic acid for valine (p.V600E) in the protein. The V600E mutation is commonly observed in melanoma. The clinical testing for this type of analysis is performed in a CLIA-certified molecular genetics or molecular pathology laboratory using technologies such as allele-specific polymerase chain reaction (PCR), Sanger dideoxy sequencing, pyrosequencing, multiplex ligation-dependent probe amplification (MLPA), or mass spectrometry (MS). Clinical testing for gene copy number and structural variants is performed in a molecular cytogenetics laboratory linked to a pathology department with fluorescence in situ hybridization (FISH) and fluorescence microscopy facility.

The more comprehensive molecular testing is based on Next-Generation Sequencing (NGS) which allows simultaneous detection of all the major types of cancer driving gene alterations, including substitutions, duplications, insertions, deletions, indels, gene copy number variations, and structural variants, including inversions and translocations. Newer, next-generation sequencing (NGS) technologies, such as massively parallel sequencing in addition allow for whole exome sequencing, which examines all protein-coding regions in the human genome or whole genome sequencing (WGS), which analyzes both protein-coding and non-coding regions in the human genome. Examples of machines used in NGS include the Illumina MiSeq and HiSeq and the Life Technologies Ion Torrent PGM and Proton. Such tests are usually outsourced to academic, or private reference laboratories like Foundation Medicine, called FoundationOneTM, providing facility for testing mutations in around 322 genes commonly altered in cancer.

17.5 Role of Pathologist in Analysis of Tumour Heterogeneity

For a long time it was believed that a tumour represented a homogeneous tumor cell population in terms of genome characteristics. This model was promoted by Vogelstein's studies on colorectal cancer, which proposed a linear stepwise progression model (Ilyas and Tomlinson 1996). In practical terms, this implied that a single sample would be representative for the entire tumor cell mass. It soon became clear, however, that this is a gross oversimplification of the dynamics of the cell populations comprised in any given tumor.

That this might not reflect the actual tumor development emerged from a seminal study looking at up to 20 samples from the same tumor. This showed co-existence of several distinct subpopulations co-existed in terms of their molecular make-up (Baisse et al. 2001). Simple attempts to reconstruct the findings in terms of clonal architecture of the tumors showed that heterogeneity was not random but clustered, suggesting the existence of distinct sub-clones. However, these clusters appeared to be partly interwoven, suggesting that clones infiltrated each other. The findings led to the following important practical conclusion:

> taking into account a significant intra-tumor genetic heterogeneity of colorectal tumors, the use of (genetic) markers for prognosis management should be reconsidered (Baisse et al. 2001).

Tumour heterogeneity describes differences between tumours of the same type in different patients, and between cancer cells within a tumour. Both can lead to different responses to therapy. Genetic and epigenetic differences between cancer cells within a tumour might explain why some tumour cells remain present in the patient after cancer treatment has finished (Fisher et al. 2013).

Several types of genetic heterogeneity have been found to be associated with cancer. The two most well-known include:

(a) Inter-patient tumor heterogeneity whereby no two patients with the same subtype of tumor behave the same clinically, with or without treatment. This may be related to host factors, such as tumor microenvironment (described next), or germ line variants influencing treatment response, together with the unique somatic mutations that can occur within the tumor of each individual patient.

(b) Intra-tumor heterogeneity can be divided into three main categories: genetic, phenotypic, and microenvironmental (Caswell-Jin et al. 2021). It is associated with distinct cellular populations with specific phenotypic features within tumors. It has been described in several tumor types (Hua et al. 2020) including lung, breast, ovarian, pancreatic, kidney, colorectal, brain and prostate cancers, as well as hematological malignancies, such as chronic lymphoblastic leukemia (CLL), and acute lymphoblastic leukemia. Metastatic lesions at different secondary sites can arise from different cellular populations within a primary tumor, resulting in heterogeneity among metastases, known as inter-metastatic heterogeneity. In addition, since metastatic lesions can acquire new mutations and evolve independently with each cell division, heterogeneity within a metastasis can also exist, known as intra-metastatic heterogeneity. The observation that some genetic aberrations are found solely in either primary or metastatic tumours lead to the proposal that further genetic divergence and evolution occurred independently at both sites after tumour dissemination. Similarly, the identification of somatic mutations present in the primary tumour or metastatic sites only or are specific to one tumour region (private mutations) provides further evidence for ongoing independent subclonal evolution within distinct and spatially separated tumour regions (Gerlinger et al. 2012).

According to a recent article by Bosman (2018) the notion of tumors heterogeneity is now well rooted in diagnostic pathology. However, the extent of this heterogeneity at the molecular level and its impact on (targeted) treatment choice are still not fully understood and therefore not included for consideration in routine pathology practice. Nevertheless pathologists are in a pivotal position to begin to contribute to solving major scientific and clinical issues related to tumor heterogeneity by developing or adopting guidelines for more standardised purposeful method for tumor sampling, in order to account for intratumor heterogeneity in the available tumor tissue samples. They should also develop or adopt guidelines and/or technology for adequately accurate documentation of sample characteristics such as percentage of tumor cells in a sample, and contribute to training of bioinformaticians in the field of cancer pathology and integrate their contribution to the analysis in the workflow leading to a final pathology report.

The analysis of the extent of intratumor heterogeneity (ITH) is quite demanding ideally requiring freshly excised snap-frozen samples with a recording of the precise site of tissue sampling which can vary from two to up to ten samples per tumour histologically confirmed. There is in addition need for non-tumor samples (including normal tissue, peripheral blood and buccal cell samples).

Genomic studies have demonstrated the complex and heterogeneous clonal landscape of tumors of different origins and the potential impact of intratumor heterogeneity on treatment response and resistance, cancer progression, and the risk of disease relapse (Jamal-Hanjani et al. 2015). However, the significance of sub-clonal mutations, in particular mutations in driver genes, and their evolution through time and their dynamics in response to cancer therapies, is yet to be determined. The necessary tools are now available to prospectively determine whether clonal heterogeneity can be used as a biomarker of clinical outcome and to what extent sub-clonal somatic alterations might influence clinical outcome. Studies that use longitudinal tissue sampling (Caswell-Jin et al. 2021), such as that based on liquid biopsies as discussed later (also see Alix-Panabieres 2020), have begun to reveal, with integration of genomic and clinical data, the subclonal composition and evolution of tumors to define the extent of genetic diversity in different tumor types and its relevance to patient outcome. Such studies are aimed to provide further evidence for drug-resistance mechanisms informing combinatorial, adaptive, and tumor immune therapies placed within the context of tumor evolution.

According to a most recent research on tumor heterogeneity (Rabbie et al. 2020), at least in part is due to the stability of multiple genomic clonal populations co-existing within the neoplasm. These seem to arise from divergent evolution of the originating cells' progeny and may be sustained by geographical isolation within the tumor and cooperation between clones. Changes in the nature and order of early driver mutations may lead to highly divergent evolution between tumors and reinforce the profound inter-tumor heterogeneity seen in human tumors. Passenger mutations in these populations may lead to altered epigenetic "attractor states" and a blurring of the boundaries between cellular phenotypes. In addition, tumor-extrinsic features of the ECM and TME may be responsible for dynamic oscillations between epigenetically regulated phenotypes. Spatial heterogeneity in TME components across a tumor may reinforce intratumor heterogeneity, whereas global changes in TME between patients may influence the development of inter-tumor heterogeneity.

17.6 Role of Pathologist in Analysis of Tumour Micro-Environment (TME)

The cancer tumour micro-environment (TME) constitutes a heterogeneous mixture of several reactive cell types and subtypes interacting with the cancer cells in a complex manner. Recently, TME has been recognized as a key contributor for cancer progression and drug resistance. This concept implies that cancer is no longer an isolated cellular population; instead, it is the consequence of collaboration of different types of dysregulated cells. An example of this the innate resistance to BRAF inhibition in BRAF-mutant tumour cell lines has been shown to be mediated by secretion of hepatocyte growth factor and its receptor, MET, by stromal cells, and it is possible to reverse the resistance by combining BRAF and MET inhibitors (Straussman et al. 2012).

Although it is possible in routine practice to analyse the above type of interaction using the routine IHC technique with antibodies specific to each cell type or subtype, applied to several parallel or serial sections taken from the same tumour tissue, there is an inevitable loss of precise spatial information pertaining to the in vivo status of the individual cancer cells in the context of the TME.

The problem with analyzing large groups of samples in traditional and manual ways by experienced pathologists, is that it is highly laborious, time-consuming, and prone to human error. To overcome this handicap it has been necessary to develop what are known as multiplex IHC methods which utilise several cell type and subtype specific antibodies sequentially or simultaneously added to the same tissue section bearing the cancerous lesion. Their binding is then revealed using a set of distinct colour or fluorescent labels or reporter molecules linked to the relevant set of secondary detection antibodies.

The resulting multiplex staining is however too complex to interpret and score visually under the light or fluorescence microscope. To overcome this difficulty it has been necessary to develop sophisticated digital image viewing systems capable of separating the individual chromogenic colours or fluorescent label signals and analysing them with computer aided algorithms (Tan et al. 2020). This approach is currently not applicable for routine diagnosis but is beginning to be applied increasingly in specialised centres for research and development towards new drug development. Also it needs to be carefully validated by pathologists to provide researchers with interpretable data which correlate clinically sufficiently well to identify new predictive or prognostic morphological characteristics or to couple them with other modalities such as genomic analysis to better stratify tumors and potential novel therapeutic targets.

Research into clinically utility of multi-immunofluoresence (mIF) analysis relates to its recent application to the analysis of clinical significance of immune cell infiltration and PD-L1 expression in early breast cancer. The SP142 assay categorizes tumors as PD-L1$^+$ if at least 1% of the tumor area is occupied by PD-L1$^+$ immune cells (ICs). While the binary designation of PD-L1 status is clinically useful its clinical utility is limited by its semi-quantitative nature and operator dependency. Similar to PD-L1 testing, sTIL is considered to be clinically useful (as it correlates with survival, chemotherapy response, and potentially immunotherapy response). However, once again suboptimal inter-observer concordance related to underlying intra-tumoral heterogeneity of sTILs limits its clinical utility as its estimation is semi-quantitative assays and requires a pathologist to visually estimate ICs, which may sometimes be present in low abundance.

The advantage of mIF is that it enables estimation of IC counts in high resolution across numerous high-powered magnification fields (hereafter called regions of interest, ROI) and therefore has the potential to produce more accurate and precise estimates of sTILs and PD-L1 expression, relative to the clinical assays. Furthermore, mIF permits more detailed characterization of IC/TC interactions via single-cell quantification of numerous phenotypic surface markers, and spatial localization of cells into various tissue compartments (i.e., tumor versus stroma). IC densities and PD-L1 expression are repeatedly sampled across multiple ROIs on a single slide, providing the opportunity to characterize spatial heterogeneity. Effort is being made with appropriate statistical modelling (Sanchez et al. 2021) based on repeated sampling of ROIs to improve both accuracy and precision of IC density and PD-L1 expression estimates. This represents an important new role for the pathologist required for selecting ROI and evaluating ROI sample size to provide sufficient statistical power to detect significant changes in ICs/PD-L1 in the context of a clinical trial and predictive diagnostic analysis.

17.7 Future Role of Pathologist in Emerging Morpho-Molecular Cancer Diagnostics

Translation of a potential biomarker identified in the laboratory to one that can be used in the clinic, based on the use of a combination of multiple biomarkers, including genomic and proteomic information, poses theoretically and practically a highly complex challenge to overcome.

However, several projects summarised below are already underway in an attempt to overcome these barriers:

1. RESPONSIFY: Genomic prediction of treatment response and resistance

   A series of projects are aimed to find genome based biomarkers to predict response and resistance to a given drug therapy in breast cancer. The index project is focused on tissue-derived predictive factors for anti-HER2 directed therapy. In addition, serum markers for response to anti-angiogenic therapy are included for evaluation. The main focus is to study immunological changes as well as mutations in tumour tissue. The project has already developed an mRNA based immune predictive test ("ImmunoPredict"), capable of monitoring changes in the immunological status in breast cancer tissue. It is planned to use this test in future clinical trials as concomitant biomarker. In addition, tumour infiltrating lymphocytes is being used as a surrogate for an active intra-tumoural immune environment since it has been found to be predictive for response to anti-HER2 as well as chemotherapy and appear to be linked to good prognosis. This has led to development of standardized approaches for TIL evaluation. Furthermore a combination tumour infiltrating lymphocytes and PIK3CA mutation have been found to be sufficiently robust biomarker indicator to be included in the German breast cancer guidelines. https://cordis.europa.eu/project/id/278659/reporting/fr

2. Proteogenomic Diagnostic Approaches into the Clinic

   NCI-funded Proteogenomic Translational Research Centers are supporting research through CPTAC and other initiatives to advance the identification and use of protein molecular markers and proteogenomic information for predicting clinical outcomes. Understanding proteins—their expression, modifications, and abnormal functions in cancer development and progression—has been critically important for developing drugs, selecting treatments, and predicting treatment response. Integration of proteomic information is the next natural step in precision oncology. The big challenge in moving proteomics into the clinic alongside genomics is collecting enough tumor tissue. The amount of tumor typically collected during a biopsy is sufficient for DNA and RNA analysis, but much more tissue is needed to analyze tumor proteins. To this effct researchers at the Broad Institute, Baylor College of Medicine, and their collaborators have developed new microscale methods of comprehensive proteomic analysis that require a smaller amount of tissue available from core needle biopsies taken from tumors after treatment with the HER2-targeted therapy. Both genomic and proteomic information was sought from these to provide insights into tumor response vs resistance. The results of proteomic analysis gave information regarding drug response and drug resistance that was not evident with genomic information alone. The study also provided evidence that proteogenomic analyses can be performed effectively on routine clinical samples.

3. Liquid Biopsies: Precision dynamic monitoring of cancer progression

   The two most well-developed biomarkers detected by liquid biopsy — circulating tumour cells (CTCs) and circulating cell-free tumour DNA (ctDNA). Both are subject to technical variability in the pre-analytical and analytical steps. A co-operative effort based on academic and industry expertise is currently taking place for the development of robust and reproducible liquid-biopsy assays.

The extent to which liquid biopsy might ultimately replace standard tissue biopsies is still unclear. For diagnosing primary tumours or determining the stage of metastatic lesions in tissues where it is difficult to extract a sample, liquid biopsy might provide a reliable alternative. Liquid biopsy could also help to avoid complications that occur after invasive tissue biopsy, such as bleeding, infections and pain. Also pre-, per- and post-treatment liquid biopsies could help to monitor persistence or increase of CTCs or ctDNA — which would indicate resistance to the chosen therapy. It also offers the potential of detecting an early relapse and provide treatment before the tumour burden becomes excessive or incurable (Alix-Panabieres 2020).

4. RNAScope: Potential for in situ single cell quantitative mRNA analysis

Tumour heterogeneity at a single cell has been difficult to resolve with PCR-based technology or immunohistochemistry. The quantitative RT-PCR is the 'gold standard' for measuring gene expression with high sensitivity and specificity. However, its sensitivity is limited when applied to heterogeneous multicellular tumour samples, and it is also prone to interference from non-cancerous cells. Immunohistochemistry (IHC) has proven to be useful studying protein expression levels in individual cell level in tissue sections for diagnostic purposes, but it is less quantitative than the RT-PCR method (Taylor et al. 2006). Furthermore, validated immunohistochemically applicable antibodies are so far available for a limited number of proteins—~25% of the proteins composing the human proteome. These limitations of PCR-based methods and IHC are resolvable to an extent through the use of laser microdissection to enrich target cells for analysis. However, this approach is both expensive and cumbersome requiring pathologist/scientist to correctly identify target cells of interest. RNAscope® produced by Advanced Cell Diagnostics, Inc. (Hayward, CA) offers a novel method capable of overcoming these barriers.

RNAscope® represents an RNA in situ hybridisation method that can detect single-molecules of mRNA in context of well-preserved cellular and tissue morphology (Wang et al. 2012). It utilises a paired probe system to ensure sensitive and selective targeting of mRNA molecules and has been successfully applied to measure gene expression in cancer cells; stem cells and circulating tumour cells. RNAscope® also offers the scope of mRNA expression measurements for individual or multiple genes in archival tumour specimens in a routine diagnostic setting. Furthermore, mRNA expression detected by RNAscope® shows a strong correlation with quantitative PCR (Morley-Bunker et al. 2019).

The clinical utility of RNAscope® has been examined in a proof of principle study for its capacity to identify poor prognostic outcomes in colorectal cancer based on in situ quantification of TNFRSF11A and/or GFI1 mRNA transcripts (Morley-Bunker et al. 2019) Further larger studies are required to confirm prognostic value of RNAScope detected GFI1 and TNFRSF11A expression and patient outcome.

References

Alix-Panabieres C. The future of liquid biopsy. Nature. 2020;579:S9.

Baisse B, Bouzourene H, Saraga EP, Bosman FT, Benhattar J. Intratumor genetic heterogeneity in advanced human colorectal adenocarcinoma. Int J Cancer. 2001;93:346–52.

Bejnordi BE, Veta M, Van Diest PJ, et al. Diagnostic assessment of deep learning algorithms for detection of lymph node metastases in women with breast cancer. JAMA. 2017;318:2199–210.

Bera K, Schalper KA, Rimm DL, Velcheti V, Madabhushi A. Artificial intelligence in digital pathology - new tools for diagnosis and precision oncology. Nat Rev Clin Oncol. 2019;16(11):703–15. https://doi.org/10.1038/s41571-019-0252-y.

Bosman F. T: tumor heterogeneity: will it change what pathologists do. Pathobiology. 2018;85:18–22. https://doi.org/10.1159/000469664.

Caswell-Jin JL, Lorenz C, Curtis C. Molecular heterogeneity and evolution in breast Cancer. Annu Rev Cancer Biol. 2021;5:79–94.

Cree IA, Deans Z, Ligtenberg MJL, for the European Society of Pathology Task Force on Quality Assurance in Molecular Pathology and the Royal College of Pathologists, et al. Guidance for laboratories performing molecular pathology for cancer patients. J Clin Pathol. 2014;67:923–31.

Dubbink HJ, Deans ZC, Tops BB, van Kemenade FJ, Koljenovic S, van Krieken HJ, Blokx WA, Dinjens WN, Groenen PJ. Next generation diagnostic molecular pathology: critical appraisal of quality assurance in Europe. Mol Oncol. 2014;8:830–9.

Dufraing K, Keppens C, Siebers AG, Kafatos G, Lowe K, et al. Pre-Analytical Challenges during RAS Testing: Tissue Quality and the Estimation of Neoplastic Cell Percentage. Biomark J. 2019;5(2).

Fisher R, Pusztai L, Swanton C. Cancer heterogeneity: implications for targeted therapeutics. Br J Cancer. 2013;108(3):479–85. https://doi.org/10.1038/bjc.2012.581.

Gerlinger M, Rowan AJ, Horswell S, Math M, Larkin J, Endesfelder D, Gronroos E, Martinez P, Matthews N, Stewart A, Tarpey P, Varela I, Phillimore B, Begum S, McDonald NQ, Butler A, Jones D, Raine K, Latimer C, Santos CR, Nohadani M, Eklund AC, Spencer-Dene B, Clark G, Pickering L, Stamp G, Gore M, Szallasi Z, Downward J, Futreal PA, Swanton C. Intratumor heterogeneity and branched evolution revealed by multiregion sequencing. N Engl J Med. 2012 Mar 8;366(10):883–92. https://doi.org/10.1056/NEJMoa1113205. Erratum in: N Engl J Med. 2012;367(10):976. PMID: 22397650; PMCID: PMC4878653.

Hamilton PW, et al. Automated tumor analysis for molecular profiling in lung cancer. Oncotarget. 2015;6(29):27938–52. https://doi.org/10.18632/oncotarget.4391.

Hua X, Zhao W, Pesatori AC, et al. Genetic and epigenetic intratumor heterogeneity impacts prognosis of lung adenocarcinoma. Nat Commun. 2020;11:2459. https://doi.org/10.1038/s41467-020-16295-5.

Ilyas M, Tomlinson IP. Genetic pathways in colorectal cancer. Histopathology. 1996;28:389–99.

Jamal-Hanjani M, Quezada SA, Larkin J, Swanton C. Translational implications of tumor heterogeneity. Clin Cancer Res. 2015;21(6):1258–66. https://doi.org/10.1158/1078-0432.CCR-14-1429.

Javey M, Reinsch C, Feldkamp M, Siemann S, Blüher A, Woestmann C, Cai L, Tran I, May T, Havnar C, Lo AA, Hinzmann B, Heilek G, Palma JF. Innovative tumor tissue dissection tool for molecular oncology diagnostics. J Mol Diagn. 2021;23(4):399–406.

Kim L, Tsao MS. Tumour tissue sampling for lung cancer management in the era of personalised therapy: what is good enough for molecular testing? Eur Respir J. 2014;44(4):1011–22. https://doi.org/10.1183/09031936.00197013.

LiVolsi V, Upton MP. The anatomic pathologist meets molecular pathology. Am J Clin Pathol. 2012;137:341–2.

Moore DA, Young CA, Morris HT, et al. Time for change: a new training programme for morpho-molecular pathologists? J Clin Pathol. 2018;71:285–90.

Morley-Bunker A, et al. Assessment of intra-tumoural colorectal cancer prognostic biomarkers using RNA in situ hybridisation. Oncotarget. 2019;10(14):1425–39. https://doi.org/10.18632/oncotarget.26675.

Nakhleh RE, Nosé V, Colasacco C, et al. Interpretive diagnostic error reduction in surgical pathology and cytology: guideline from the College of American Pathologists Pathology and Laboratory Quality Center and the Association of Directors of Anatomic and Surgical Pathology. Arch Pathol Lab Med. 2016;140:29–40.

Nass SJ, Cohen MB, Nayar R, Zutter MM, Balogh EP, Schilsky RL, Hricak H, Elenitoba-Johnson KS. Improving cancer diagnosis and care: patient access to high-quality oncologic pathology. Oncologist. 2019;24(10):1287–90.

Rabbie R, Ansari-Pour N, Cast O, et al. Multi-site clonality analysis uncovers pervasive heterogeneity across melanoma metastases. Nat Commun. 2020;11:4306. https://doi.org/10.1038/s41467-020-18060-0.

Rosai J. Why microscopy will remain a cornerstone of surgical pathology. Lab Investig. 2007;87:403–8.

Sanchez K, Kim I, Chun B, et al. Multiplex immunofluorescence to measure dynamic changes in tumor-infiltrating lymphocytes and PD-L1 in early-stage breast cancer. Breast Cancer Res. 2021;23:2. https://doi.org/10.1186/s13058-020-01378-4.

Straussman R, Morikawa T, Shee K, Barzily-Rokni M, Qian ZR, Du J, Davis A, Mongare MM, Gould J, Frederick DT, Cooper ZA, Chapman PB, Solit DB, Ribas A, Lo RS, Flaherty KT, Ogino S, Wargo JA, Golub TR. Tumour micro-environment elicits innate resistance to RAF inhibitors through HGF secretion. Nature. 2012 Jul 26;487(7408):500–4. https://doi.org/10.1038/nature11183. PMID: 22763439; PMCID: PMC3711467.

Sun L, Pfeifer JD. Pitfalls in molecular diagnostics. Semin Diagn Pathol. 2019;36(5):342–54.

Tan WCC, et al. Overview of multiplex immunohistochemistry/immunofluorescence techniques in the era of cancer immunotherapy. Cancer Commun (Lond). 2020;40(4):135–53. https://doi.org/10.1002/cac2.12023.

Taylor CR, Levenson RM. Quantification of immunohistochemistry–issues concerning methods, utility and semiquantitative assessment II. Histopathology. 2006 Oct;49(4):411–24. https://doi.org/10.1111/j.1365-2559.2006.02513.x. PMID: 16978205.

Vnencak-Jones C, Berger M, Pao W. Types of molecular tumor testing. My Cancer Genome; 2016. https://www.mycancergenome.org/content/molecular-medicine/types-of-molecular-tumor-testing/. Updated 8 Feb 2020.

Volynskaya Z, Chow H, Evans A, Wolff A, Lagmay-Traya C, Asa SL. Integrated pathology informatics enables high-quality personalized and precision medicine: digital pathology and beyond. Arch Pathol Lab Med. 2018;142(3):369–82. https://doi.org/10.5858/arpa.2017-0139-OA.

Wang F, Flanagan J, Su N, Wang LC, Bui S, Nielson A, Wu X, Vo HT, Ma XJ, Luo Y. RNAscope: a novel in situ RNA analysis platform for formalin-fixed, paraffin-embedded tissues. J Mol Diagn. 2012;14:22–9. https://doi.org/10.1016/j.jmoldx.2011.08.002.

Part IV

Digital and Computational Pathology and Their Role in Precision Oncology

18 Introduction to Digital and Computational Pathology

One of the challenges of modern precision oncology is to deal with increasing complexity of modern tissue diagnostics. The concept of "predictive biomarker" has been firmly established in precision oncology as well as its increasing discovery and clinical utility for different therapies, including novel immunotherapies, its combinations in immune-oncology (IO/IO) or with small molecular respectively advanced therapeutics (IO/non-IO). This might require the analysis of multiplex immunofluorescence of proteins and its associated spatially resolved genetic information even on a single slide, the integration of other multi-omics information including molecular data from next-generation sequencing (NGS), the quantification of 3D-images and the integration of individual patient data from related areas like radiology, liquid biopsies and the entire diagnostic portfolio.

The topics of the previous parts and chapters hold even more true and relevant for the dawning computational future of diagnostic medicine and precision oncology when the implementation of artificial intelligence will be introduced clinically on a routine scale. Thus, the standardization of processes to ensure high and reproducible quality of clinical decisions is even more critical for the development, implementation and use of novel diagnostic technologies. This inevitably applies to the preparation of tissue samples, the image acquisition processes, its interpretation as well as any data-generation technology such as NGS, proteomics, transcriptomics and the use of nanomicroscopy and machine intelligence. The bigger and more complex the available and accessible data source for further analysis and decision-making is, the more we have to ensure their robustness and quality.

Until recently, the conventional role of the pathologist has been to present anatomical pathology findings on various specimens, particularly as a written report or at interdisciplinary and molecular tumor boards. However, in the emerging age of precision medicine and molecular diagnostics, the responsibilities of pathologist have greatly expanded especially in their cancer-related work dealing with an increasing level of complexity. The knowledge base of histopathologic diagnoses that usually lead to therapeutic decisions is no longer sufficient in the emerging world of molecular and precision oncology, because its holds too many different and sometimes inconclusive implications for distinct types and subtypes of cancers related to their diagnosis and treatment options on the individual patient level.

Modern pathology driving precision oncology is getting increasingly more complex and can only be adequately assessed by specially trained pathologists, even if they comply with the already ambitious continuous professional development and education plans. Therefore, specialist training and technical education and support on an interdisciplinary level is urgently needed.

The previous Parts II and III have demonstrated the legacy of today's best practice of

B. Jasani et al., *Precision Cancer Medicine*, https://doi.org/10.1007/978-3-030-84087-7_18

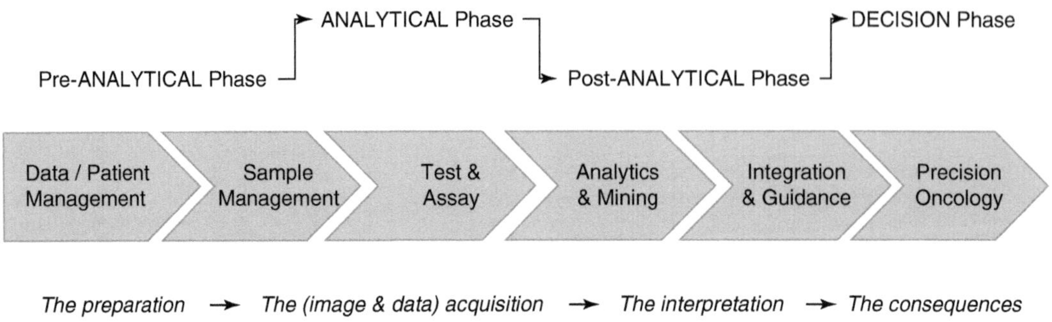

Fig. 18.1 Overview on the entire workflow and process steps in Precision Oncology to ensure clinically relevant and robust decisions supported by digitization, data integration and machine intelligence. Each analytical step is crucial for success and requires a robust and diligent quality management process. Engineering calls this "Quality-by-design"

pathology and are of crucial importance to the clinical success of Computation Pathology in Precision Oncology and the introduction of artificial intelligence (Fig. 18.1). Until today, it has been rather an evolution from describing the gross or histomorphological changes in diseased organs and tissues and connecting the dots between a distinct morphology and the understanding of the underlying cause of disease and possible therapeutic options (Chaps. 1, 2, and 3). Generations of pathologists have added multiple layers of experience, collected knowledge and expert wisdom to reach a general diagnosis including a prognostic assessment for a group of diseases or similar disorders and eventually predicting the best available and least-toxic treatment for an individual patient. Pathologists have gradually assumed their role in guiding therapies in the treatment of most cancers.

Accurate and timely diagnosis of cancer is critical for deciding on the best right treatment for the right individual patient at the right time. In cancer care, diagnostic tests are critical also to inform prognosis, prediction, and assessment of treatment response, disease progression, and recurrence. As described in Part III, pathologists are essential physicians on the oncology care team because they have specialized knowledge to inform diagnostic test selection, performance, and interpretation at the highest quality level, as well as the communication of results and the implications for subsequent care decisions.

The field of artificial intelligence and machine-learning algorithms offers a wide array of diagnostic and therapeutic decision support. One of the prerequisite technologies is directed towards scanning a whole microscopic slide (whole slide imaging = WSI) into a high-quality digital image and apply artificial and machine intelligence–driven algorithms or solutions for further analysis. This might provide an even more precise, robust and reproducible anatomic assessment, leading to an even more robust diagnosis and a sustainable prediction of the best treatment option with a high degree of accuracy and confidence. It is "remarkable" how a computer can already "read" and "interpret" a digitized slide and usually "deliver" a more accurate and quantitative interpretation than just through eyeballed microscopic viewing. Yet, machine-based decision tools either require a comprehensive training of the algorithms and many possible iterations using big sets of data or human experts (pathologists) to create heuristic rule sets. However, for the time being and until a broader acceptance of computational pathology in the oncology community, it remains also legally necessary to confirm any machine-supported diagnosis through a highly skilled and well-trained pathologist and to provide a plausibility check on the accuracy of the computer-assisted decision. This applies even more to any prediction and treatment recommendation, which also relies on the appropriate pre- and post-analytical quality of the tissue sample and the analytic process.

With the evolution of precision oncology, the role for precision diagnostics guiding the patient treatment and care management decisions is growing fast. The potential for harm or at least inadequate treatment must be considered when patients lack access to high-quality oncology pathology, advanced diagnostic solutions and expert decision boards that are supported by computational solutions. Policy makers and leaders in pathology and oncology need to take action addressing these critical gaps in cancer care. There is a need for a new integrative medical specialty in diagnostic oncology, with training in pathology, radiology, cancer biology, and new computational methods for developing cancer-specific diagnostic expertise.

There has been a proceeding evolution through the gradual implementation of novel technologies such as molecular and genomic testing, which has become a true digital revolution on how we will practice medicine in the future; on how we may diagnose diseases and on how we will select the best possible therapeutic option as part of a "precision medicine".

With the availability of big data from real-world-evidence (RWE), computer-assisted data analysis and artificial-/machine- intelligence tools, it is now possible to start the heuristic quest into the yet unknown without the proven pre-existing hypothesis provided by generations of practicing pathologists. New comprehensive sets of data are suggesting novel diagnostic entities with unique molecular and phenotypic signatures eventually demanding alternative treatment modalities. Computer-assisted decisions are further supported by methodologies like "systems medicine" and bottom-up *in-silico* simulation approaches. The alternative however, is to start top-down based on existing hypothesis that drive and direct computational and AI-based solutions refining existing diagnosis and therapies commensurate to what is already known and plausible to an existing group of medical experts.

Artificial intelligence (AI) is a powerful technology, but many pathologists do not yet know how it could be applied in their daily clinical work (van der Laak et al. 2021). Yet pathologists must participate in the development of AI-based solutions to remain professionally relevant in the digital future and guiding the generation of algorithms through their existing knowledge and experience (Fig. 18.2).

The implementation and execution of precision medicine, which will be the medicine of the twenty-first century, will inevitably "call for pathologists as their leaders embracing digital and computational pathology".

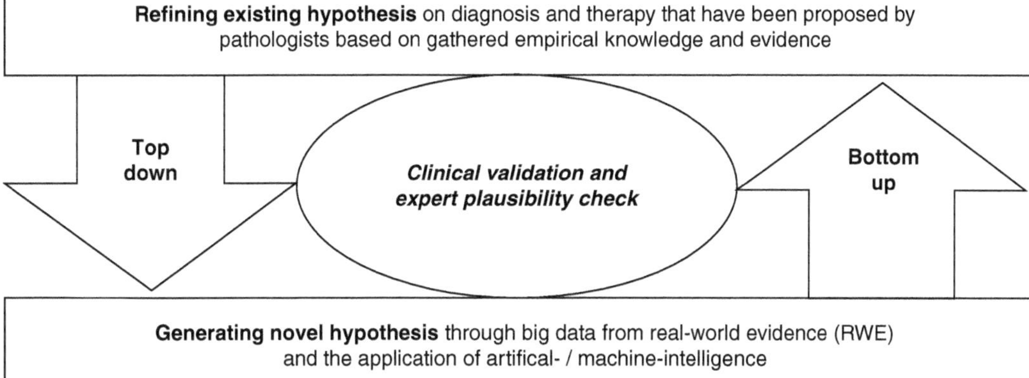

Fig. 18.2 There are different approaches to generate novel hypothesis on the diagnosis and therapy of cancer. The disruptive revolution provided by AI and machine intelligence in general is to start "bottom-up" without existing assumptions to generate novel hypotheses, which have to undergo an expert plausibility check and thorough clinical validation. However, it remains an iterative process to continuously refine existing hypothesis and to integrate well-curated and cleaned real-world evidence

To enable precision oncology, the practice of pathology has to evolve along the following lines:

- Building awareness on the required quality measures for the entire workflow from sample and data management towards data mining, interpretation and decision making
- Identifying the opportunities and challenges to utilize machine or artificial intelligence to standardize workflow quality, implement the robust quantification of single-slide respectively whole slide imaging (WSI) including multiplexing as well as complex spatial readouts and the integration of multi-*omics*;
- Defining the role of computer-assisted solutions to support and guide the pathologists in their role in precision oncology including the quantification of tissue-based biomarker;
- Developing the clinical utility of digital and artificial and machine intelligence technology for more effective assessment of tumor heterogeneity and the role of the tumor microenvironment in cancer progression and treatment resistance allowing more accurate and reproducible predictive analysis;
- Publishing illustrative case examples on digital technology leading precision oncology;
- Working towards regulatory approval of computer-assisted decision support systems and implementing training and educational programs for students and peers.

There is still an enormous or at least a substantial fear among pathologists to embrace such novel technologies that increase the level of automation and standardization in their subject domain. Given the increasing scarcity of expert pathologists in the future and the almost overwhelming demand to report complex diagnosis that are of immediate relevance to the individual treatment of advanced-stage patients, it becomes quite apparent why anatomical pathology is a great lead example how modern technologies will revolutionize and change the practice of medicine in the future (Pantanowitz and Parwani 2017).

The challenge posed by a vast number of practicing anatomical and surgical pathologists is increasing with a high demand for complex diagnosis using various and expensive techniques. In addition, physicians and especially oncologists on behalf of their cancer patients but also the diagnostic industry are demanding the retrieval of more information from less material and the integration of all available data from many different sources to guide the treatment as part of the routine clinical approach. Furthermore, all relevant information and data are increasingly required to be available in real-time, at any time and at every remote place. This also calls for the application of relevant related information technologies or alternative (cloud) solutions to protect data integration and patient data privacy.

To achieve robust and comparable readouts, all different sources of variabilities from the beginning to the end need to be understood and addressed. The development and application of sustainable image analysis solutions, algorithms and diagnostic decision trees heavily depend on established pre- and post-analytical quality control (QC) processes (Chap. 12) that include the sufficient and standardized preparation of the specimens, the absence of any technical artifacts, continuous staining quality checks, etc. Each technology that provides data into a common pool of data are also a source of error, missing interfaces, unreadable formats and different levels of robustness. While genomic data are usually quite reliable and clean (based on available standardized platform technologies), transcriptomic and translational pathway readout data are more influenced by environmental and outside factors, which albeit represent part of the natural heterogeneity in tissues. Any technically prone error will weaken or falsify the results and misguide diagnostic decisions.

The challenges mentioned above explain the current problems facing modern pathology, but they equally encourage anatomical pathologists to accept the role as "digital pathologists" applying artificial and machine intelligence as well as computer science to guide and lead precision oncology in the future (Bui et al. 2019).

References

Bui MM, Asa SL, Pantanowitz L, et al. Digital and computational pathology: bring the future into focus. J Pathol Inform. 2019;10:10. https://doi.org/10.4103/2153-3539.255259.

Pantanowitz L, Parwani A. Digital pathology. Chicago, IL: American Society of Clinical Pathologists Press; 2017.

van der Laak J, Litjens G, Ciompi F. Deep learning in histopathology: the path to the clinic. Nat Med. 2021;27:775–84.

19 AI in the Pre-Analytical Phase

19.1 The Workflow Design

In the following pages various examples and issues on the use and implementation of digital and computational pathology into clinical practice will be listed and discussed. Attempts to be detailed and comprehensive must fail because it is a very fast moving and growing field as any technology market, and any strive for completeness will remain unsuccessful. However, the reader is encouraged to read the original literature or to contact other domain experts in the field of digital and computational pathology to design the best possible solution for each personal and laboratory situation.

Figure 19.1 conveys the evolution of digital pathology and the necessary steps towards its implementation. Along this path the integration of the laboratory information system (LIS) and its connectivity with even "simple" telepathology tools will start addressing disparities in the practice of pathology. However, such a scenario allows pathology labs to go fully digital, establish attractive new business models, implement guidelines to be developed to standardize workflow and promote best pathology practices. This will feed many AI and machine learning projects to generate decision support solutions. The digital revolution is enabling pathology to meet the demands of modern medicine and is connecting pathologists with the rest of healthcare system which has already undergone a digital transformation. Digital pathology is contributing significantly to emerging fields in medicine such as immuno-oncology and the future use of combination therapies. It is intended to beckon pathologists to add these new tools to their toolbox. In so doing, digital pathology will help catapult them into a future where every patient can gain access to an expert pathology opinion and all pathologists can count on computer aided diagnostic tools.

There is currently no "one-stop-shop" available for automated and digital pathology diagnostics and many attempts by laboratory and technology suppliers have failed so far. The main reason is the current availability of "stand-alone-solutions" either because it is still the "business model of choice" like with OEM (Original Equipment Manufacturer) or the unintentional or deliberate incongruity of different workflow components. As a result, there is a definite move by manufacturers, and approval agencies (FDA, CE), towards a modular 'plug and play' approach, with different components often from different suppliers, requiring separate validation of each module with integration and final validation of the completed system. The onus falls upon the user laboratory to select and then achieve functional connectivity and interoperability of the different modules and systems that are necessary to complete an entire diagnostic workflow. This task is a challenge and usually requires domain specific expertise in each pathology lab or section.

Work from several studies exemplify different aspects of a possible path towards a

B. Jasani et al., *Precision Cancer Medicine*, https://doi.org/10.1007/978-3-030-84087-7_19

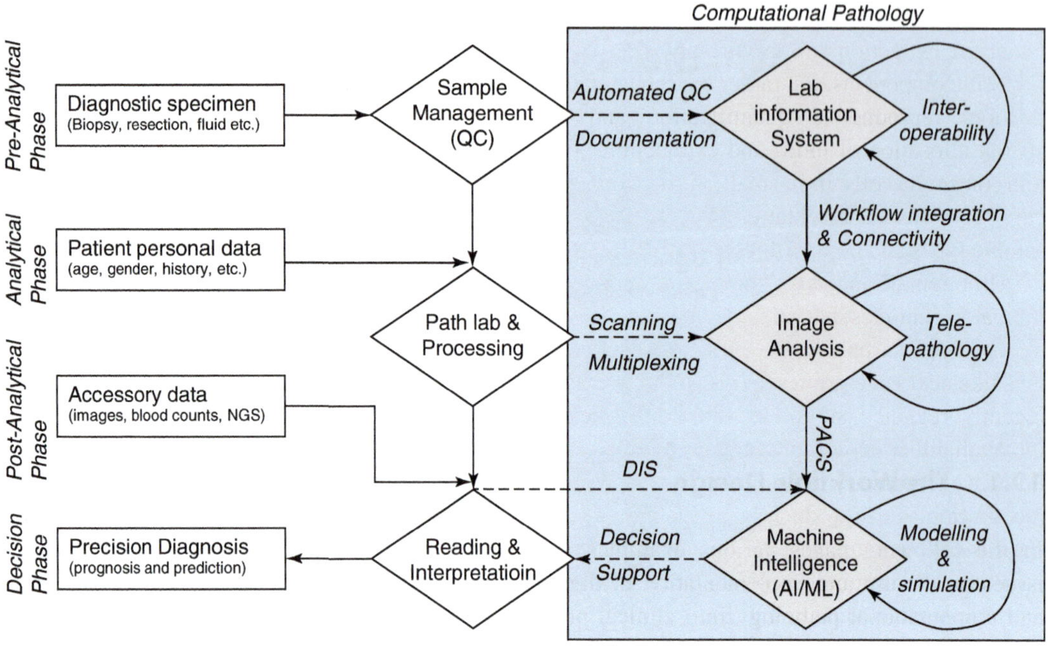

Fig. 19.1 The evolution and integration of a computational pathology toolbox is a revolution for Precision Oncology. However, it is not sufficient to add one tool after the other but rather ensure the connectivity and interoperability of the different solutions. Open interfaces and standardized formats are crucial for a complete and successful workflow, leveraging each component and the availability of patient data. (*DIS* Digital Imaging System, *PACS* Picture Archiving Communication System)

"computer-assisted diagnosis for pathologists" and provide a theoretical framework for automating pathology work for pathologists. Essential technical components like whole slide imaging (WSI) and annotation techniques will also be discussed as a pivotal part of the image analysis in the digital pathology workflow as well as the connectivity of the laboratory information system (LIS) and other data platforms and repositories.

All this will eventually allow the use and application of artificial or machine intelligence to model and simulate the heterogeneity of cancer tissue and its consequences for treatment decisions in precision oncology.

19.2 Sample and Quality Management

As already discussed in Part II (Chaps. 5, 6, and 7), the standardized preparation of the tissue or cytology specimens is of crucial importance to allow a robust and reproducible use of image-based artificial and machine intelligence to make sustainable decision on a clinical level in precision oncology. Over the past decades, we have learned to acknowledge the importance of a correct sample management to yield the best results in the field of molecular pathology. Many approved predictive biomarkers are based on DNA- or RNA-analytics and the isolation of genetic material from biopsies, fine needle aspirates or cytology specimens is already a challenge of its own. However, the necessary techniques are well established in the meantime and platform solutions are proved by molecular pathology suppliers usually on an affordable scale.

On the contrary, the comprehensive analysis of images supported by machine-assisted object detection and classification/segmentation tools along with mathematical algorithms that model or simulate the biology of individual cancers require even higher standards on the sample quality. Computational pathology is not necessarily about the extraction and in-vitro analysis of cellular subcomponents, but rather the robust identification, reproducible quantification and the spatial allocation of intra- and extracellular proteins on single cells, or in small biopsies or surgical specimens, representative of different tissue sample types and compartments.

Although the analysis of proteins by immunological techniques has a long history and has almost been surpassed by molecular technologies like next generation sequences (NGS), it has recently regained significant attention through the availability of complex analytical tools like fluorescence-based multiplexing with spatial recognition, the introduction of machine-learning based image analysis and the clinical implementation of immunotherapies. The latter require the almost exact quantification of proteins like checkpoint molecules, e.g. PD-L1 in different cellular subtypes, e.g. tumor cells versus immune cells. However, many attempts have failed to harmonize the reading and reporting of the checkpoint status because different pharmaceutical companies use different commercial suppliers with different antibodies to report the biomarker at different thresholds. While there is literature to support the automated and harmonized analysis of PD-1/PD-L1 expression using artificial and machine intelligence with a higher precision and concordance than manual reading, pathologists still need to receive training to improve the intra- and interobserver variability in reporting the expression of checkpoint inhibitors (Jasani et al. 2020).

Eventually pathologists start to acknowledge the practical importance and value to harmonize the entire diagnostic workflow and implement a robust and sustainable "quality management process". This starts with the sample management including whole-workflow documentation, appropriate fixation times, specimen handling, automated staining procedures and validated image analysis followed by data integration and mining. This is discussed in different parts of the book.

19.3 Quality Control and Validation

Comparable readouts across different assays and indications including all different sources of variability (see previous parts of the book) need to be understood and considered to start an early and inevitable quality control (QC) process to develop image analysis and machine-assisted decision making in precision oncology. A robust QC process along the entire diagnostic workflow makes a significant impact on the clinical acceptance of any automated decision-making tool. It starts with the investigation of the input data, comprising the identification of missing or inadequate quality images by the pathologist or an experienced lab personal including the visual assessment of the preparation quality. However, there are already first successful attempts to automate this pivotal task by machine intelligence. Unfortunately, it is not uncommon to fix or recreate slides or image files during the QC process without proper documentation. Quality-by-design (QbD) is an industrial measure to maintain, optimize and improve quality standards during an automated production or manufacturing workflow, which should also be implemented into diagnostic pathology, especially in the context of precision oncology. Valuable, well acknowledged and even mandatory steps are of course certification processes and the implementation of standard operation procedures (SOPs).

In these regards, we have learned a lot from toxicological pathology. Veterinarian pathologists are already using digital tissue imaging to extract large, complex and quantitative data sets. But like in precision oncology, the quality of generated results is dependent on a well-designed quality control system for the entire digital pathology workflow. Like in anatomical and surgical pathology, the toxicologic pathologists is responsible for reported data and therefore needs to ensure that it is correct (Zuraw et al. 2021).

The process of algorithm development for future clinical decision-making tools as well as its application in clinical practice and output review in precision oncology is still based on constant iterations of reviewing steps, at which the expert pathologist can intervene at any stage if the quality is unacceptable and/or the results are not plausible (Huss and Coupland 2020).

19.4 CIS, LIS, DIS and PACS

The clinical and laboratory information systems (CIS/LIS) are hard- and software solutions that are designed to collect, store, manage and retrieve clinical and laboratory data usually in a regulated healthcare environment. CIS/LIS are the technical backbone in managing patient data including the reimbursement from payor and health insurance. While it has been and still is at the core center of any CIS/LIS system to protect critical and personal data and maintain data privacy (according to US HIPAA, the British data protection act or the European General Data Protection Regulation) as a trusted stronghold of individual patient rights, CIS/LIS systems are sometimes seen as the obstacle to open up to modern science and digital innovation. However, modern CIS are key to clinical decision support (CDS), electronic medical records (EMR) and training and research for physicians and clinical researchers. Such CIS allow easy access to patient data, to query and retrieve structured data and even improve patient safety through monitoring prescriptions and the course of any disease. To realize the huge potential of clinical and laboratory data in any CIS/LIS, its operational integration is a significant issue in the move to full digital adoption for clinical diagnostics. This is based on the fact that the digital imaging system (DIS) should be tied to the CIS/LIS and will be integral in housing/viewing/managing the images and/or the workflows. Modern CIS/LIS or associated communication server (specialized or virtualized computer systems) can function as a passive bystander (middleware) that connects the CIS/LIS and the DIS together seamlessly. The awareness of the importance of a seamless workflow integration of any pre-existing or newly acquired systems is crucial to the success of the adoption of digital pathology and to identify the strengths and weaknesses of automated diagnostic workflows.

The adoption of digital/computational pathology (see below) offers benefits over labor-intensive, time-consuming and error-prone manual processes. However, because most workflow and lab transactions are centered on the existing CIS/LIS, adoption of digital/computational pathology ideally requires the seamless integration within the CIS/LIS. This does not stop at the connectivity of CIS/LIS with DIS (data integration systems as part of a data integration/transfer center), but also with PACS (Picture archiving and communication system) as part of RIS (Radiology information system) to ensure full interoperability.

19.5 Workflow Integration, Connectivity and Interoperability

Given Radiology's inherent two to three-decade lead time in acquiring substantial operational experience from the generation, curation and use of diagnostic digital imagery, it is beneficial to learn from this experience, which approaches and methodologies have been effective and which ones have not. Understanding the trajectory of both Radiology's and Pathology's digital imaging utilization for both routine diagnostics as well as more advanced computational use-cases, such a machine learning, CAD (computer-aided diagnosis) and CDS (clinical decision support) tools will allow us to expedite the implementation of functioning workflows into the routine clinical practice. However, in the context of precision oncology and the quantification of predictive biomarker, those solutions have impact on the patients' well-being and their survival of a devastating disease. Therefore, this requires the involvement of notified bodies and regulatory agencies to approve any such "medical device" outside the imminent control of a pathologist.

Are regulations friend or foe of innovation and how and if regulations and standards such as DICOM could have an impact on interoperability? Where are the hurdles today and can we overcome them in the future? This is especially important to enable and open digital pathology for precision medicine. Analytical algorithms, either developed under the traditional learning or deep learning, need to be able to be safely and effectively run on every file format. How could regulations and standards bring the future into focus?

What does it mean for conventional H&E pathology? The majority of histological examination are still conducted on H&E stained sections—a treasure to be lifted by data companies. There are many attempts to use and apply AI/ML retrieving more information from conventional H&E images which are the standard "working horse" of pathologists worldwide. Many such attempts by information giants like Google or IBM hiring more or less experienced pathologists have underestimated the practical implications. What is quite obvious to experienced pathologist is still a trap for a computer scientist only being used to transfer algorithms developed in an in-silico model. While models can be helpful, they might be totally misleading in clinical reality. Patients have different (epi)genetic backgrounds and have undergone quite different previous treatment regimens depending on the line of therapy. Those pretreatment conditions will inevitably modulate and change the individual tumor microenvironment (TME), which is almost impossible to modulate in mice or in-silico models. Alternatively, and due to a lack of pathology expertise, this is why some companies focus on the evaluation of "real world data" (RWD) or "real world evidence" (RWE), which however requires access to big and well curated data.

However, it is also misleading to assume that H&E images always come at the same quality, since their manufacturing are yet not by any means standardized. Also, the reading and interpretation are far from being harmonized. During their education and training, pathologists learn how to use H&E slide to identify certain characteristic features in tissue and cytology specimen but HE-based robust quantification and measurable spatial relationships usually do not exist.

Even in advanced and IVD-approved IHC-based assays like the Hercept ® test, there are good reasons why pathologists still report "weak" or "moderate" or "strong" staining patterns. One of the reasons is the lack of standardization and the heterogeneity of different staining patterns in the tissue. This intra-tumor heterogeneity of predictive biomarker has been considered for quantification as represented by the Immune reactive score (IRS) for hormone receptor in breast cancer or the Gleason-Score in prostate cancer.

Today, highly multiplexed IHC is a powerful technique for probing complex interactions in the tumor microenvironment (compare previous sections). Applying this technique to large sample sets requires an organized workflow and an underlying infrastructure of hardware and software. This generates data to be stored and retrieved from virtual repositories for comparison like an electronic pathologist's textbook (e.g. virtual slide repository with annotations and comments).

An integrated system using special image analysis software coupled with an image database and slide-sharing environment can be established on virtual computers in a cloud environment outside or in parallel to on-premises storage devices. One of the main reasons is the regulatory framework and legal requirements by national legislations. Multiple virtual machines network to provide image storage, image processing and database hosting. Additional processes are being developed to streamline pre-processing of multispectral images and automatically fuse multiple component images into a whole slide fluorescent image. Projects with the associated images are created for image management and to allow pathology support to be rendered remotely without the need for specialized hardware (Fuchs and Buhmann 2011).

A highly integrated and automated network is necessary to facilitate the analysis of large sets of images: a system of web-based file transfer, image analysis software, project management software for pathologist review, and data storage retrieval. These may be used to determine concordance in staining pattern and algorithm scoring across all methods. There is an enormous need for standardization in the pre-analytical process but also during image analysis possibly applying validated app solutions (see further below). Currently there are serious attempts to utilize the existing international HL7 (Health level 7) respectively FHIR (Fast Healthcare Interoperability Resources) standards.

A powerful and efficient digital pathology workflow for evaluating and scoring highly multiplexed IHC images can be created by leveraging multiple technologies and coupling it with pathology support. The combination of cloud storage services, application software and custom APIs (application program interfaces) may be connected into a system which efficiently and securely manages a complex digital pathology workflow environment which couples the efficiency of automation and the necessity of algorithm development and validation. Steps are taken to ensure data integrity and preservation of source files for archival purposes and to ensure availability for future use and review.

References

Fuchs T, Buhmann J. Computational pathology: challenges and promises for tissue analysis. Comput Med Imaging Graph. 2011;35(7–8):515–30.

Huss R, Coupland SE. Software-assisted decision support in digital histopathology. J Pathol. 2020;250(5):685–92. https://doi.org/10.1002/path.5388.

Jasani B, Bänfer G, Fish R, Waelput W, Sucaet Y, Barker C, Whiteley JL, Walker J, Hovelinck R, Diezko R. Evaluation of an online training tool for scoring programmed cell death ligand-1 (PD-L1) diagnostic tests for lung cancer. Diagn Pathol. 2020;15(1):37. https://doi.org/10.1186/s13000-020-00953-9.

Zuraw A, Staup M, Klopfleisch R, Aeffner F, Brown D, Westerling-Bui T, Rudmann D. Developing a qualification and verification strategy for digital tissue image analysis in toxicological pathology. Toxicol Pathol. 2021 Jun;49(4):773–83. https://doi.org/10.1177/0192623320980310.

20 AI in the Analytical Phase

20.1 Overcoming Variabilities

As one prime example, the variability in the visual inspection of medical images by pathologists is a well-known problem. Both inter- and intra-observer variability may affect image assessment and subsequently the ensuing diagnosis. A large body of work have reported high rates of diagnostic inaccuracy as a result of major discordance among participating physicians with respect to case diagnoses and propose a combination of "routine second opinions" and "directed retrospective peer review". As most proposed AI-driven solutions for digital pathology focus on the concept of object classification, it appears that algorithmic decision-making may not necessarily contribute to supporting concordance by providing a framework for consensus building. Most capable classification schemes trained with immense effort are supposed to be used for triaging cases in the pathology laboratory (e.g. detecting region-of-interest = ROI), and not for direct and immediate assistance in the pathologist's office. In contrast, instantly retrieving multiple recently diagnosed cases from a virtual repository with histopathologic and diagnostic similarity to the patient's biopsy about to be diagnosed offers a new generation of decision support that may even enable "virtual" peer review. This warrants the establishing "centers of excellence" (CoE) that will lead such initiatives and provide the technical and conceptual groundwork before a broader roll-out to the medical community.

20.2 Telepathology

As stated before, remote access to image and data files and distant case sign-out has become one of the major lessons during the COVID-19 crisis and many departments have not been ready for this challenge and opportunity. Telepathology is one of the oldest disciplines in digital and computation pathology, allowing second opinions and case referencing across longer distances since the early 1960s. With the global availability of the world wide web, telepathology should become available everywhere and connect pathologists even in very remote places. However, sending images and sensitive patient data through electronic wires requires high regulatory standards to protect individual patient rights and data integrity, which has the highest priority in developed countries. Nevertheless, the implementation of a world-wide telematic infrastructure is one pivotal task to improve patient care through connecting experts everywhere in the world for reference statements and expert opinions. But there are also still areas in the world where no pathologist is physically available and telepathology allows remote access to such capabilities. In the future and given the increasing scarcity of expert pathology knowledge, machine-based algorithms will assist the management of pathology workflows and the decision making of diagnosis as well as the stratification of patients not only to their best possible treatment but also to the only treatment available, which is sometimes their best option.

B. Jasani et al., *Precision Cancer Medicine*, https://doi.org/10.1007/978-3-030-84087-7_20

20.3 Standardization, Harmonization and Concordance

The facilitation of information interoperability in pathology requires the tracking of specimens, the structuring and coding of all data sources including images and ensuring the consistency of results for clinical applications. Currently the collecting and sharing of data are still not standardized to provide diagnostic and prognostic information crucial to standard patient care and clinical research. Different healthcare organizations at an international level, need to join efforts to provide accepted methodologies and standardized tools to define international implementation guides, especially in the domain of cancer pathology and precision oncology. This is not limited to software and algorithms, but also includes hardware tools and cloud solutions.

Computational and digital pathology will largely if not exclusively benefit from their inherently interdisciplinary work bringing together clinicians, basic scientists, computational engineers, mathematical wizards, hands-on physicists etc. (Pantanowitz et al. 2015). However, one major and initial hurdle is finding the same language to agree on common tasks: imagine what the word "solution" means to all of them in a different way and context. Today's medical revolution will be triggered from open innovations and external techniques coming from the outside (like the first X-ray beam applied in medicine) rather than from an evolution from the inside. Technical solutions become available to the broader community of practicing pathologists, one of the first is whole slide imaging (WSI) necessary for modern telepathology and digital/computational pathology. WSI has already demonstrated accuracy in the interpretation of permanent and frozen sections in surgical pathology.

A pilot study in New York suggests that WSI is as accurate as light microscopy (LM) in determining tumor presence on a single slide containing cutaneous frozen sections prepared *en face*. One promising aspect of telepathology is the expansion of access to intraoperative subspecialty expertise. With newer and approved WSI technology, the process of slide scanning is now largely automated, which enables the scanning of large number of slides feasible.

Remote assessment of fine needle aspiration (FNA) adequacy using telecytology is in high demand given its important impact on diagnostic quality of FNA materials and disperse nature of cytology practice. The performance of using a robotic digital microscope (RDM) and whole slide imaging (WSI) as potential substitutes for FNA onsite adequacy evaluation was successfully explored in a different study. The diagnostic industry now offers automated solutions combining WSI and machine learning algorithms alleviating the burden on cytology pre-screening activities.

20.4 Scanning and Whole Slide Imaging

As we have already seen above, the advent of WSI technology is a catalyst for change. There is a proposal for a set of systems (actors) and critical activities (transactions) that will help facilitate interoperability and value of vended digital pathology solutions including the pathology-LIS, image scanners, and image archives/PACS. There is more to digital pathology than just supporting WSI and associated instrumentation or algorithms, although it is noted that this innovation is a catalyst for change and has enabled a significant evolution of workflow and advancement of the field.

In previous chapters, we have already begun to discuss that digital pathology methods are of growing value for studying fluorescent-labeled samples, to obtain quantitative expression measures and to take advantage of multiple markers. At the same time, multiplexed immunofluorescence (mIF) labeling techniques and multispectral imaging systems have made it practical to measure many colors per specimen, enabling insights into complex samples such as are present in immuno-oncology studies (Laurinaviciene and Dasevicius 2011). The inclusion of optimized dyes, software, and a scanner that performs rapid WSI multispectral imaging along with viewing and analysis tools for handling multispectral analysis allows the use of established digital pathology interactions and workflows. This further enables studying cell-to-cell interactions over multiple spatial scales and especially measuring heterogeneity in immune response across the tumor microenvironment (Ronneberger et al. 2015).

It was the Dutch company Philips who introduced WSI as an FDA-approved, standardized process by which conventional glass slides are scanned and converted into digital images. This technology can be utilized to improve the efficiency of workflow, better integrate images into laboratory information systems, and, when utilized properly, may offer substantial cost savings. These advantages have prompted the recent exponential growth of WSI platform usage. Indeed, some labs have moved towards the complete digitization of all tissue slides, and the breadth of WSI technologies approved by the U.S. Food and Drug Administration (FDA) for diagnostic use continues to widen. As with traditional glass slides, digital slides can be annotated for region of interest (ROI). Annotation of ROI is essential for communication amongst pathologists and other functions in various diagnostic, educational, and research settings. Digital annotation offers obvious advantages to the marking of glass slides with ink, namely in its ability to preserve the integrity of the annotation over time and distance. Traditionally, a hand-held mouse and desktop monitor are used for digital annotation. In addition to the barriers of poor ergonomics and lack of familiarly of the user with imaging software, this approach may lack the speed and precision of hand-drawn annotation. Thus, some pathologists are still hesitant to embrace digital annotation. Technology capable of replicating hand-drawn annotation, namely touchscreen personal computers with stylus capabilities, may be a means of surmounting the latter impediment. These tools have increasingly been embraced by other professions (graphic design, architecture, etc.), in many instances supplanting pencil and pen entirely, but their value in the generation and modification of scientific images has yet to be fully explored.

20.5 Image Analysis

The extraction of biological and histomorphological data from virtual slides is the foundation for the identification of known or novel patterns and features that are usually difficult to quantify or simply not amendable to assessment by the human eye and mind. After the digitization of tissue slides from formalin-fixed, fresh frozen sections or FNA, various image analysis solutions can be applied to highly multiplexed or even multidimensional tissue techniques such as immunofluorescent detection of DNA probes, RNA or proteins, co-registered serial sections or even imaging mass cytometry of >>100 variables/cell.

Novel patterns may comprise spatial relationships of single cells, cell populations or geometric properties of specific tissue architectures, even in the context of different tissue compartments and genomic hot spots. Related rich data sets can be analyzed by cognition-based and pathologist-guided solutions to possibly integrate machine learning or deep learning approaches. In the end it is the aim to generate explainable imaging results suitable for anatomical and surgical pathology (Campbell et al. 2013).

However, image analysis cannot be leaned upon unless resolving any inconsistencies caused by pre-analytical variables as discussed in the previous parts of this book. Therefore, proper sample handling, processing, staining and scanning are as important as the curation of data and the development of robust algorithms. Limited ischemia time, appropriate type of fixative and fixation time, automated processing, skilled sample embedding and sectioning (or future alternatives, e.g. 3D-imaging), the use of staining automation are all necessary to generate the required consistency and robustness of images prior to any sustainable analysis and feature extraction (Yamamoto et al. 2017). Quality control (QC) of all images and tissue processing steps should be performed ideally by the pathologist, throughout the entire workflow, something to be copy-pasted from the automotive and computer chip industry (compare also Sect. 19.2).

Image analysis is at the core of digital and computational pathology and requires special expertise and competencies by expert pathologists and an active interdisciplinary collaboration with computer and data scientists as well as software engineers (Gurcan and Boucheron 2009). The body of literature and informative textbooks on this topic are steadily growing with the advancement of associated hardware technologies, data storage and processing capabilities as well as machine and deep learning techniques (Binnig et al. 2018). As stated before, the objective of image mining is the discovery and description of features with diagnostic, prognostic and possibly predictive features relevant for the future practice of precision oncology (Dobson and Conway 2010). The increasing amounts of patient-specific data from images and other (*−omics*) sources are used to augment the understanding of an individual disease and to generate hypothesis around diagnostic and other cancer-related biomarkers (Fig. 20.1). In the field of oncology, the ability to complement genetic and transcriptomic data with clinical characteristics and tissue image-based data will facilitate a deeper understanding of clonal heterogeneity within tumors and across patient populations and allow a comprehensive exploration of the tumor microenvironment (Akbar and Jordan 2015).

20.6 Advanced Microscopy

Novel technologies such as multiplexing immunofluorescence or mathematical model like algebraic topology now allow the extraction of deeper insights into the biology, retrieve accurate contextual information and describe spatial relationships of important tissue components (Nazeer et al. 2017). While transmission/scanning electron microscopy has established itself in some niche applications, atomic force microscopy (AFM), super-/high-resolution (nano) microscopy, cryo-electron microscopy or Raman spectroscopy are overcoming the limits of light diffraction and generate novel data sets in ana-

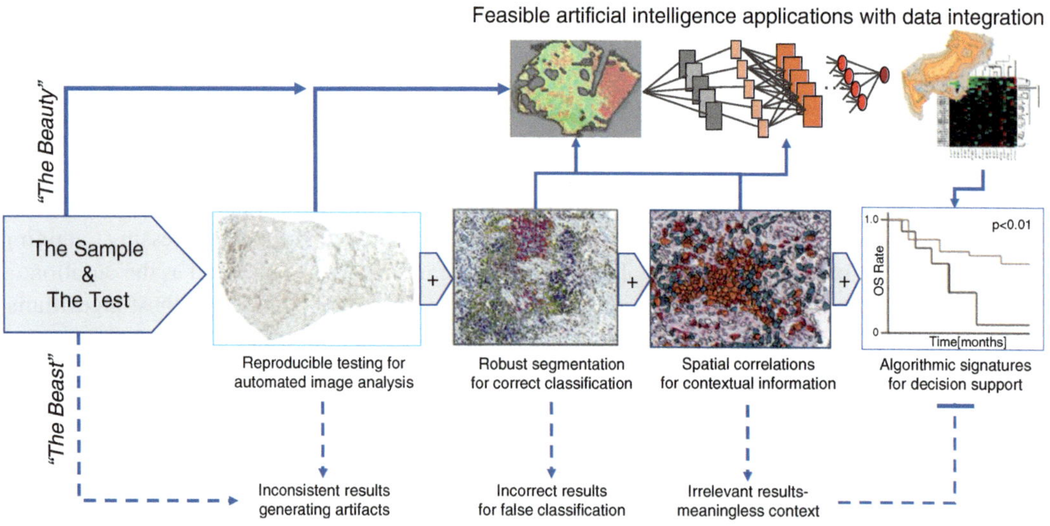

Fig. 20.1 The beauty of a robust and reproducible pre-analytical sample processing and test execution allows feasible AI applications, while the beast of inconsistencies, artifacts, false classification will lead to misleading and uninterpretable data. Automated image analysis is the basis for a robust and correct segmentation of objects (e.g. nuclei, cells, tissues, compartments) and the proper classification of objects (e.g. lymphocytes, tumor cells, invasive margin) to quantify tumor antigen or checkpoint molecule expression as well as their spatial relationships and functional interactions. The use of a comprehensive quality assessment and control measures along the entire computational pathology workflow will eventually generate algorithms and signatures for a reliable decision support on the prognosis of an individual disease and the correct patient stratification for a personal treatment (Binnig et al. 2018)

tomical pathology (Walsh et al. 2012; Sreedhar et al. 2016). Another future milestone might be the implementation of 3D-visualization of tissue specimens, e.g. using light sheet microscopy (Baker et al. 2018).

The in-situ assessment of protein expression ("spatial proteomics") in any dimension has long be plagued by inaccuracy or technologies that work on some tissues but not others. Years of effort in this field, and the recent introduction of new software and new approaches is improving the accuracy, but we are still not there yet. However, major progress is currently on it way and clinical validation will follow (Baker et al. 2014).

With the success of immuno-oncology treatment strategies as one of the leading examples of precision oncology, there is an increasing need to investigate response—resistance mechanisms in order to optimize therapeutic regimens and develop combination strategies. Multiplexed and multi-dimensional immunohistochemistry enables translational researchers to characterize immune cell populations within patient tumor samples to further our biological understanding into response/resistance profiles.

References

Akbar S, Jordan L. Comparing computer-generated and pathologist-generated tumour segmentations for immunohistochemical scoring of breast tissue microarrays. Br J Cancer. 2015;113(7):1075–80.

Baker MJ, Trevisan J, Bassan P, Bhargava R, Butler HJ, Dorling KM. Using fourier transform IR spectroscopy to analyze biological materials. Nat Protoc. 2014;9:1771–91.

Baker MJ, Byrne HJ, Chalmers J, Gardner P, Goodacre R, Henderson A. Clinical applications of infrared and Raman spectroscopy: state of play and future challenges. Analyst. 2018;143:1735–57.

Binnig G, Huss R, Schmidt G. Tissue phenomics – profiling cancer patients for treatment decisions. PAN Stanford; 2018.

Campbell WS, Foster KW, Hinrichs SH. Application of whole slide image markup and annotation for pathologist knowledge capture. J Pathol Inform. 2013;4:2.

Dobson L, Conway C. Image analysis as an adjunct to manual HER-2 immunohistochemical review: a diagnostic tool to standardize interpretation. Histopathology. 2010;57(1):27–38.

Gurcan M, Boucheron L. Histopathological image analysis: a review. IEEE Rev Biomed Eng. 2009;2:147–71.

Laurinaviciene A, Dasevicius D. Membrane connectivity estimated by digital image analysis of HER2 immunohistochemistry is concordant with visual scoring and fluorescence in situ hybridization results: algorithm evaluation on breast cancer tissue microarrays. Diagn Pathol. 2011;6(1):87–96.

Nazeer SS, Sreedhar H, Varma VK, Martinez-Marin D, Massie C, Walsh MJ. Infrared spectroscopic imaging: label-free biochemical analysis of stroma and tissue fibrosis. Int J Biochem Cell Biol. 2017;92:14–7.

Pantanowitz L, Farahani N, Parwani A. Whole side imaging in pathology: advantage, limitations, and emerging perspectives. Pathol Lab Med Int. 2015;7:23–33.

Ronneberger O, Fischer P, Brox T. U-Net: convolutional networks for biomedical image segmentation. In: Medical image computing and computer-assisted intervention (MICCAI), LNCS, vol. 9351. Springer; 2015. p. 234–41.

Sreedhar H, Varma VK, Gambacorta FV, Guzman G, Walsh MJ. Infrared spectroscopic imaging detects chemical modifications in liver fibrosis due to diabetes and disease. Biomed Opt Express. 2016;7:2419–24.

Walsh MJ, Reddy RK, Bhargava R. Label-free biomedical imaging with mid-IR spectroscopy. IEEE J Sel Top Quantum Elec. 2012;18:1502–13.

Yamamoto Y, Saito A, Tateishi A, Shimojo H, Kanno H, Tsuchiya S. Quantitative diagnosis of breast tumors by morphometric classification of microenvironmental myoepithelial cells using a machine learning approach. Sci Rep. 2017;7:46732.

21 AI in the Post-Analytical Phase

21.1 Dealing with Complexity

With the challenges to deal with more and complex data sets and the increasing demand from the field of precision oncology, solutions are needed to extract relevant and robust knowledge and actionable information from any type of tissue or cell suspension. Multi-dimensional and multi-color images together with NGS data etc. from a single piece of tissue are such a complex task to yield a decision on best treatment option for every individual patient. Machine intelligence denotes a set of methodologies for addressing these needs which also includes topological data analysis.

21.2 Artificial Intelligence, Machine Learning and Topology

Machine intelligence (MI) is considered an extension of Machine Learning (ML) and implies also artificial intelligence (AI), a branch of computer science that assists humans in making decisions and providing alternative interpretations and interactions. Although, there are sometimes different and conflicting definitions (none of them being absolutely true or false), ML is usually not the same thing as AI, both being different techniques to create machine cognition (Kainz 2017). To a large degree, AI depends on human experts ("conventional expert knowledge") to create heuristic rule sets in order to support decision making. AI's ability to solve a problem is dependent on having a human expert describing a current problem or anticipating a future problem in advance (Campion and Carlsson 2017). Instead, ML uses stochastic methods to analyze big and complex data sets creating its own rules. ML is simply an attempt to substitute for human experience and expert knowledge and heavily relies on good data input. However, there are also different definitions naming AI as the heading for ML, of which DL is another subdiscipline.

MI goes beyond the "black box" nature of ML and includes techniques such as neural networks and Deep Learning (DL). The output allows the capture of the full complexity of features and communication networks in heterogenous and multiplexed tissue specimens and provides explanations of the results for pathologists' consumption and use (Badrinarayanan et al. 2017). In this pursuit, expert pathologists still need to verify the agreement between the MI-based decisions and any ground-truth (expert) knowledge (Fig. 21.1). Therefore, explainable AI (X-AI) has developed as a field of MI/AI, focused on exposing complex MI/AI models to humans in a systematic and interpretable manner. X-AI tries to rationalize decision rules in analogy to what is known by (pathology) experts. Naturally, painfully acquired human expert knowledge during many years of training and education and the use of MI is an area of conflict (compare also Fig. 21.1). Both approaches converge in the clinical validation of

B. Jasani et al., *Precision Cancer Medicine*, https://doi.org/10.1007/978-3-030-84087-7_21

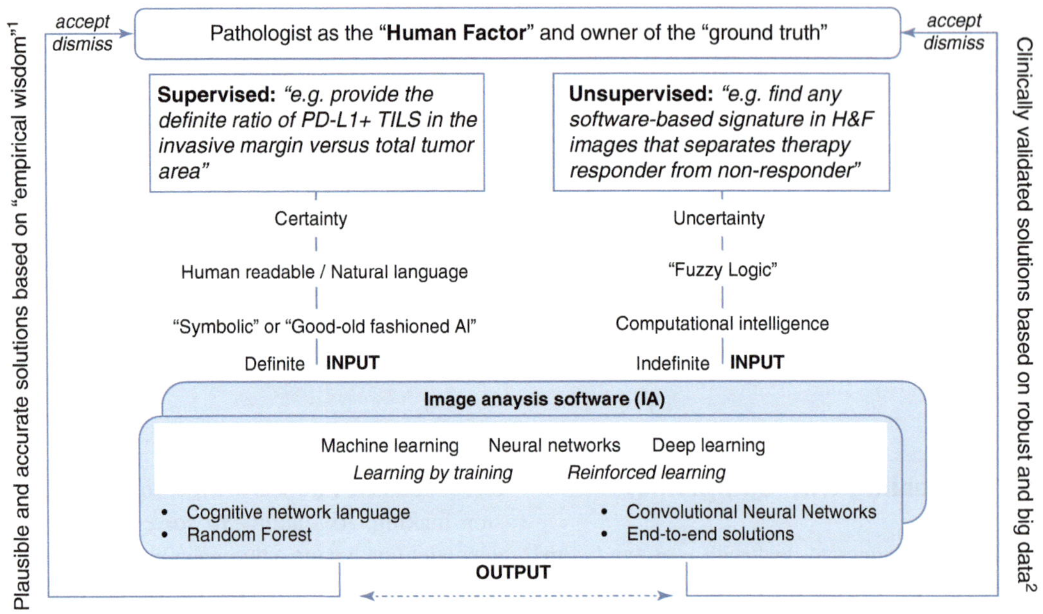

Fig. 21.1 With the pathologist supervising the development of software algorithms based on their "empirical wisdom" (path 1) or alternatively reviewing the results of unsupervised solutions (path 2), there are different but certainly overlapping AI solutions to generate relevant output from image analysis. Symbolic or "good old fashioned AI" (GOFAI) repeats the work of the "human pathologist" in a robust and reproducible manner, being rather certain about the computational task. The use of weak or unsupervised learning, applying deep learning or end-to-end solutions has a higher degree of uncertainty and might demand for "explainable AI" (X-AI) to trust the output generated by computational pathology. By any means, the pathologist is still at the center of the clinical utility of AI, owning the ground truth (at least for now) and still having the competence and responsibility to accept or dismiss any digital solution

automated rule sets, proving the sustainable correctness of machine-based decisions in pathology and medical practice.

Machine learning (ML) is a collection of mathematical and computer science techniques for the extraction of relevant data from large data sets trained and explained by human experts or in this case by expert pathologists. Therefore, ML can substitute or support the human factor, mostly by performing difficult and tedious tasks. An automated ML method will read a multiplex immunohistochemistry image always in the same reliable and robust manner, yielding the identical result over and over again. This allows a global comparability of complex and larger data sets without significant inter- and intra-observer variability. ML algorithms may include decision trees, Bayes' networks, clustering solutions, regression solutions, also depending on whether the solution is rather (weakly) supervised or unsupervised (Xu et al. 2014; Meier et al. 2020). With the advent of convolutional neural networks in recent years, ML is becoming increasingly accessible to researchers from non-computer science background. However, preparing data for machine learning remains a crucial step which requires hands-on expertise.

One other important topic for the development of robust ML/AI especially in the context of clinical practice and decision making is the use of correct data. Incorrect or inconsistent data lead to false conclusions. Besides the use of big and real-world data, the cleaning or cleansing of data has a high impact on the quality of results. This should also become a part of the standard quality management and control workflow.

Creating graphical shapes and visual representations have been used for centuries to allow the understanding of complex data as well as extracted information and non-domain experts (e.g. pathologists) the rationale behind MI-based decision rules. To also visualize complex MI-based solutions, topological data analysis (TDA) makes it possible to understand multidimensional data sets more easily. With the emergence of immune and combination therapies in the field of precision oncology, a multitude of markers (different cell types, receptors, pathway molecules, genetic mutations etc.) will be potential numerators or denominators of the same equation. The use of topological networks (sometimes also called graphs, e.g. t-SNE plots) can also intuitively describe spatial relationships between different checkpoint molecules, immune effector cells or inhibitory factors (Dundar et al. 2010).

21.3 Computational Pathology

Advances in machine learning have propelled computational pathology research. Machine intelligence is able to do what humans respectively pathologists can, but in a more reliable and in a standardized way. Today, computer systems approach the diagnostic reality achieved by humans for certain well-defined tasks in pathology. At the same time, pathologists are faced with an increased workload both quantitatively (numbers of cases) and qualitatively (the amount and complexity of work per case; with increasing treatment options, the data delivered by pathologists is also expected to become more fine-grained).

In this section, the potential of machine learning techniques will be addressed and discussed how these may alleviate the challenges of pathologists. Possible solutions range from computer aided support for relatively straightforward tasks to discovery of innovative prognostic and predictive biomarkers (Rana et al. 2020). The most basic applications deal mostly with simple dichotomous detection problems such as presence of lymph node metastases or not; or counting the density of mitotic or Ki-67 positive tumor cells. They have the potential to increase efficiency and precision of the pathological diagnostic workflow. Expectedly, the first algorithms of this "simple kind" are already commercially available and viable. At the other end of the spectrum are models that can assess sub-visual morphological information, potentially playing a role in personalized medicine and precision oncology like cancer pathway analysis (Szegedy et al. 2016). With the increasing complexity of the applications comes an increasing demand for large (big or augmented), well-curated and clean datasets. This poses challenges for researchers and algorithm developers, as data collection is cumbersome and expensive. Still, the potential for computational pathology is large and applications will definitely play a role in the future of pathology (Jegou et al. 2010).

Computational pathology (CP) will leverage mathematical tools and implement data-driven methods as a center for data interpretation in modern tissue diagnosis (Fig. 21.2). The value proposition of CP as well as digital pathology to some extent, will require working with institutional administrations, regulatory offices, other departments, and pathology colleagues. CP will also foster the training of future computational pathologists, those with both pathology and non-pathology backgrounds, who will eventually decide that CP will serve as an indispensable hub for data-related research in a global health care system.

21.4 The Science of Data or Data Science

Data science or the science of data is one of the fastest growing fields in biomedical research and medicine. It involves the automated use of mathematical methods and integrated computer sciences to solve real world problems. The different required tasks involve the cleaning of data, analyzes of the cleaned data (i.e. applying software tools and artificial intelligence), the processing and storage of cleaned, raw or analyzed (anonymized) data with the appropriate hardware in data lakes or data warehouses and the visualization of even high-dimensional results to allow the understanding and implementation into the daily histopathological practice. In recent years, the

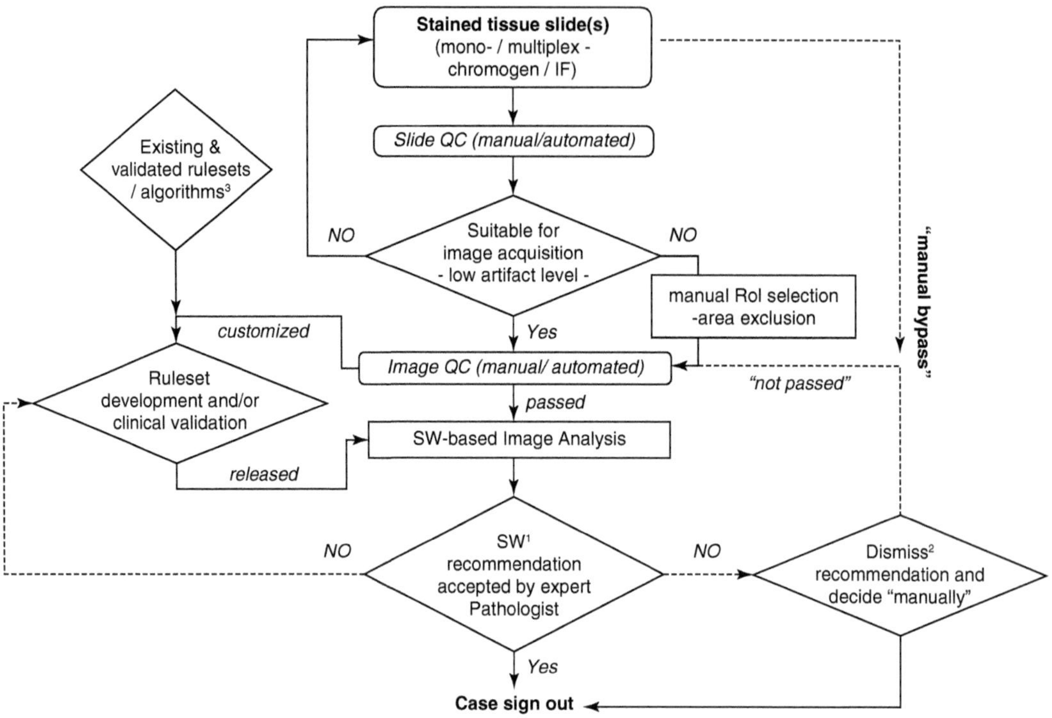

Fig. 21.2 Continuous quality control by pathologists during the entire computer-supported image analysis. The pathologist can dismiss or accept any digital recommendation at any stage of the workflow (reprinted with permission from Wiley & Sons: Huss and Coupland 2020)

collection of very large amounts of data from tissue specimens has increased dramatically. Technologies like next-generation sequencing (NGS), single-cell genomics and transcriptomics, (phosphor-) proteotyping, mass spectroscopy, natural language processing (NLP), digital pathology etc. allow the extensive characterization of individual cancers. Such a multi-omics data integration will advance the mechanistic insights of a patient's tumor, and enable prognostic and predictive biomarker discovery, and has the potential to support clinical decision making in precision oncology (Chen et al. 2020).

Next-Generation Sequencing (NGS) has already revolutionized diagnostic molecular testing. Accordingly, many pathology labs today either offer NGS or send out their samples for molecular testing to reference laboratories. Not surprisingly, there are various ways in which NGS techniques and the need for extracted genetic material has also started to influence WSI. For example, WSI offers a mechanism to "immortalize" slides that otherwise get sacrificed for molecular testing. Unfortunately, many labs still rely on manual methods instead of digital tools to designate which regions need to be tested or employ image analysis to automate tumor analysis for molecular testing ("annotations"). Image-driven laser capture dissection is a one mechanism that can be employed to address this problem, as well as automate and scale up NGS testing. NGS data also has great potential when used to help develop deep learning algorithms for digital pathology.

Deep learning algorithms hold promise for pathology but usually require very large datasets for building accurate prediction models that need to be clinically validated. Obtaining annotations at large scales is challenging given constraints on pathologist time, particularly when carefully delineating histologic structures. Most previous applications of crowdsourcing in histopathology were limited to small-scale IHC scoring tasks and malaria diagnosis, and there has been little attention to scalable generation of H&E annotations of histopathology. Online tools are important for facilitating crowdsourced histopathology annotation (Alialy et al. 2018). Organizing volunteers by experience can help scale annotations and leverage volunteers who are enthusiastic but less experienced. Not surprisingly, one study showed that women who survived breast cancer very diligently annotated breast cancer specimens and reliably scored Her2/neu expression after initial training by expert pathologists.

21.5 Algebraic Pathology

Mathematical and theoretical (algebraic) pathology employs theoretical analysis, appropriate mathematical models and abstractions to investigate the principles that govern the structure, development and hidden information also of tissue specimens. The field is close to the discipline of bioinformatics and aims at the mathematical representation and modeling of pathological conditions, using techniques and tools of applied mathematics and statistics. Discrete components of biological systems arise from state transitions (e.g. from healthy to abnormal / malignant tissues), abstractions and approximations, nonlinear effects, and the presence of inherently discrete processes, often observed in systems governed by one, few and many different events in a single cell or a complex tissue. Here applied mathematics can be useful in both theoretical and practical applications also in anatomical and surgical pathology. Algebraic topology including spatial modeling, swam behavior, pattern formation etc. includes tools from abstract algebra to study topological spaces. The goal is to find algebraic invariants from all complex data sources that classify topological spaces. Although algebraic topology primarily uses algebra to study topological problems, application to other problems is sometimes also possible. Algebraic topology, for example, allows for a modeling of cohort studies, i.e. clinical trials. Cohort studies are a convenient method attempting to understand correlations between particular attributes of a subject and an outcome. An example could be to determine whether the number and spatial distribution of certain immune cells and their proximity to each other and the tumor cells have an association with the response to immune stimulating agents and whether this can be predicted directly from tissue specimen analysis.

21.6 Encoded Pathology

Standardized processes are an inevitable prerequisite for the development and implementation of AI-based rule sets during the entire digital pathology workflow. Only through robust procedures and sustainable protocols which ensure consistent quality, machine intelligence will generate legitimate and enduring confidence throughout the community of pathologists (Colling et al. 2019). The "input" from tissue specimens, images and associated data has to be structured (and sometimes curated) to extract useful digital information and to generate also clinically relevant algorithms. "Encoded pathology" also uses the available semantic information from structured and standardized pathology reports. However, the extraction of knowledge and clinical insights is one of the last steps of the diagnostic (digital) workup but should contain—by definition and demanded by almost all pathological and medical societies—all relevant diagnostic, prognostic and possible predictive information of an individual disease. While there are still many unsolved issues with incompatible IT-interfaces (especially with CIS, LIS etc.), the semantics of a spoken and written language is usually homogenous but not necessarily using generally accepted terms or expressions. The use of "natural language processing algorithms" demands a "structured input" similar to the application of hierarchical patterns in image analysis to allow a quantitative and qualitative recognition and assessment of the available pathology reports (Kersloot et al. 2020). There are now corresponding recommendations for best practice in encoded pathology by the respective societies (Abels et al. 2019).

21.7 Disease Modelling and Simulation

This section is about discussing disease in-silico modeling and simulation. For decades, pathology had an experimental branch to model many types of diseases (infections, malignancies etc.), but with advances in computer and tissue imaging technologies, the assembly of detailed models has become a relatively easy process and may lead to more available resources for researching the biology also relevant for the modeling of individual cancers. Models are potentially powerful tools in the research process, but they will expand the inductive and deductive abilities by removing the task of dealing with details and by stressing clarity in conceptualization. It will bridge more conceptual and theoretical hypotheses to clinically applicable and diagnostic solutions in pathology (Xu et al. 2012).

The author once discussed modeling the immune system with a Nobel laureate in Physics, who was excited about the progress made by a computational network language applied to a univariant model. But most problems in human cancer biology are not only about a single and linear problem, but rather understanding the entire complexity of a diseases, an approach increasingly utilized in systems medicine.

Computer models can help to understand and go beyond the current view of understanding through a multitude of simulation, even the unexpected and yet unknown. But it is about a "computer" to assist medical science and pathologists and not to give a new meaning and reason to existing machine learning and AI (Fig. 21.3).

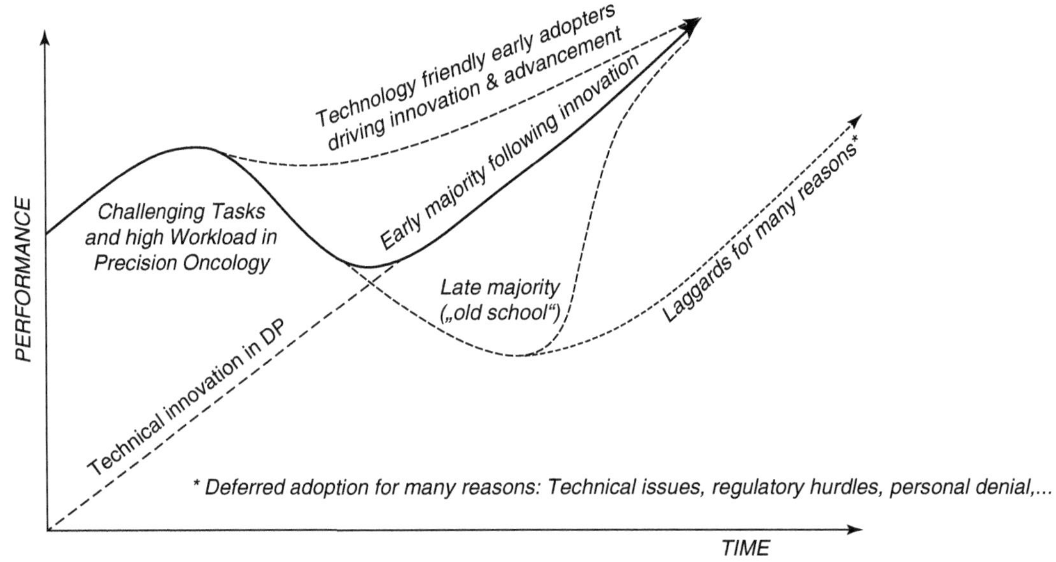

Fig. 21.3 Naturally, for existing human expert (pathologists') knowledge and the use of MI is an area of conflict. Classical change management process following the rules of innovation can also be applied to digital pathology (DP). While the technical innovation advances in a linear regression (an assumption for illustration purposes), the adoption depends on the willingness and individual capabilities of the pathologist. Some pathologists will adopt change early and become drivers of innovations, others will lag behind for some time ("late majority) or for good ("laggards")

References

Abels E, Pantanowitz L, Aeffner F, Zarella MD, van der Laak J, Bui MM, Vemuri VN, Parwani AV, Gibbs J, Agosto-Arroyo E, Beck AH, Kozlowski C. Computational pathology definitions, best practices, and recommendations for regulatory guidance: a white paper from the Digital Pathology Association. J Pathol. 2019;249(3):286–94. https://doi.org/10.1002/path.5331.

Alialy R, Tavakkol S, Tavakkol E, Ghorbani-Aghbologhi A, Ghaffarieh A, Kim SH. A review on the applications of crowdsourcing in human pathology. J Pathol Inform. 2018;9:2.

Badrinarayanan V, Kendall A, Cipolla R. SegNet: a deep convolutional encoder-decoder architecture for image segmentation. IEEE Trans Pattern Anal Mach Intell. 2017;39(12):2481–95.

Campion FX, Carlsson G. Machine intelligence for healthcare. 1st ed. CreateSpace; 2017.

Chen RJ, Lu MY, Wang J, Williamson DFK, Rodig SJ, Lindeman NI, Mahmood F. Pathomic fusion: an integrated framework for fusing histopathology and genomic features for cancer diagnosis and prognosis. IEEE Trans Med Imaging. 2020; https://doi.org/10.1109/TMI.2020.3021387.

Colling R, Pitman H, Oien K, Rajpoot N, Macklin P, CM-Path AI in Histopathology Working Group, Snead D, Sackville T, Verrill C. Artificial intelligence in digital pathology: a roadmap to routine use in clinical practice. J Pathol. 2019;249(2):143–50. https://doi.org/10.1002/path.5310.

Dundar M, Badve S, Raykar V, Jain R, Sertel O, Gurcan M. A multiple instance learning approach toward optimal classification of pathology slides. In: International conference on pattern recognition. IEEE; 2010. p. 2732–5.

Huss R, Coupland SE. Software-assisted decision support in digital histopathology. J Pathol. 2020;250(5):685–92. https://doi.org/10.1002/path.5388.

Jegou H, Douze M, Schmid C, Pérez P. Aggregating local descriptors into a compact image representation. In: Computer vision and pattern recognition. IEEE; 2010. p. 13–8.

Kainz P. Segmentation and classification of colon glands with deep convolutional neural networks and total variation regularization. PeerJ. 2017;5:e3874. https://doi.org/10.7717/peerj.3874.

Kersloot MG, van Putten FJP, Abu-Hanna A, Cornet R, Arts DL. Natural language processing algorithms for mapping clinical text fragments onto ontology concepts: a systematic review and recommendations for future studies. J Biomed Semant. 2020;11(1):14. https://doi.org/10.1186/s13326-020-00231-z.

Meier A, Nekolla K, Hewitt LC, Earle S, Yoshikawa T, Oshima T, Miyagi Y, Huss R, Schmidt G, Grabsch HI. Hypothesis-free deep survival learning applied to the tumour microenvironment in gastric cancer. J Pathol Clin Res. 2020;6(4):273–82. https://doi.org/10.1002/cjp2.170.

Rana A, Lowe A, Lithgow M, Horback K, Janovitz T, Da Silva A, Tsai H, Shanmugam V, Bayat A, Shah P. Use of deep learning to develop and analyze computational hematoxylin and eosin staining of prostate Core biopsy images for tumor diagnosis. JAMA Netw Open. 2020;3(5):e205111. https://doi.org/10.1001/jamanetworkopen.2020.5111.

Szegedy C, Vanhoucke V, Ioffe S, Shlens J, Wojna Z. Rethinking the inception architecture for computer vision. In: 2016 IEEE conference on computer vision and pattern recognition (CVPR). IEEE; 2016.

Xu Y, Zhu JY, Chang E, Tu Z. Multiple clustered instances learning for histopathology cancer image classification, segmentation and clustering. In: IEEE conference on computer vision and pattern recognition. IEEE; 2012. p. 964–71.

Xu Y, Zhu JY, Chang E, Lai M, Tu Z. Weakly supervised histopathology cancer image segmentation and classification. Med Image Anal. 2014;18(3):591–604.

AI in the Decision Phase

22

22.1 Examples of Clinical Utility

Digitization is transforming healthcare in general and precision oncology in particular. The ability to collect and analyze images and data will be the gatekeeper of a new era in pathology. Collecting all available information about a patient's individual cancer and the prediction of the (immune) response to therapy is the next step in precision oncology. The information should include biomarkers with known clinical relevance and should also be broad enough to be relevant across multiple options (one test, many drugs and their possible combination). Genetic information on cancer (mutations, rearrangements, translocations, mutational load etc.) has known prognostic and predictive value. However, densities and locations of different immune cells in the TME are also known to be associated with outcomes and therapy response.

The consistent profiling of an individual patient's immune therapy response is already possible but still less well established than genomic profiling. A current limitation for systematic profiling in pathology routine is the conventional visual assessment of tissue biomarkers. Trained pathologists are very skilled at detecting and interpreting clues in the tissue morphology and protein expression but less so at providing consistent quantification (e.g. PD-L1). A standardized set of tissue biomarkers with corresponding detection and quantification algorithms can determine a unique fingerprint of a patient's response to treatment.

22.2 Prognosis of Cancer

A prognostic biomarker informs about a likely cancer outcome regardless of what treatment a patient has received (including no treatment), reflecting the natural course of a disease. A biomarker is prognostic when there is a correlation with any event (progression or survival) regardless of any treatment. Usually, a proper diagnosis, tumor classification and staging according to the WHO- or other guidelines provides already a prognostic assessment, e.g. glioblastoma multiforme generally has a poor prognosis, while there may be still individual variants in the course of the disease.

22.3 Predicting Treatment Outcomes

Predicting cancer outcomes from histology and genomics using deep learning usually relate to an available treatment including the possibility to surgically remove the tumor and metastases or the availability of effective treatment regimens. A biomarker is predictive when the treatment effects differ for biomarker-positive and biomarker-negative patients. However, the differ-

B. Jasani et al., *Precision Cancer Medicine*, https://doi.org/10.1007/978-3-030-84087-7_22

ence may sometimes be only marginal (reflected in the hazard ratio) or is only reflected in the overall survival in larger cohorts.

A new approach was developed that combines deep learning algorithms with conventional survival modeling techniques to predict the clinical outcomes of patients diagnosed with glioma using histology images and genomic biomarkers. They compared these models to WHO classification based on genomic testing and manual histologic grading performed by pathologists using whole-slide images, genomics, and overall survival data from 769 gliomas in The Cancer Genome Atlas (TCGA). To gain insights into deep learning survival models, they also developed a visualization framework to examine the histologic and molecular patterns that these models associate with poor clinical outcomes. This approach surpassed the prognostic accuracy of human experts using the current clinical standard for classifying diffuse gliomas. Visualization revealed that deep learning survival models recognize important histologic structures and molecular biomarker status that are related to prognosis, and that are used by pathologists in grading and molecular classification. These results highlight the emerging role of deep learning in precision diagnostic oncology and suggest an expanding utility for computational analysis of histology and genomics in the future practice of pathology.

22.4 Clinical Decision Support Through Applications

Accurately predicting the clinical outcomes of patients diagnosed with cancer is essential for effective treatment. Despite advances in genomics, prognostication often relies on a small number of molecular biomarkers and subjective manual histologic analysis. Computational analysis of digital pathology and high-dimensional genomic data present opportunities to improve prognostic accuracy, however, significant challenges exist in creating algorithms to learn prognostic patterns from this data, and in integrating histology and genomics into a unified prognostic model. The amount and quality of images and data available differ in various cancer types. This depends not only on the incidence and prevalence of cancer in different population, but also on the general attention and scientific/clinical interest as well as the available funding. Hereinafter are a few examples and spotlights on the most recent developments in the field of applied digital and computational pathology, referring however to the appropriate and steadily growing body of literature.

22.4.1 Colorectal Cancer

One of the most prominent examples supported by sound science is the ImmunoScore developed by Jerome Galon and colleagues (Angell et al. 2020). They used a computer-based algorithm to quantify spatially resolved immune cells in different tumor compartment (invasive margin versus tumor center). Unfortunately, it only proved its prognostic relevance in stage 2 colo-rectal cancer and did not add significantly more information than other surgical and pathological features like membrane integrity, TNM stage, grading, budding index or microsatellite instability (MSI). With the increasing complexity and multitude of variables as biomarkers, the design of clinical trials becomes even more challenging. However, at the same time with the advent of genetic profiles for disease classification like MSI-H cancer, we will see also more classifications based on the machine algorithms that predict prognosis and therapy outcome in the future. This already started with signatures for immunologically "hot", "cold", "excluded" or "deserted" tumors, describing the individual TME (Galon and Bruni 2019), but is obviously still insufficient to make significant prognostic claims. Recently Schiele et al. (2021) described a weakly supervised algorithm that identified rulesets for the invasive margin just based on plain H&E images. In the near future, complex and n-dimensional analysis of clinical information, multiplexed images and augmented (−omics) data will change the clinical trial design and execution.

22.4.2 Lung Cancer

Among the conventional tumor histology, lymph node metastasis plays an important role to evaluate stages, treatment and prognosis of lung cancer. Using a deep learning algorithm to detect metastasis in lymph nodes has attracted much attention but there are still errors due to cancer mimickers such as "reactive" lymphoid follicles, and "macrophage clusters". There is still the hypothesis that lymphoid follicles are the most error-causing factor, therefore using double steps deep learning can reduce mistake and increase accuracy in detection of lymph node metastasis with the first step to exclude lymphoid follicles and the following step to detect tumor. These attempts are ongoing and heavily depend on pre-analytical standards like serial sections, high quality staining and high-resolution image acquisition to also detect micro-metastasis or isolated tumor cells (ITC). However, there are already many more examples and applications of ML/DL in the diagnosis and therapy prediction on lung cancer.

22.4.3 Melanocytic Lesions

As already discussed, whole slide images are a rich source of biomedical imaging data. The use of automated systems to classify and segment whole slide images has recently come to forefront of the pathology research community. While digital slides have obvious educational and clinical uses, another exciting potential lies in application of quantitative computational tools to automate search tasks, assist in classic diagnostic classification tasks, and improve prognosis and prediction. An essential step in enabling these advancements is to apply advances in machine learning and artificial intelligence from other fields to previously inaccessible pathology data sets, thereby enabling the application of new technologies to solve persistent diagnostic challenges in pathology. A Convolutional Neural Network (CNN) was applied to differentiate between two forms of melanocytic lesions (Spitz and Conventional). Large sections of tissue were curated by an expert dermatopathologist from 100 Hematoxylin and Eosin (H&E) slides each containing Conventional or Spitz nevi.

Slides were digitized and used to train and validate the deep CNN using the TensorFlow framework. Models were trained using pretrained weights and also entirely from scratch. Classifications where the classification probability was at least 10% higher than the next likely class were used as votes, with the classification label for the entire slide assigned by simple majority (Spitz or Conventional, others being intentionally ignored). Accuracy for the WSI-label predictions were then assessed for binary classification accuracy. The gold standard for the correct classification was the diagnosis made by the dermatopathologist. Treating 'Spitz' classification as the positive class and 'Conventional' as negative, the classification accuracy of whole slides was 92.5%. Sensitivity was 87% with a specificity of 98%. When further exploring the false positive calls, a strong edge effect was observed around the decision boundary, meaning that the incorrect calls were primarily driven by small differences in the expected versus observed classes. The manual curation, though tedious for the clinician (deploying conventional expert knowledge), proved to be a valuable contribution to optimizing model performance. By pre-selecting representative examples of Spitz and conventional nevi—along with providing examples for non-diagnostic areas such as hair follicles, sweat glands, tissue artifacts etc.—the model was able to learn faster and have an overall higher accuracy on the training and validation sets with fewer examples. The number of images used from the curated images was 16× less than a non-curated approach but were more focused on learning the salient features for discrimination in less time, taking only 50 h to train versus 800.

22.4.4 Lymphoid Aggregates

Inflammatory processes are involved in various patterns of immune cell recruitment and distributions. Like in many cancer types, lymphoid aggregates (LA) are also observed in patients with kidney allografts and may be indicative of acute kidney rejection (Kayler et al. 2007). Histological slides of kidney biopsies from patients with kidney allografts were digitized at 40× magnification. The ground-truth labels for normal tissue regions and LA regions in each slide were provided by a board-certified pathologist. A deep convolutional neural network based on U-Net was trained. The final model was able to accurately segment lymphoid aggregates (Dimitropoulos et al. 2017).

The successful identification of lymphoid aggregates provides a quantifiable measure of inflammation in digitized histological slides. The visualization tools that display regions of high lymphoid aggregate density (so called "hot spots), may be of potential use to clinicians investigating inflammatory processes in kidney allografts. Similar approaches have also been applied to the investigation of renal and gastric cancer (Kather et al. 2019; Schraml et al. 2019).

22.4.5 Bladder Cancer

There is an increasing number of examples on the use of machine and deep learning algorithms in different diagnostic challenges. As already discussed, the questions answered through computational pathology are sometimes limited due to the insufficient availability of good-quality images or inappropriate data. Therefore, it is quite popular to combine different existing insights to address problems in other areas. Brieu et al. (2019) used existing immune features to predict the survival of bladder invasive cancer, therefore establishing further prognostic subgroups in pT2a/b bladder cancer.

22.4.6 Renal Biopsies

Complete evaluation of a renal biopsy is a complex process usually requiring a highly skilled renal pathologist examining multiple serial sections of tissue by light microscopy, immunohistochemistry, and electron microscopy (Walker et al. 2004). The process to obtain an adequate biopsy sample requires a trained observer, the pathology resident or renal pathologist, assessing samples under light microscopy in real-time for sufficient glomerular content and the presence of renal cortex and medulla (Varma et al. 2018; Rosenberg 2016). The pathologist is not always immediately available to assess the sample and delays in patient care may arise as a result of scheduling conflicts between the pathologist and interventional radiologist performing the procedure. Digital pathology has already proven to be a suitable platform in nephropathology for renal biopsy evaluation and presents a potential solution through the use of telepathology for real-time transmission of image data between remote devices. The application of telepathology for expert assessment of renal cortex is a practical methodology to obtain adequate tissue for triaging, comparable to conventional light microscopy. Telepathology facilitates the centralization of assessment, increasing efficiency and making better use of the pathologist's time and expertise.

22.4.7 Breast Cancer

During the visual examination of the biopsy specimen of the tissue, breast pathologists look for certain features that can help them predict disease prognosis. The grading of the invasive breast carcinoma is usually classified into a three-point scale (Elston and Ellis 1991). However, the visual qualitative assessment is a labor and time-consuming task and still results in significant inter- and intra-observer variability, i.e., different pathologists may come up with discordant interpretations, leading to different prognostic evaluations, or the same pathologist may provide different gradings of the biopsy at different times for the same set of histological images. Various methods of automatic breast cancer grading have been proposed in the literature in order to increase the accuracy and reproducibility of diagnosis. In most of the cases the main challenges are the accurate segmentation and detection of histologic primitives, such as nuclei, as well as the extraction of a number of suitable textural or spatial features in order to model the pathologist's knowledge used in clinical practice. On the other hand, other approaches have used deep-learning techniques aiming to address the problem by extracting knowledge directly from the data (Khan and Mohammed 2014).

One recently proposed method considers leveraging the abundance of Hematoxylin and Eosin (H&E) stained breast cancer histological image as a set of multidimensional spatially evolving signals that can be efficiently represented as a cloud of points in a non-Euclidean space (Anand et al. 2020) By taking advantage of the geometric properties of the space in which these points lie, each image allows the identification of the grading of invasive breast carcinoma through the manifold of order in each image.

Published algorithms for the assessment of HER/neu expression are usually evaluated according to how well they correlate with expert-generated classifications, though it seems that each research group has its own dataset of images, whose scores are based on the subjective opinion of only one, two or three experts. With non-public datasets, direct comparison between competing algorithms is a very difficult task (Spanhol et al. 2016a, b). It would be desirable to have a HER2 assessment ground-truth, as it would represent the absolute truth, but it seems impossible because of the subjectivity of the task (Press and Sauter 2005). Alternatively, it can be correlated with the mRNA expression level or gene amplification (Perez et al. 2014). The main goal is to generate a reliable public breast cancer gold-standard, to be used as training/testing dataset in future developments of machine learning methods for automatic HER2 assessment. Also, it is expected to evaluate intra- and inter-variability of the experts. This will be a very significant contribution to the scientific community, because at present there is no accepted public gold-standard for HER2 assessment (Veta et al. 2014). Such a solution can also be transferred to other predictive biomarkers, such as PD-1/PD-L1.

22.4.8 Prostate Cancer

In order to ensure accurate and rapid diagnosis, and to provide an additional quality control measure researchers and companies develop algorithms for cancer diagnostics. Some start off validating software that enables identification of various cell types and features within whole slide images of prostate cancer, including cancerous glands (Gleason patterns 3, 4 and 5), high-grade PIN and inflammation, to support the pathologist in his diagnosis. Most studies are designed to raise alerts when encountering discrepancies between the automated analysis and the pathologist diagnosis, prompting a second pathologist review. Retrospectively, some of the algorithm identified missed cancers. Prospectively, deployment of the algorithm identified a case of low-grade cancer diagnosed by the pathologist as benign. AI-based diagnosis in prostate cancer can increase diagnostic speed and accuracy and has demonstrated some clinical utility.

Beyond the diagnostic scope of this approach, others are using deep learning to identify novel predictive signature that might open up prostate cancer as a target for combined immunotherapy (Harder et al. 2018).

22.4.9 Thyroid Cancer

Thyroid follicular neoplasms (FN) can be detected based on preoperative thyroid fine needle aspirations (T-FNA) using subjective cytomorphologic criteria which frequently lead to poor diagnostic precision and suboptimal patient management. Using T-FNA evaluated in liquid-based preparations (LBP) with standardized processing, there are studies ongoing to design an automated digital image analysis (DIA) algorithm to improve FN detection. There are actually DIA algorithm that can distinguish FN from benign T-FNAs with better precision than a cytopathologist. Current work is further trying to refine the algorithm to incorporate other thyroid lesions and whole slide imaging technology (Li et al. 2021). However, there are still major challenges to be met, e.g. the distinction of thyroid follicular cancer from thyroid follicular adenoma or to differentiate non-invasive follicular thyroid neoplasms with papillary features from classic papillary thyroid carcinoma. Maybe a solution similar to prostate cancer could be a preliminary solution, i.e. the identification of "area-at-risk" that require special attention by the expert pathologist.

22.4.10 Cytology

One other approach in screening exfoliative or effusion fluid cytology slides is to find if the smears contain malignant cells instead of identifying every single malignant cell. This would fit in the framework of multi-instance learning (MIL) to develop ML algorithms to screen fluid cytology effectively (once again identifying regions of interest = ROI). An approach could be a nucleus segmentation algorithm based on hierarchical multilevel thresholding (geometry, pixel intensity and textures) to extract such ROI. Some medical device manufacturers have taken this already to clinical utility not only for PAP smears but also for general cervical cancer screening, HPV testing or infection detection.

22.4.11 Biobanking

The amount of available material and images poses an additional challenge for management, quality control, and information retrieval. Digital Pathology is proving an invaluable tool to document surgical pathology specimens in large scale and in a cost-effective way. The evolution of molecular analysis technology is helping to enhance quality assurance practices for biobanks. Until now, the documentation of the microscopic analysis of tissue adequacy was based solely on descriptive criteria like tumor, necrosis and inflammation percentage. Digital Pathology allows the digitization of the glass slide, thus adding visual documentation of the specimen stored and avoiding the unnecessary preparation of new HE slides and allowing the archiving and retrieval of images and the potential use of image analysis and artificial intelligence to enhance and automate this process. The integration of digital whole slide (WSI) images as part of a biobank's database is a feasible approach and can be part of the routine work with minimum impact in the workflow of the pathology department. A simple and effective way to generate WSI is to gather the frozen section slides prepared to assess the specimen adequacy and scan all material on a daily basis (if permitted by the responsible authorities and notified bodies) (Wei and Simpson 2014).

Digital pathology potential uses are growing and expanding to all areas that use microscopy at a faster pace. The main advantages of digital pathology applied to biobank histology samples include permanent image documentation and access, proper selection of areas of interest by visual inspection and by image analysis and/or AI tools, thus enhancing cost-effectiveness and minimizing risks and costs of storing inadequate material (Lewis et al. 2016).

Pathologists, researchers and ML/AI experts have developed sophisticated and imaginative tools for analysis, interrogation and discovery. To fully experience the power and utility of these applications, there is an expectation for seamless image collaboration and exchange between users who desire a simple yet comprehensive workflow that integrate their applications of choice. Commercial vendors have started to undertake the challenge to provide such simplicity from a complex array of technologies. Platform providers need to share their image collaboration innovations through the perspective of their clients and provide integration tools and allow solutions for collaboration workflows, security and de-identification, cloud versus on premise deployment, appropriate staffing and other topics that are on the checklist of any organization looking to implement a digital pathology solution to their laboratory (Meredith et al. 2015).

Large archives of digital scans in pathology are slowly becoming a reality. The amount of information in such archives is still not only overwhelming but also not easily accessible yet. Fast and reliable search engines, customized for histopathology to perform content-based image retrieval (CBIR), are urgently needed to exploit the evidence-based knowledge from past cases and make them available to the pathologist for a more efficient and more informed decision making. Through an ensemble approach, a reliable search engine prototype is warranted that exploits the strengths of both handcrafted and deep features for image characterization.

22.5 Opportunity for Discovery of Novel Biomarker

Digital pathology and image analysis have become cornerstones of translational research, transforming tissue pathology-based biomarker strategies for drug development or repurposing (Gutman et al. 2017). In some cases, the speed of technological innovation in the tissue biomarker space has outpaced data managers and clinical teams working to bring new drugs to market. At this interface between research and the clinic, the deployment and standardization of image analysis methods and the adoption of end-to-end digital pathology is necessary to preserve data integrity and deliver new and effective medicines to patients quickly and safely.

The multi-faceted approach enables the validation and delivery of quantitative tissue biomarker data to support secondary and exploratory biomarker endpoints for phase I and II clinical trials across diverse therapeutic areas. Harmonization of IHC/ISH assay validation with digital image algorithm validation along with the validation of multiplex and other specialized algorithms need to already receive attention in the early clinical trial design.

The adoption of digital workflows allows greater adherence to GCP (good clinical practice) and the timely delivery of high-quality clinical data, as well as improving transfer of tissue biomarker methods from preclinical discovery to clinical trials. Standardization of digital image analysis facilitates more quantitative tissue biomarker endpoints for clinical trials allowing clinical teams to make more informed decisions. Digital pathology enables quantitative image analysis that is now the standard for tissue biomarker data delivery for clinical trials, but continual refinement of workflows and implementation of new biomarker technologies that will further inform clinical teams is ongoing (Kalra et al. 2020).

References

Anand D, Kurian NC, Dhage S, Kumar N, Rane S, Gann PH, Sethi A. Deep learning to estimate human epidermal growth factor receptor 2 status from hematoxylin and eosin-stained breast tissue images. J Pathol Inform. 2020;11:19. https://doi.org/10.4103/jpi.jpi_10_20.

Angell HK, Bruni D, Barrett JC, Herbst R, Galon J. The immunoscore: colon cancer and beyond. Clin Cancer Res. 2020;26(2):332–9. https://doi.org/10.1158/1078-0432.CCR-18-1851.

Brieu N, Gavriel CG, Nearchou IP, Harrison DJ, Schmidt G, Caie PD. Automated tumour budding quantification by machine learning augments TNM staging in muscle-invasive bladder cancer prognosis. Sci Rep. 2019;9(1):5174. https://doi.org/10.1038/s41598-019-41595-2.

Dimitropoulos K, Barmpoutis P, Koletsa T, Kostopoulos I, Grammalidis N. Automated detection and classification of nuclei in PAX5 and H&E stained tissue sections of follicular lymphoma. Signal Image Video Process. 2017;11(1):145–53.

Elston CW, Ellis IO. Pathological prognostic factors in breast cancer. I. the value of histological grade in breast cancer: experience from a large study with long-term follow-up. Histopathology. 1991;19(5):403–10.

Galon J, Bruni D. Approaches to treat immune hot, altered and cold tumours with combination immunotherapies. Nat Rev Drug Discov. 2019;18(3):197–218. https://doi.org/10.1038/s41573-018-0007-y.

Gutman DA, Khalilia M, Lee S, Nalisnik M, Mullen Z, Beezley J. The digital slide archive: a software platform for management, integration, and analysis of histology for cancer research. Cancer Res. 2017;77:e75–8.

Harder N, Athelogou M, Hessel H, Brieu N, Yigitsoy M, Zimmermann J, Baatz M, Buchner A, Stief CG, Kirchner T, Binnig G, Schmidt G, Huss R. Tissue phenomics for prognostic biomarker discovery in low- and intermediate-risk prostate cancer. Sci Rep. 2018;8(1):4470. https://doi.org/10.1038/s41598-018-22564-7.

Kalra S, Tizhoosh HR, Shah S, et al. Pan-cancer diagnostic consensus through searching archival histopathology images using artificial intelligence. NPJ Digit Med. 2020;3:31.

Kather JN, Pearson AT, Halama N, Jäger D, Krause J, Loosen SH, Marx A, Boor P, Tacke F, Neumann UP, Grabsch HI, Yoshikawa T, Brenner H, Chang-Claude J, Hoffmeister M, Trautwein C, Luedde T. Deep learning can predict microsatellite instability directly from histology in gastrointestinal cancer. Nat Med. 2019;25(7):1054–6. https://doi.org/10.1038/s41591-019-0462-y.

Kayler LK, Lakkis FG, Morgan C, Basu A, Blisard D, Tan HP, McCauley J, Wu C, Shapiro R, Randhawa PS. Acute cellular rejection with CD20-positive lymphoid positive lymphoid clusters in kidney transplant patients following lymphocyte depletion. Am J Transpl. 2007;7:949–54.

Khan A, Mohammed A. A novel system for scoring of hormone receptors in breast cancer histopathology slides. In: 2nd IEEE Middle East conference on biomedical engineering. IEEE; 2014. p. 155–8.

Lewis C, McQuaid S, Hamilton PW, Salto-Tellez M, McArt D, James JA. Building a 'repository of science': the importance of integrating biobanks within molecular pathology programmes. Eur J Cancer. 2016;67:191–9.

Li LR, Du B, Liu HQ, Chen C. Artificial intelligence for personalized medicine in thyroid cancer: current status and future perspectives. Front Oncol. 2021;10:604051. https://doi.org/10.3389/fonc.2020.604051.

Meredith AJ, Slotty A, Matzke L, Babinszky S, Watson PH. A model to estimate frozen tissue collection targets in biobanks to support cancer research. Biopreserv Biobank. 2015;13:356–62.

Perez EA, Cortés J, Gonzalez-Angulo AM, Bartlett JM. HER2 testing: current status and future directions. Cancer Treat Rev. 2014;40(2):276–84. https://doi.org/10.1016/j.ctrv.2013.09.001.

Press M, Sauter G. Diagnostic evaluation of HER-2 as a molecular target: an assessment of accuracy and reproducibility of laboratory testing in large, prospective, randomized clinical trials. Clin Cancer Res. 2005;11(18):6598–607.

Rosenberg AZ. The application of digital pathology to improve accuracy in glomerular enumeration in renal biopsies. PLoS One. 2016;11(6):e0156441.

Schiele S, Arndt TT, Martin B, Miller S, Bauer S, Banner BM, Brendel EM, Schenkirsch G, Anthuber M, Huss R, Märkl B, Müller G. Deep learning prediction of metastasis in locally advanced colon cancer using binary histologic tumor images. Cancers (Basel). 2021;13(9):2074. https://doi.org/10.3390/cancers13092074.

Schraml P, Athelogou M, Hermanns T, Huss R, Moch H. Specific immune cell and lymphatic vessel signatures identified by image analysis in renal cancer. Mod Pathol. 2019;32(7):1042–52. https://doi.org/10.1038/s41379-019-0214-z.

Spanhol FA, Oliveira LS, Petitjean C, Heutte L. A dataset for breast cancer histopathological image classification. IEEE Trans Biomed Eng. 2016a;63(7):1455–62.

Spanhol FA, Oliveira LS, Petitjean C, Heutte L. Breast cancer histopathological image classification using convolutional neural networks. In: International joint conference on neural networks 2016 Nov:24–29. IEEE; 2016b.

Varma VK, Kajdacsy-Balla A, Akkina S, Setty S, Walsh MJ. Predicting fibrosis progression in renal transplant recipients using laser-based infrared spectroscopic imaging. Sci Rep. 2018;8:686.

Veta M, Pluim JP, van Diest PJ, Viergever MA. Breast cancer histopathology image analysis: a review. IEEE Trans Biomed Eng. 2014;61(5):1400–11.

Walker PD, Cavallo T, Bonsib SM. Practice guidelines for the renal biopsy. Mod Pathol. 2004;17(12):1555.

Wei BR, Simpson RM. Digital pathology and image analysis augment biospecimen annotation and biobank quality assurance harmonization. Clin Biochem. 2014;47:274–9.

Index

B. Jasani et al., *Precision Cancer Medicine*, https://doi.org/10.1007/978-3-030-84087-7

GPSR Compliance

The European Union's (EU) General Product Safety Regulation (GPSR) is a set of rules that requires consumer products to be safe and our obligations to ensure this.

If you have any concerns about our products, you can contact us on ProductSafety@springernature.com

In case Publisher is established outside the EU, the EU authorized representative is:

Springer Nature Customer Service Center GmbH
Europaplatz 3
69115 Heidelberg, Germany

Batch number: 10732809

Printed by Printforce, the Netherlands